SIXTH EDITION

PEDIATRICS REVIEW

CORE

CURRICULUM

Book 2 of 5

Topics in this volume:

Infectious Disease

Allergy & Immunology

Dermatology

Robert A. Hannaman, MD
Editor in Chief

Disclaimers

NOTICE: Medicine and accepted standards of care are constantly changing. We at MedStudy do our best to review and include in this publication accurate discussions of the standards of care and methods of diagnosis. However, the editor in chief, the reviewers, the section editors, the publisher, and all other parties involved with the preparation and publication of this work do not guarantee that the information contained herein is in every respect accurate or complete. We recommend that you confirm the material with current sources of medical knowledge whenever considering presentations or treating patients.

A note on editorial style: MedStudy uses a standardized approach to the naming of diseases. The previous method of naming was to use the possessive form that adds "'s" to the names of diseases and disorders, such as Lou Gehrig's disease, Klinefelter's syndrome, and others. In MedStudy material, you will see the non-possessive form when the proper name is followed by a common noun; e.g., "This patient's symptoms warrant a workup for Crohn disease." Possessive form will be used, however, when an entity is referred to solely by its proper name without a following common noun; e.g., "The symptoms are classic for Crohn's." The *AMA Manual of Style*, *JAMA*, *Scientific Style and Format,* and *Pediatrics* magazine are among the publications now using the non-possessive form.

MEDSTUDY
1455 Quail Lake Loop
Colorado Springs, Colorado 80906
(800) 841-0547

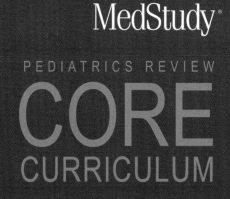

MedStudy®

PEDIATRICS REVIEW

CORE
CURRICULUM

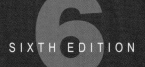

SIXTH EDITION

INFECTIOUS DISEASE

Section Editor:

Sue Jue, MD, FAAP
Associate Professor of Pediatrics
Greenville Hospital System
Greenville, SC

Reviewers:

Claire Elizabeth Bocchini, MD, FAA P
Assistant Professor
Department of Pediatrics,
Section of Infectious Disease
Baylor College of Medicine
Texas Children's Hospital
Houston, TX

Table of Contents
Infectious Disease

BACTERIA

GRAM-POSITIVE BACTERIA

Staphylococcus aureus

Staphylococcus aureus is a common inhabitant of skin and mucous membranes. It can cause localized disease, such as impetigo or serious, life-threatening infections. Bacteremia is especially common among those with indwelling catheters, IV drug users, and hemodialysis patients. *S. aureus* is also a cause of 3 toxin-mediated syndromes: toxic shock syndrome (TSS), staphylococcal epidermal necrolysis, and staphylococcal scalded skin syndrome (SSSS). Pathogenicity (which is not the same as resistance to antibiotics!) is associated with production of entero- and exotoxin, coagulase, and Panton-Valentine leukocidin. *S. aureus* colonizes the skin and mucous membranes in 30–50% of healthy children and adults; frequent sites of colonization include the anterior nares, throat, axilla, perineum, vagina, or rectum.

The percentage of methicillin-resistant *S. aureus* (MRSA) infections has grown substantially due to the previous indiscriminate use of methicillin and similar antibiotics. In many hospitals, a majority of *S. aureus* isolates are MRSA. Unfortunately, MRSA is now frequently seen in community-acquired infections as well, known as CA-MRSA. The gene that confers methicillin resistance is *mecA*.

In carriers, *S. aureus* is difficult to eradicate. You can try topical mupirocin ointment (Bactroban®, Centany®) and oral rifampin or clindamycin, but, even with these, it still recurs. Some experts recommend improved skin hygiene, Hibiclens®, or bleach baths in an attempt to decontaminate the skin.

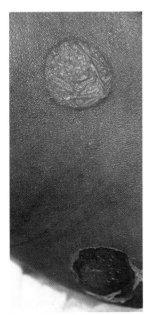

Image 5-1: Bullous impetigo

In all cases of bacteremia and serious infection with MRSA, vancomycin is the only drug of choice—although there are newer agents such as linezolid, daptomycin, quinupristin-dalfopristin, and a 5th generation cephalosporin, ceftaroline. Linezolid (Zyvox®) is quite expensive and generally should be reserved for patients intolerant of vancomycin; daptomycin (Cubicin®), quinupristin-dalfopristin (Synercid®), and ceftaroline (Teflaro®) are not yet approved for use in children. Additional antibiotics such as trimethoprim/sulfamethoxazole (TMP/SMX) or clindamycin are used in less severe MRSA infections, such as skin and soft tissue infections.

For empiric therapy for life-threatening *Staphylococcus aureus* infections (when there is a risk of MRSA), vancomycin + nafcillin are recommended because nafcillin is more effective against MSSA (methicillin-sensitive *S. aureus*) than vancomycin is. When final culture and sensitivity results return, MSSA is treated with nafcillin and MRSA with vancomycin.

Skin infections are common with *Staphylococcus aureus*, especially impetigo, which also is due to *Streptococcus pyogenes*. This presents as red-crusted papules and pustules, often at the site of a prior insect bite. "Bullous impetigo" is usually staphylococcal in origin; it presents as flaccid, coalescent pustules with bullae on previously normal skin (Image 5-1). Uncomplicated impetigo can be treated with topical antibiotics only. *S. aureus* is the usual cause of furuncles (boils) and carbuncles.

The 2012 Red Book has published an algorithm for management of skin and soft tissue infections caused by suspected community-acquired *S. aureus*.

First, if the lesion is a boil or abscess, begin with incision and drainage and send for culture and susceptibility testing.

Next, evaluate the severity of the infection.

Mild: If the infection is mild, incision and drainage alone are likely adequate. Or, if necessary, begin an oral antibiotic (TMP/SMX if group A *Streptococcus* is unlikely; clindamycin if there is little clindamycin resistance in the community; or doxycycline if > 8 years of age).

Note: The D-test determines if there is macrolide-inducible clindamycin resistance. It must be done when the *S. aureus* isolate shows both clindamycin sensitivity and erythromycin resistance. If the D-test is positive, all recommendations are to not use clindamycin as a treatment.

Moderate disease includes those with fever but who were previously healthy. Patients can be managed either as mild cases or if the area of involvement is extensive; if they have systemic symptoms or compliance is an issue, they may require hospitalization.

Severe: For those with severe disease (toxic, immunocompromised, or limb-threatening infection), admit and perform emergent incision and drainage, and start empiric vancomycin or clindamycin (with negative D-test). For those critically ill, the recommendations are to treat with vancomycin plus nafcillin +/– other agents.

Additionally, cases of vancomycin-intermediately susceptible *S. aureus* (VISA) and vancomycin-resistant *S. aureus* (VRSA) have been reported—although they are exceedingly rare in children. Exam questions typically do not ask you how to treat these cases, but you could be asked about infection control for these types of patients!

Table 5-1: Infection Control for Preventing Spread of Highly Resistant *Staphylococcus aureus*

Isolate patients in private room
Gown and gloves (contact precautions)
Wear mask/eye protection or face shield if performing a procedure that might produce splash or splatter
Hand washing with soap and water or alcohol-based hand sanitizer
Dedicate nondisposable items for patient use
Consult with local health department and CDC before discharging and/or transferring the patient

See Table 5-1—Infection Control for Preventing Spread of Highly Resistant *Staphylococcus aureus* (i.e., those with decreased susceptibility to vancomycin).

If a child has *S. aureus* bacteremia, be very suspicious of endocarditis or osteomyelitis. (*S. aureus* is the most common cause of osteomyelitis, except in patients with sickle cell!) Also, *S. aureus* bacteremia frequently "seeds" many sites in the body. Deep vein thrombosis and septic pulmonary emboli are also common (especially in children with indwelling catheters or osteomyelitis). If a catheter is involved, you must remove it—in addition to treating with antibiotics.

S. aureus CNS infections are unusual. Children with cyanotic congenital heart disease have an increased risk of staphylococcal brain abscesses (especially in the setting of endocarditis and septic emboli). Also, children who undergo neurosurgical procedures, especially shunt revisions, are at increased risk for staphylococcal infections.

Other things to remember:

- There is an increased incidence of empyema with *S. aureus* pneumonia.
- Influenza infection can predispose children to *S. aureus* pneumonia.
- *S. aureus* is the most common cause of bullous impetigo, furuncles, bacterial parotitis, and bacterial tracheitis! It is also a frequent cause of lymphadenitis.

Table 5-2: Criteria for Diagnosis of Toxic Shock Syndrome

Temp > 38.9° C (102.02° F)
Systolic blood pressure < 90 mmHg (or < 5th percentile for age < 16 years)
Rash with subsequent desquamation (palms/soles especially)
Involvement of > 3 organ systems: GI, muscular, mucous membranes, renal, liver, blood, CNS
Negative serology for RMSF, leptospirosis, measles

- Infections are associated with foreign bodies (intravascular catheters, ventriculoperitoneal [VP] shunts, prosthetic joints).
- Children with increased risk for severe *S. aureus* disease include those with diabetes mellitus, cirrhosis, an immunodeficiency (e.g., HIV, chronic granulomatous disease, hyper-IgE syndrome), nutritional disorders, surgery, and a transplantation.

Toxic Shock Syndrome (TSS)

Staphylococcal TSS is a toxin-mediated disease caused by strains producing TSS toxin-1 or other related enterotoxins. It is characterized by generalized red skin (erythroderma), hypotension, fever, diarrhea, and signs of multiorgan system involvement. Desquamation (especially of palms, soles, fingers, and toes) occurs 1–2 weeks after onset of illness. Although 50% of cases of staphylococcal TSS occur in menstruating females using tampons, nonmenstrual TSS cases can occur after childbirth or abortion, after surgical procedures, and in association with cutaneous lesions. It can also occur in males and females without a defined focus of infection. People with TSS, especially if menses-related, are at risk of a recurrent episode.

Any time there is a postsurgical toxic shock, any device implanted during the surgery must be immediately removed (prosthetic device, implant, etc.). See Table 5-2—Criteria for Diagnosis of Toxic Shock Syndrome. Treatment includes fluid management, nafcillin (substitute vancomycin in regions where MRSA infections are common) + clindamycin (decreases toxin production) +/– IVIG.

Another cause of TSS is *Streptococcus pyogenes*, which typically results from a progressive skin infection—especially post-op and with chicken pox! Note: In staphylococcal TSS, blood cultures are usually negative; whereas in streptococcal TSS, blood cultures are generally positive!

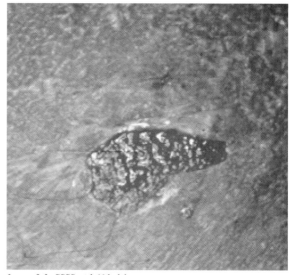

Image 5-2: SSSS with Nikolsky sign

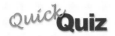

Quick Quiz

- If a child presents with bacteremia due to MRSA, what is effective therapy?
- What organisms commonly cause impetigo?
- Half of staphylococcal TSS cases are associated with what?
- List the criteria for the diagnosis of toxic shock syndrome.
- What is Nikolsky sign?
- In staphylococcal scalded skin syndrome, what 2 things should you watch out for?
- What is the most common cause of food poisoning in the U.S.?
- What is the most common organism found in catheter-related and VP-shunt infections?
- Which types of patients are at highest risk for pneumococcal sepsis?

Treatment is the same as staphylococcal TSS except substitute penicillin for nafcillin.

Staphylococcal Scalded Skin Syndrome (SSSS)

S. aureus can cause a desquamative dermatitis mediated by exfoliative toxins A and B. In young infants, it is known as Ritter syndrome. Bacteremia may or may not be present. Fever is common, and minimal friction applied to the skin results in removal of the superficial layers of epidermis; this is known as Nikolsky sign (Image 5-2). Extensive sloughing of skin can occur (like in a burn patient), so watch out for dehydration and superinfection. Older children can have a similar syndrome without the skin sloughing; it presents with red, tender skin that looks like group A *Streptococcus* scarlet fever.

Staphylococcus aureus Food Poisoning

S. aureus is the most common cause of food poisoning in the United States. Eating preformed enterotoxin from food that is contaminated is the cause. Incubation period is < 4–6 hours, and the patient presents with abrupt-onset nausea, vomiting, abdominal cramps, and often diarrhea. Low-grade fever rarely occurs. Most have a self-limited disease (1–2 days), but some children can have severe dehydration. Treatment is supportive only. This is typically associated with sliced meats, salad dressings, poultry, and cream-filled baked goods. Short incubation, brevity of illness, and lack of fever help to distinguish this from most other types of food poisoning—except maybe food poisoning due to *Bacillus cereus*, which is associated mainly with fried rice left at room temperature!

Coagulase-Negative Staphylococci

S. epidermidis and *S. saprophyticus* are examples of coagulase-negative staphylococci. *S. epidermidis* is almost always methicillin-resistant. It is the most common cause of both catheter-related bacteremia and bacteremia occurring post-op when anything foreign was left in the body; e.g., prosthetics, including heart valves and joints, pacemakers, CNS shunts. Especially be on the lookout for VP-shunt infections with this organism. Treat with vancomycin +/− rifampin +/− gentamicin.

S. saprophyticus causes UTIs in adolescent females and should be treated. Treat with TMP/SMX, nitrofurantoin, or cephalothin. Note that 2nd and 3rd generation cephalosporins are not effective against *S. saprophyticus*.

S. epidermidis is responsible for ~ 1/3 of the bacteremias in children receiving chemotherapy for childhood malignancies; it also accounts for the majority of bacteremias in neonates in NICUs. The key factor for both is the presence of an intravascular catheter.

Additionally, *S. epidermidis* is a common "contaminant" in blood and other cultures. A single blood culture that is positive for *S. epidermidis,* without an underlying prosthetic device or risk factors, is usually the result of a contaminant. However, this is more difficult to discern in NICUs where, generally, a positive culture must be initially treated if there is suspicion of infection. Coagulase-negative staphylococci are the most common cause of late-onset bacteremia/septicemia among preterm infants (especially with birth weights < 1,500 grams).

Streptococcus pneumoniae

Remember: You need a functioning spleen and functioning antibodies to defend against the encapsulated *S. pneumoniae* (as well as the other encapsulated organisms *Neisseria meningitidis* and *H. influenzae*)—so all 3 infections are seen more often in:

- Asplenic patients (anatomically or functionally asplenic, including those with sickle cell disease)
- Very young and old patients
- Patients with hypogammaglobulinemia (i.e., any antibody dysfunction or decrease)

Additional children at high risk for invasive pneumococcal disease include:

- Children with HIV infection
- Children with cochlear implants (increased risk of meningitis)
- Alaska Natives who are < 2 years of age
- Native Americans who are < 2 years of age

Children with congenital immunodeficiency, chronic cardiac/pulmonary/renal disease, CSF leaks, DM, or on immunosuppressive therapy are also presumed to be at increased risk.

S. pneumoniae is the most common cause of otitis media (OM). High-dose (80–90 mg/kg/day) amoxicillin is the drug of choice for acute otitis media (AOM). If patients fail to respond within 48 hours, broaden coverage to include penicillin-resistant *S. pneumoniae* and beta–lactamase-producing *Haemophilus influenzae* and *Moraxella catarrhalis*, such as amoxicillin-clavulanate or a 2nd or 3rd generation cephalosporin. Complications of OM include mastoiditis.

In 2013, the AAP published new guidelines for the diagnosis and management of uncomplicated AOM in children 6 months–12 years of age. These guidelines base initial treatment with antibiotics on age (6 months–2 years vs. > 2 years), severity of symptoms, unilateral vs. bilateral disease, and presence of otorrhea. For children 6 months–2 years of age with unilateral AOM without otorrhea and for children ≥ 2 years with unilateral or bilateral OM without otorrhea, you can simply observe—but only if you ensure close follow-up and start antibiotics if the child worsens or fails to improve within 48–72 hours from onset.

Pneumococcus is the most common bacterial cause of bacteremia, meningitis, and pneumonia. In children, "occult bacteremia without a focus" used to account for ~ 60% of all pneumococcal invasive disease. This "syndrome" classically occurred in febrile children 3–36 months of age. In the 1990s, it occurred in 3% of all children in this age group with a temperature > 39° C (102.2° F). However, the introduction of heptavalent pneumococcal conjugate vaccine (Prevnar®, PCV7) in 2000 has resulted in a 99% decrease in vaccine-type invasive pneumococcal infections and overall decrease of 77% of invasive disease in children < 5 years of age. Despite this success, invasive disease caused by non-vaccine serotypes has increased.

Pneumococcus serotype 19A has become the most common cause of invasive disease in PCV7-immunized children, and 19A is also associated with increased antibiotic resistance. In 2010, PCV7 was replaced by PCV13, which includes serotype 19A. In 2013, the Advisory Committee on Immunization Practices (ACIP) of the CDC expanded its recommendations for use of PCV13. It now recommends that children 6–18 years of age with immunocompromising conditions, functional or anatomic asplenia, CSF leaks, or cochlear implants who have not previously received PCV13 be given a single dose of PCV13—regardless of whether they have received PCV7 or the pneumococcal polysaccharide vaccine (PPSV23).

S. pneumoniae is the most common cause of bacterial pneumonia in children older than 1 month of age. (Viruses, however, cause more pneumonia than any other etiology!) In children with documented pneumonia, 1–3% will have a positive blood culture. Complications are rare but empyema can occur.

Complicated invasive *S. pneumoniae* disease is the 2nd most common cause of hemolytic uremic syndrome (after *E. coli* O157:H7!).

In infants > 2–3 months of age, pneumococcus is the most common cause of bacterial meningitis and has the highest rate of complications—30% have hearing loss. The mortality rate in children is estimated at 8%; ~ 1/3 have severe morbidity with neurologic sequelae. Meningitis is discussed later in this section.

Depending on the geographic location, 10–60% of those with *S. pneumoniae* develop some degree of resistance to penicillin (PCN), usually by alterations in PCN-binding proteins. (This is not the same as β-lactamase resistance as seen in *S. aureus*.) For bacteremia without evidence of meningitis, use ceftriaxone or cefotaxime until PCN susceptibility is known. Empiric treatment of presumed *S. pneumoniae* meningitis should always include both vancomycin and cefotaxime or ceftriaxone until susceptibility is known.

For outpatients with otitis media or pneumonia and who are allergic to PCN, give a cephalosporin, clindamycin, doxycycline (for adolescents), or quinolone.

Remember: Post-splenectomy pneumococcal sepsis can be rapidly fatal and can present with flu-like symptoms, purpura, and DIC and may have Howell-Jolly bodies on peripheral smear.

Because of PCV7 and now PCV13, there has been a drop in cases of pneumococcal disease; however, it is important to remember that pneumococcal disease can still occur in those who are vaccinated, especially with serotypes not covered by the vaccine.

Streptococcus pyogenes (Group A Streptococcus)

S. pyogenes is the only species in group A beta-hemolytic *Streptococcus*. It may cause 1 or more of the following:

- Pharyngitis/Retropharyngeal abscess
- Scarlet fever
- Impetigo, erysipelas, perianal cellulitis
- Streptococcal TSS
- Rheumatic fever
- Acute glomerulonephritis

The major protein on its cell surface is the "M protein." The M protein occurs in > 80 antigenically distinct types and defines which strains are rheumatogenic, which cause glomerulonephritis, which are toxigenic for toxic shock syndrome, etc.

Pharyngitis

Streptococcal pharyngitis (usually from *S. pyogenes*) is more likely with each of these 3 findings:

1) Temperature > 100° F
2) Tender cervical lymphadenopathy
3) Exudative tonsils

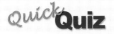

Quiz

- How do you treat otitis media?
- What is the empiric therapy for pneumococcal meningitis?
- How may a toddler with *S. pyogenes* infection present?
- Describe the rash of scarlet fever.
- What areas of the body are commonly affected by impetigo?

If you don't find any of these, the chance of *Streptococcus* is < 3%; 1 finding = 20%; 3 findings = 50%. In children > 2 years of age who have cough, rhinorrhea, hoarseness, oral ulcers or other symptoms of URI with "sore throat," it is not streptococcal infection but more suggestive of a viral etiology! Headache, nausea, vomiting, and abdominal pain may also be present. Toddlers do not present with pharyngitis, but rather with thick, purulent, nasal discharge, low-grade fever, and decreased feeding (known as streptococcosis). Streptococcal disease is most commonly seen in the winter and spring—and in children > 3 years of age.

Just because the throat is red, has exudates, and "looks like strep" does not mean it is. Conduct a rapid diagnostic test or throat culture in children you suspect of having streptococcal pharyngitis. Rapid diagnostic tests have a sensitivity of ~ 90%, and a specificity approaching 100%. Recent optical immunoassay has shown to be even more sensitive. If using a rapid test and the test is negative, the 2012 Red Book recommends a throat culture. Culture is the gold standard and takes 1–2 days for results. It is perfectly appropriate to wait on culture results before giving antibiotic therapy. The risk of rheumatic fever is alleviated as long as you start antibiotics within 9 days of infection, so waiting 1–2 days is not going to be a problem.

Suppurative complications of pharyngotonsillitis include otitis media, sinusitis, cervical lymphadenitis, and peritonsillar/retropharyngeal abscesses (covered in Respiratory Disorders, Book 4). Nonsuppurative complications include acute rheumatic fever and acute glomerulonephritis.

Scarlet Fever

Scarlet fever in a child presents with a fine, diffuse, red rash with acute streptococcal pharyngitis. The rash is due to streptococcal pyrogenic exotoxins (SPE, specifically SPE A, B, C, and F).

The rash usually appears 24–48 hours into the illness but can appear as the 1st sign. The rash has a "sandpaper" quality, begins on the neck and upper chest, and spreads (Image 5-3).

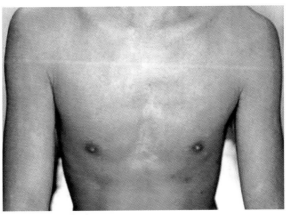

Image 5-3: Scarlet fever

The rash is especially prominent in the flexor skin creases of the antecubital fossa and produces what are known as Pastia lines; these lines are pathognomonic for scarlet fever. Also, the mouth area is pale and described as "circumoral pallor." The rash lasts ~ 1 week, and then fades with desquamation of the trunk, hands, and feet (Image 5-4).

Impetigo (Superficial Pyoderma) and Erysipelas

Impetigo, a.k.a. superficial pyoderma, is the most common form of skin infection caused by *S. pyogenes*. It is common after minute injuries to the skin such as insect bites, scabies, or minor trauma. The child is usually afebrile and does not have pain. Impetigo is most common in children 2–5 years of age. It also is common for other family members to become infected.

The lesions of impetigo are "honey-crusted" and may be oozing purulent material (Image 5-5). The lesions most commonly occur around the mouth, nose, and extremities. Several serotypes, including 49, 55, 57, and 59, are highly associated with the development of post-streptococcal glomerulonephritis, but not rheumatic fever.

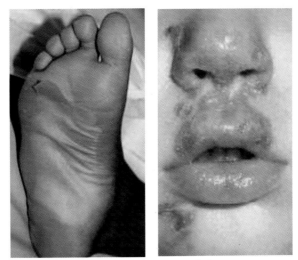

Image 5-4: Strep desquamation   *Image 5-5: Impetigo*

Erysipelas (Image 5-6) is an acute streptococcal infection of the deeper layers of skin and underlying connective tissues. It is rare in children. In contrast to impetigo, the skin is tender. It is common to see and feel a well-demarcated line between infected and uninfected skin. Lymphangitis can also occur. "Leading-edge" cultures may be useful for detecting the organism.

Cellulitis from group A *Streptococcus* can be very serious; in some cases, it can become deep-seated and lead to necrotizing fasciitis, which is infection that causes destruction down to the subcutaneous tissue level. There is severe pain and swelling, and the skin becomes bluish and dusky in appearance. After 4–6 days, frank gangrene can occur. Surgical debridement is the treatment of choice, along with IV PCN and clindamycin. Recent/concurrent varicella infection is an identified risk factor. Note that cellulitis due to *S. pyogenes* can also be responsible for post-streptococcal glomerulonephritis, but not rheumatic fever.

As noted above, *S. pyogenes* can cause toxic shock syndrome. Remember: With streptococcal toxic shock, blood cultures are more likely to be positive!

Perianal streptococcal dermatitis/perirectal cellulitis is a brightly erythematous, sharply demarcated rash that is painful and often itchy. It most commonly occurs in children 6 months–10 years of age.

Rheumatic fever and acute post-streptococcal glomerulonephritis are discussed in Rheumatology, Book 5, and Nephrology, Book 5.

Treatment

Penicillin is the drug of choice for *S. pyogenes* infection. For streptococcal pharyngitis, use PCN V. Generally, most use 400,000 U (250 mg) 2–3 times a day x 10 days for children < 27 kg and 800,000 U (500 mg) bid x 10 days for those > 27 kg. The most common reason for PCN failure is nonadherence. If compliance is an issue, administer a single IM dose of benzathine PCN G 600,000 U for children weighing < 27 kg (60 lb) or 1.2 million U for children weighing ≥ 27 kg.

Even in compliant patients, eradication of *Streptococcus* does not occur in 15% of cases. Most believe that many of these failures occur in *S. pyogenes* "carriers."

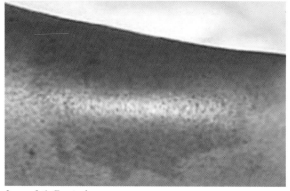

Image 5-6: Erysipelas

If the child is PCN-allergic, use cephalexin, cefadroxil, or other cephalosporins. Oral erythromycin or azithromycin is acceptable for those allergic to both PCNs and cephalosporins. However, it recently has been reported that ~ 5–10% of *S. pyogenes* are resistant to erythromycin or azithromycin. Most do not recommend using azithromycin if the child can tolerate PCN.

Management of patients who have recurrent episodes of pharyngitis associated with positive laboratory tests for group A streptococci can be a problem and may represent pharyngeal carriage.

Antibiotics are not usually indicated for strep carriers except in certain situations:

- Local outbreak of acute rheumatic fever (ARF) or post-streptococcal glomerulonephritis
- Outbreak of GAS in a closed community
- Family history of ARF
- Multiple ("ping-pong") episodes of pharyngitis in the family despite appropriate antibiotic therapy.

To try to eradicate the carrier state, the most effective drug is clindamycin (20 mg/kg/day in 3 divided doses x 10 days). Very few may require tonsillectomy.

Treatment of impetigo generally involves treating for both *S. pyogenes* and *S. aureus* infection, commonly with cephalexin. If MRSA is suspected, then clindamycin is commonly used or, if severe, linezolid. Topical therapy may work for small areas with mupirocin or retapamulin.

Skin strains of *S. pyogenes* may cause acute glomerulonephritis, even with treatment, but cannot cause rheumatic fever.

Note: Pharyngeal strains of *S. pyogenes* can cause both glomerulonephritis (not prevented with therapy) and rheumatic fever (prevented with therapy).

A clue to help differentiate the cause of hematuria that develops after an *S. pyogenes* skin infection is that the latency is generally 21 days for *S. pyogenes* GN vs. < 5 days for IgA nephropathy. (Pharyngitis has a latency of 10 days, on average, for developing hematuria.)

In children with a history of acute rheumatic fever or rheumatic cardiac disease, use 1.2 million U of benzathine PCN G IM every 3–4 weeks, or oral PCN, or sulfadiazine daily (for those PCN-allergic). Additionally, some recommend treating all household contacts of a case of rheumatic fever or post-streptococcal glomerulonephritis to rid the household of the potentially offending strain— but a majority of experts recommend only targeted chemoprophylaxis in household contacts ≥ 65 years of age or those who have other risk factors for potentially invasive *S. pyogenes* disease (HIV, varicella, DM, chemotherapy, etc.).

Quick Quiz

- How does erysipelas differ from impetigo?
- What is a risk factor for necrotizing fasciitis due to *S. pyogenes* infection?
- What is the drug of choice for *S. pyogenes* infection? If a child has anaphylaxis to penicillin and you are uneasy about using cephalosporins, what is an acceptable alternative therapy?
- In what situations would you treat a group A strep carrier?
- Differentiate "early-onset" and "late-onset" group B streptococcal disease.
- What type of streptococci are common organisms in endocarditis?

Streptococcus agalactiae (Group B Streptococcal Infection)

S. agalactiae (group B) is a common cause of infection in the newborn and young infant. It is a major cause of newborn pneumonia, bacteremia, and meningitis. (This is why ampicillin is included in the empiric treatment for meningitis; ampicillin is also used for *Listeria* and enterococci in this age group.) *S. agalactiae* is associated with UTIs in pregnant women and is also a cause of postpartum endometritis and bacteremia. It can originate from a GI or GU reservoir.

There are "early-" and "late-onset" group B streptococcal infections in the newborn/early infancy period.

Things to know about early onset:

- Onset occurs within 7 days of birth.
- Obstetric complications are common.
- Prematurity is common.
- Septicemia is the most common presentation (45%).
- Pneumonia is next most common (40%).
- Meningitis occurs in < 10%.
- The most common serotypes are Ia, Ib, II, III, and V.
- Case fatality rates are 5–15%.

Things to know about late onset:

- Range of onset is 7 days–3 months.
- Bacteremia without a focus is the most common presentation (50%).
- Meningitis is next most common (40%).
- Osteomyelitis (especially proximal humerus) and septic arthritis (hip, knee, ankle) occur in < 10%.
- Cellulitis-adenitis syndrome (unilateral, cervical, genital, or inguinal areas) occurs in up to 4%; nearly all are bacteremic and require lumbar puncture; many are deceivingly well-appearing with concomitant bacteremia.

- Serotype III is responsible for 90%.
- Case fatality rates are 2–6%.

There is a "late-late onset," which occurs > 3 months out. This typically occurs in premature infants as bacteremia without a focus. The case fatality rate is < 1%.

Do not use antigen detection in urine or blood. Blood/CSF cultures are the gold standard; but if the infant has been/is on antibiotic therapy, antigen detection in CSF may be helpful.

A newborn with presumed bacterial sepsis should initially be treated with ampicillin + gentamicin. On confirmation of group B *Streptococcus* as the etiology, penicillin G alone (or ampicillin) can be used for 10 days for pneumonia and sepsis, and 14–21 days minimum for meningitis. Septic arthritis or osteomyelitis requires 3–4 weeks. Treat non-meningitis cases with 200,000 U/kg/day and meningitis with 400,000–500,000 U/kg/day.

For bacteremia, repeat blood cultures 24–48 hours into therapy. For those with meningitis, some experts repeat lumbar puncture 24–48 hours into therapy. (Some recommend repeat lumbar puncture at the end of therapy to document resolution of inflammatory response.) If, on the repeat lumbar puncture, there are still significant numbers of neutrophils or an elevated protein, many continue treatment for another week and then repeat the lumbar puncture. With meningitis, most also recommend a CT/MRI with contrast before completion of therapy.

Prevention of group B strep infection with maternal prophylaxis is reviewed in The Fetus & Newborn, Book 3. Maternal prophylaxis prevents early-onset disease but has no effect on late-onset disease. Because of the reported increased risk of infection, siblings of a multiple birth index case should be evaluated and monitored closely for signs of illness.

β-hemolytic Group C, G, Non-hemolytic Group D (*Streptococcus bovis*), and Viridans Streptococci

These organisms are normal flora of the mouth, GI tract, and female genital tract. Viridans (Latin for "green") streptococci refer to a group of 18+ species, which now are subdivided into *Streptococcus anginosis* (previously *milleri*), *mitis*, *salivarius*, and *mutans*. Viridans streptococci are not particularly pathogenic, but, because they are frequently present in transient bacteremia episodes after dental procedures or mucous membrane injury, they can cause disease. 20–40% of all toothbrushing leads to bacteremia! In particular, *S. mutans*, *S. sanguis*, and *S. mitis* adhere more easily to damaged heart valves.

Viridans streptococci are the most common cause of endocarditis in children. They make up ~ 1/3 of cases. The majority of children who have endocarditis also have some underlying congenital heart defect—or have had rheumatic fever. These organisms are also frequent causes of bacteremia/sepsis in neutropenic leukemia patients.

Group C streptococci cause pharyngitis, particularly in college student outbreaks. Numerous case reports show that groups C and G streptococci may occasionally cause bacteremia, pneumonia, epiglottitis, osteomyelitis, endocarditis, UTIs, and other systemic infections. They are also associated with foodborne outbreaks.

Group D *Streptococcus* (*S. bovis*) rarely causes disease in children, although some cases of meningitis, bacteremia, and endocarditis have occurred in infants and neonates. It is more common (although still rare) in adults. If found in adults, search for colon cancer.

Groups C, non-hemolytic D, and G are susceptible to PCN. Viridans streptococci have increased rates of resistance, and you must guide therapy for endocarditis by susceptibility testing. Vancomycin is the drug of choice if the organism is PCN-resistant.

For endocarditis, viridans streptococci, or *S. bovis* (MIC ≤ 0.1 µg/mL) that is highly susceptible to PCN, treat with 4 weeks of IV PCN or ceftriaxone. For MICs between 0.1–0.5 µg/mL, use PCN and gentamicin for 2 weeks, followed by PCN alone for 2 more weeks. For resistant viridans streptococci (MIC ≥ 0.5 µg/mL), use 4–6 weeks of PCN or ampicillin plus gentamicin, or use vancomycin alone.

Remember that pharyngitis due to streptococci other than *S. pyogenes* (group A *Streptococcus*) does not cause acute rheumatic fever!

Enterococcus

2 species of *Enterococcus* are responsible for the majority of infections in humans—*E. faecalis* and *E. faecium*. *E. faecalis* is responsible for ~ 90% of infections. The source of these organisms is usually either the GI or urinary tract. ~ 50% of newborns become colonized with enterococci by the 1st week of life. The organism is easily spread by fomites, especially in the hospital setting. Fomites are inanimate objects (e.g., toy, doorknob, dish, clothing) that can be contaminated with infectious organisms and serve in their transmission.

There are 3 main types of infection in children/infants:

1) UTI
2) Polymicrobial abdominal infections
3) Bacteremia/Sepsis

Few enterococci infections occur in "normal" infants. Most neonatal enterococcal infections are nosocomial and occur after the 2nd week of life, typically with bacteremia due to line infection or necrotizing enterocolitis. Common symptoms include bradycardia, fever, apnea, and abdominal distention.

Enterococci are uniformly resistant to cephalosporins and penicillinase-resistant PCNs—and moderately resistant to the aminoglycosides. *E. faecium* is one of the few organisms resistant to imipenem and is causing great problems with rapidly emerging, strong resistance to vancomycin ("VRE").

If sensitive, ampicillin and vancomycin are only inhibitory, but an aminoglycoside + ampicillin or vancomycin is effective treatment. So you must treat sensitive enterococcal sepsis, meningitis, or endocarditis with ampicillin or vancomycin in addition to gentamicin. Resistance to these antibiotics is increasing, so it is imperative that you do sensitivity testing. Linezolid is recommended for treating VRE infections in children.

Listeria monocytogenes

Listeria monocytogenes infections are associated with decreased cellular immunity syndromes like solid organ transplants (especially renal), immunodeficiency, lymphoma, and leukemia, but you may also see them in neonates and pregnant women. The highest incidence occurs in infants < 1 month of age, and is associated with maternal amnionitis, brown-staining of the amniotic fluid, preterm birth, pneumonia, septicemia, and an erythematous rash with papules called "granulomatosis infantisepticum." The case fatality rate of listerial meningitis is variable depending upon age and associated risk factors; some sources list mortality rates as high as 5–15%. Most texts still consider *S. pneumoniae* meningitis as having a higher fatality rate at 8%. Case fatality rates for the other common meningitis organisms: *H. influenzae* is 6%, *N. meningitidis* is 3%, and group B *Streptococcus* is 7%.

Neonates generally get the infection from their colonized mothers postnatally, transplacentally via premature rupture of membranes, or via fecal contamination from the mother at the time of birth. Environmental sources of the organism include sheep, goats, other livestock, and poultry. Infection can occur with direct contact with contaminated milk products (especially goat cheese!), meats, deli meats, hot dogs, soft cheeses, smoked salmon, tofu, or vegetables soiled with manure.

On the examination, be careful of a neonate for whom you are told the laboratory has preliminarily identified an organism from blood or CSF as "diphtheroids." Remember: *Listeria* is a gram-positive rod and can mimic the appearance of contaminant "diphtheroids." Outside of the neonatal period, *Listeria* still causes bacteremia/meningitis but can also cause rhombencephalitis (brain stem encephalitis), brain abscess, and endocarditis.

Like *Enterococcus*, *Listeria* is resistant to cephalosporins. (Again, this is why ampicillin is included in the empiric treatment for meningitis in the elderly or neonates.) Also, as with enterococci, PCN and ampicillin are only inhibitory; however, an aminoglycoside in combination with either of these is very effective treatment, usually given for 2–3 weeks.

So, although most mild-to-moderate cases of listeriosis do not require an aminoglycoside, treat resistant or serious cases with PCN or ampicillin in combination with an aminoglycoside; vancomycin or TMP/SMX if the patient is allergic to PCN. Because aminoglycosides do not penetrate the CSF well, use very high-dose PCN or ampicillin to treat listerial meningitis. Again:

- Mild-to-moderate listeriosis: ampicillin
- Serious/resistant: ampicillin + aminoglycoside
- Listerial meningitis: high-dose ampicillin +/– aminoglycoside

Corynebacterium

Corynebacterium diphtheriae causes diphtheria. Tonsillopharyngeal diphtheria is an upper respiratory infection with a gray-white pharyngeal membrane (Image 5-7), hoarseness, sore throat, and a low fever (< 101° F)! Again, low fever! See Image 5-8, showing the conjunctivitis and classic "bull neck" seen with diphtheria infection. The incubation period is 2 days. Laryngotracheobronchial diphtheria occurs in ~ 10% of patients and results in hoarseness, stridor, and respiratory compromise. Nasal diphtheria is more common in infants and younger children. These children have a profuse, mucoid, grayish discharge. It is the mildest type and rarely causes toxic manifestations.

Toxic effects include myocarditis with possible cardiac failure, renal effects, and polyneuritis. 10% of patients with diphtheria develop myocarditis, which typically occurs in the 1st week of infection. Arrhythmias are common. Renal failure is rare, but proteinuria, cylindruria, or microscopic hematuria is common. Usually, the neural involvement includes isolated peripheral nerve palsies or a Guillain-Barré–like syndrome.

You can treat based on clinical diagnosis only. Treatment for diphtheria is a specific equine antitoxin. Patients should also receive erythromycin, mainly to render the patient noncontagious, as opposed to being therapeutic. 2nd choice is PCN. Also, after recovery, immunize patients with diphtheria toxoid.

Corynebacterium jeikeium (JK) is especially a problem in neutropenic patients and bone marrow transplant units, where it is a cause of IV catheter-related infections. JK is resistant to most drugs. Vancomycin is the only effective agent, and you must remove the catheter.

Arcanobacterium haemolyticum

Arcanobacterium haemolyticum (previously *Corynebacterium haemolyticum*) causes a pharyngitis similar to that of *S. pyogenes* with fever, a desquamative scarlatiniform rash, and lymphadenitis; but palatal petechiae and strawberry tongue are absent. Respiratory tract infections that mimic diphtheria, including membranous pharyngitis, sinusitis, pneumonia, and skin and soft tissue infections have been reported. Invasive infections, including sepsis, meningitis, endocarditis, osteomyelitis, and peritonsillar abscess, have also been described.

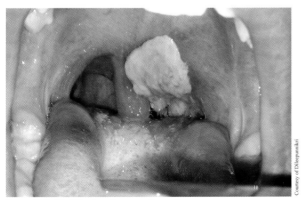

Image 5-7: Diphtheria; pharyngeal membrane

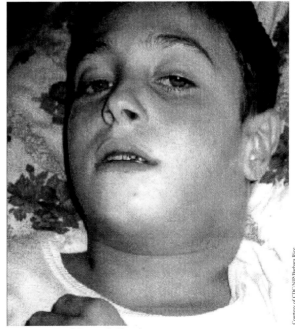

Image 5-8: Diphtheria; bull neck, conjunctivitis

Most commonly, the infection occurs in the adolescent age group.

Erythromycin is the drug of choice. Treatment with penicillin may fail.

Bacillus anthracis

Bacillus anthracis is a large, gram-positive rod (bacillus) that causes anthrax. There are 3 types of anthrax: **cutaneous** (95%, see Image 5-9), **gastrointestinal**, and **pulmonic** ("woolsorters' disease"). Inoculation occurs from handling contaminated hides/wool or—less naturally—via malicious contamination, such as in the mail. The cutaneous form of anthrax starts as a painless papule that vesiculates and forms a painless ulcer, then a painless black eschar, and often with a lot of nonpitting, painless induration and swelling. *B. anthracis* produces a tripartite exotoxin, consisting of edema factor, protective antigen, and lethal factor. Both edema factor and lethal factor require protective antigen to be active.

Treatment of choice for anthrax is ciprofloxacin or doxycycline; use penicillin G only if organism is susceptible.

Prophylaxis for exposures is ciprofloxacin or doxycycline for 30–60 days, unless the MICs of the organism indicate PCN susceptibility (then use high-dose amoxicillin). There is also an anthrax vaccine (BioThrax®) used in adults as part of postexposure prophylaxis; this vaccine has not been studied in children.

Bacillus cereus

Bacillus cereus is a close relative of *Bacillus anthracis*. It can cause 2 forms of gastroenteritis:

1) A short incubation (1–6 hr) emetic type, due to preformed heat stable toxin
2) A longer incubation (8–16 hr) diarrheal type, due to heat-labile enterotoxin production *in vivo* in the GI tract

The emetic form is associated with fried rice left at room temperature. This gastroenteritis is self-limited and necessitates only symptomatic treatment.

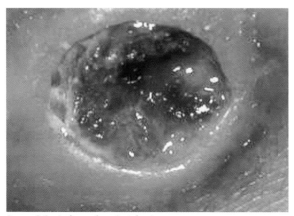

Image 5-9: Anthrax ulcer (painless)

Diagnosis is usually clinical, but you can look for *B. cereus* spores from stool or emesis—or by isolating the toxin from the suspected food item.

B. cereus is an occasional cause of infection in contact lens wearers, after a traumatic eye injury, and is a possible cause of wound infections and IV catheter-related infections. *B. cereus*-contaminated 70% alcohol pads have been associated with nosocomial outbreaks. Treat serious disease with vancomycin.

Clostridium Species

Overview

Clostridium is a strict anaerobic, gram-positive rod.

Clostridium difficile is associated with GI disease as well as asymptomatic carriage. Manifestations include colitis (commonly antibiotic-associated), pseudomembranous colitis, and toxic megacolon.

Clostridium botulinum causes botulism—the most potent toxin known! It blocks presynaptic acetylcholine release. This is discussed further in Neurology, Book 3.

Clostridium perfringens is one of the most common causes of food poisoning in the U.S. It presents as a 24-hour (or less) diarrheal illness and is associated with contaminated meat and poultry.

Clostridium septicum: The majority of patients with *C. septicum* sepsis have an associated GI malignancy—this is seen mostly in adults.

Clostridium tetani is the cause of tetanus.

Clostridium difficile

As mentioned above, antibiotic-associated colitis is caused by *Clostridium difficile.* (Antibiotic-associated diarrhea is typically just a side effect of the medicine.) Symptoms can occur up to 3 weeks after the antibiotics are stopped. Community-acquired *C. difficile* is becoming more virulent and can occur even without antibiotic exposure. So, think about *C. difficile* in any patient with prolonged bloody diarrhea!

Diagnosing *C. difficile* is based on the presence of diarrhea + laboratory evidence of *C. difficile* toxins in the stool specimen. Stool cultures are not useful. The enzyme immunoassay (detects toxins A and B) is the most commonly used testing method, but has low sensitivity. *C. difficile* PCR assays are now preferred as they have good sensitivity and specificity as well as rapid turnaround time. Remember: Test only symptomatic patients because 5% of healthy persons have *C. difficile* in their stools. Also, *C. difficile* carriage (without symptoms) is common in newborn infants and in children < 1 year of age.

Treatment: Stop precipitating antibiotics and give at least 10–14 days of metronidazole. Oral metronidazole is the drug of choice for the initial mild-to-moderate *C. difficile* infection. Oral (+ rectal if severe infection)

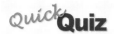

Quick Quiz

- Fried rice left out unrefrigerated may grow this bacteria, which can cause a self-limited gastroenteritis. What is the bug?

- What is the treatment for the 1ˢᵗ recurrence of *C. difficile* diarrhea?

- How do you treat tetanus?

vancomycin should be used for children with severe disease. Fidaxomicin has been approved in adults.

Initial recurrences should be treated with metronidazole if disease remains mild to moderate, but metronidazole should not be used past the 1ˢᵗ recurrence (due to concern for neurotoxicity). Treatment of the 2ⁿᵈ or greater recurrence should be with oral vancomycin and should include a tapered regimen.

For the exams, use metronidazole for the initial *C. difficile* infection and for the 1ˢᵗ reccurrence. If they relapse again, use oral vancomycin. Infection control is very important to stop nosocomial spread of *C. difficile* infections. Gowns and gloves are required, and hand washing is generally preferred over alcohol-based hand hygiene products (because spores are not inactivated by alcohol). Exercising meticulous hand hygiene, proper handling of contaminated waste, disinfecting fomites, and limiting the use of antimicrobial agents are all important in the prevention of *C. difficile* transmission.

Gas Gangrene

Cellulitis and gas gangrene can be caused by *C. septicum, perfringens, tetani, sordellii,* or *novyi*. Most gas gangrene is due to *C. perfringens*, usually after contamination of a wound. "Alpha toxin" is the main toxin in Clostridia. Symptoms can include severe pain, swelling, and crepitus.

For acute antibiotic treatment of *C. perfringens*, use PCN (clindamycin, metronidazole, or meropenem if patient is PCN-allergic). Prompt surgical debridement is essential.

Clostridium tetani

Tetanus is an acute illness due to the neurotoxin produced by *C. tetani*. This *Clostridium* is commonly found in soil and in normal human fecal flora 2–30% of the time. The highest incidence occurs in people who live on farms. Tetanus in children is rare in the U.S. However, in developing countries, it kills 60,000–200,000 neonates yearly.

4 forms of tetanus are observed:

1) **Generalized**, with widespread distribution of toxin

2) **Local**, with toxin only near the portal of entry

3) **Cephalic**, with dysfunction of the cranial nerves (associated with head and neck wounds)

4) **Neonatal**, generalized tetanus in newborn infants

In children, the generalized form is more common. The incubation period is 3–21 days (most cases occur within 8 days). The portal of entry, typically a wound, appears to be inconsequential. The infection begins with increasing stiffness of muscles of the neck, jaw, and large muscles of the back and lower extremities. Usually, by 24 hours into the illness, there is marked stiffness of the jaw and neck. The spasms of tetanus are characteristic: Stimuli (e.g., a loud noise, a touch, a flashing light) can cause paroxysmal contraction of the whole body that lasts for 5–10 seconds. The body is rigid like a board, the head is pulled back, the back is arched, the fists are clenched, and the thumbs are abducted (Image 5-10). The child's jaw is completely immobile, and the face has a tonic expression known as "risus sardonicus": raising of the eyebrows, narrowing of the palpebral fissures, downward/outward moving of the angles of the mouth, and pressing of the upper lip to the teeth. The affected person does not lose consciousness. Death results from eventual respiratory failure.

Neonatal tetanus, a.k.a. tetanus neonatorum, is more common in developing countries where women are not routinely immunized and nonsterile umbilical cord practices (such as placing manure on the stump) are routine. The illness starts on day 4–14 of life and presents with the child crying excessively and unable to suck. Quickly ensuing are trismus (persistent contraction of the masseter muscles), tonic contractions, spasms, and seizures. Death occurs from hypoxia, exhaustion, and lack of calories. Mortality rates approach 75%.

Diagnosis is clinical. Aim treatment at providing a quiet, stimulus-free environment. Manage with continuously administered neurologic blocking agents and mechanical ventilation. It is vital to use parenteral fluids and careful nutritional support.

Human tetanus immune globulin (TIG) is required. (When TIG is not available, equine tetanus antitoxin is used—but this is no longer available in the U.S.) Metronidazole is now the preferred antibiotic, although PCN G is also acceptable.

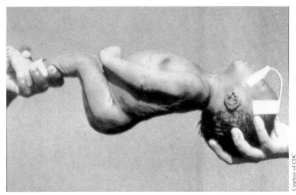

Image 5-10: Tetanus in newborn

What about tetanus prophylaxis for routine wound management? [Know this!] Let's consider some cases involving a girl named Marla:

- Marla has a staple injury (a clean, minor wound). She has had either an unknown number of tetanus immunizations or a known number < 3. Give her Tdap (or DTaP if < 7 years of age).
- Marla has a staple injury (a clean, minor wound). She has had ≥ 3 prior tetanus immunizations, with the last immunization < 10 years ago. She requires no further immunization at this point.
- Marla has a staple injury (a clean, minor wound). She has had ≥ 3 prior tetanus immunizations, and her last immunization was > 10 years ago. She requires a booster Tdap today.
- Marla steps on a dirty nail with cow feces on it. Her dog licks the foot after the injury. She has an unknown number of immunizations or a known number < 3. Give her Tdap (or DTaP if she's < 7 years of age) and human TIG.
- Marla steps on a dirty nail with cow feces on it. Her dog licks the foot after the injury. She has had ≥ 3 tetanus immunizations in the past, with the most recent < 5 years ago. She requires no vaccine.
- Marla steps on a dirty nail with cow feces on it. Her dog licks the foot after the injury. She has had ≥ 3 tetanus immunizations in the past, and her last immunization was 5.5 years ago. She requires Tdap (or DTaP if she is < 7 years old).

Here, then, are the protocols [Know]:

- Wound is dirty and either the child has had < 3 tetanus immunizations or the immunization history is unknown—use TIG + immunize.
- Wound is clean and immunizations are up to date (most recent < 10 years)—no treatment.
- Wound is dirty and immunizations are up to date (most recent immunization < 5 years)—no treatment.
- Recognize that Tdap is now OK for those between age 7 and 10 who need a booster; even though it is not FDA-approved as of 2013, it is recommended by the major immunization groups.
- Adolescents 10–18 years of age who require tetanus vaccine as wound prophylaxis should get Tdap instead of just Td if they have not had Tdap before.
- Pregnant women who require tetanus toxoid for wound prophylaxis should also get a dose of Tdap if they have never had one before. They have waning immunity to pertussis and it protects their newborn.

GRAM-NEGATIVE BACTERIA

Neisseria meningitidis

Neisseria meningitidis (meningococcus) is a gram-negative diplococcus that is an occasional, ordinary inhabitant of the upper respiratory tract. Carrier rates normally are 2–30% in normal populations. In an epidemic, the carrier rate approaches 100%! Meningococcus usually does not cause disease because specific antibodies (humoral defense) and complement lyse the organisms as they enter the bloodstream. There are 5 clinically significant serogroups based on the antigenic differences between their capsular polysaccharides. These groups are A, B, C, W-135, and Y. In the U.S., serogroups B, C, and Y each account for 30% of the cases reported.

Meningococcus is now the leading cause of meningitis in children and adolescents. The highest incidence of infection is seen in children < 2 years of age, the period of waning maternal IgG antibodies. A 2nd increase in incidence occurs in adolescents ages 15–19. Highest rates occur in the winter and early spring. Most adults have developed natural immunity against meningococcus.

Meningococcemia presents with fever, hypotension, diffuse purpuric lesions, and DIC. Of the patients with meningococcemia, > 60% have a petechial rash (Image 5-11).

Patients with terminal complement deficiency (C5–C9), or those deficient of properdin, are especially prone to meningococcemia. Ensure that all patients with bacteremia or meningitis have a CH50 or CH100 assay. Depending on the study, 1–17% of children with systemic meningococcal disease are found to have a complement deficiency.

Penicillin G is the treatment of choice; for the PCN-allergic, give fluoroquinolones (to adults) or 3rd generation cephalosporins—if rash only—to children. If the child is allergic to PCN and cephalosporin, meropenem or chloramphenicol is the drug of choice. With prompt treatment, the mortality rate from meningococcemia is 10%. Sequelae associated with meningococcal disease, including hearing loss, neurologic disability, digit or limb amputation, skin scarring, and renal failure, occur in 11–19% of survivors.

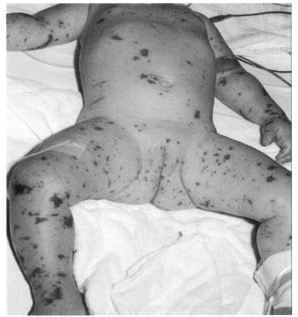

Image 5-11: Meningococcemia

Quick Quiz

- Know the tetanus scenarios listed for Marla in the text.
- What age groups have the highest incidence of meningococcal infection?
- What laboratory test is recommended in children with meningococcemia to screen for an immunologic deficiency?
- What is the treatment for meningococcemia?
- After exposure to a child with meningococcemia, who in the community should receive prophylaxis?
- After exposure to a child with meningococcemia, which health care workers should receive prophylaxis?
- Who should receive the meningococcal vaccine?
- What age group is most commonly affected by gonococcal ophthalmia?
- What is responsible for eye discharges if they occur within 48 hours after delivery? 2–7 days after delivery? 7–14 days after delivery?

Who should receive prophylaxis? Household, day care, close intimate contacts, and passengers seated directly next to an index case during airline flights lasting more than 8 hours. "Close intimate contacts" are defined as household members, especially children < 2 years of age, and children attending child care/preschool with the ill child anytime in the 7 days prior to illness onset. This also includes direct exposure to patient secretions such as eating, drinking, kissing, or sleeping under the same roof during the 7 days prior to illness onset. Do not prophylax individuals with indirect contact or with casual contact (e.g., school or work)! Give rifampin 10 mg/kg (max dose 600 mg) q 12 hours x 2 days, or ceftriaxone 125 mg IM for children < 15 years, or 250 mg IM for children ≥ 15 years as an alternative. Ceftriaxone is the drug of choice for an exposed pregnant woman. You can give a one-time dose of ciprofloxacin (500 mg) in adults > 18 years. These drugs are better than PCN for eradicating the carrier state because they concentrate in the throat mucosa. Give prophylaxis regardless of immunization status. (Vaccine is not 100% effective and does not cover serogroup B!) Give prophylaxis to patients with meningococcus before they leave the hospital. (Obviously, if they received ceftriaxone or cefotaxime for treatment, they are covered.)

What about the nurse who took the blood pressure when the patient came in? Or, you're the physician who spent 30 minutes in the room with the patient before making your astute diagnosis? You do not take prophylaxis unless you have close intimate contact such as with intubation or mouth-to-mouth resuscitation. This is different from what most people do in the "real world," where ciprofloxacin is given out like candy on Halloween. But for the examination, as the provider, you take prophylaxis only under those circumstances involving contact with oral secretions!

There are 2 tetravalent meningococcal polysaccharide-protein conjugate vaccines, MCV4 (Menactra®, Menveo®) available for serogroups A, C, Y, and W-135.

Remember: 30% of infections are due to serogroup B, so you are still missing a good chunk of infections. There is also a bivalent meningococcal-Hib combination vaccine, Hib-MenCY-TT, approved in June 2012. This vaccine includes serogroups C and Y, and is approved for use in infants ≥ 6 weeks of age. Routine vaccination of persons ≥ 2 months of age at increased risk for meningococcal disease is now recommended (as of March 2013). High-risk children include those who are splenectomized or have functional asplenia (children with sickle cell), complement or properdin deficiency, or who travel or are residents of countries where meningococcal disease is hyperendemic.

MCV4 is routinely administered to all 11–12-year-olds with a booster dose at 16–17 years. MCV4 is also given to all military recruits and college freshmen living in campus dormitories. More information on the meningococcal vaccine recommendations and dosing intervals can be found in Growth and Development/Preventive Pediatrics, Book 1.

Neisseria gonorrhoeae

Sexually Transmitted Disease

Neisseria gonorrhoeae is a common cause of sexually transmitted disease. It is a gram-negative organism that is usually found as diplococci. The penicillinase-producing strains of *N. gonorrhoeae* now account for 50% of cases in many areas of Asia and Africa and are also common in the U.S. The sexually transmitted disease aspects (cervicitis, PID, urethritis, etc.) are discussed in Adolescent Health and Gynecology, Book 1, as is disseminated gonococcal infection in adolescents—which is very important to know for the exams!

In all prepubertal children beyond the newborn period and in nonsexually active adolescents, suspect sexual abuse.

Gonococcal Ophthalmia

Gonococcal ophthalmia can occur at any age (presumably from self-inoculation). Most cases occur in the newborn as the infant passes through an infected birth canal. The use of 1% silver nitrate, 0.5% erythromycin, or 1% tetracycline ointment significantly reduces incidence.

Infants present 2–7 days after delivery with bloody, green, or serosanguineous discharge from the eyes. If this occurs, the first thing to do is a Gram-stained smear and culture for *N. gonorrhoeae*! If the discharge occurs within 48 hours of delivery, it is almost always due to a chemical reaction to the prophylaxis. If it occurs 7–14 days post-birth, it is almost always due to *Chlamydia trachomatis*. In infants with presumed gonococcal conjunctivitis, do a blood culture and lumbar puncture, evaluate for joint disease/focal infection, and consider working up for *C. trachomatis*, syphilis, HIV/HBV.

Complications of gonococcal ophthalmia can include iridocyclitis and corneal ulcerations.

Ceftriaxone 50 mg/kg IM or IV x 1 is sufficient for treating ophthalmia neonatorum; however, many receive antibiotics for 2–3 days until blood and CSF cultures are confirmed negative.

Bordetella pertussis

There are 3 well-known stages of infection with *Bordetella pertussis*. Pertussis, or whooping cough, begins as a mild respiratory tract infection very similar to the common cold (**catarrhal stage**). It then advances to a cough associated with paroxysms and an inspiratory whoop (**paroxysmal stage**). Symptoms gradually improve over weeks to months (**convalescent stage**). Fever is usually absent or slight. Duration is 6–10 weeks in children, but a majority of adolescents cough for > 10 weeks. Main complications are seen in children < 6 months of age, preterm, and unimmunized infants; these complications include pneumonia, seizures, and death.

Diagnosis is by culture (gold standard) of the nasopharyngeal region. PCR testing is increasingly used; no FDA-licensed PCR test is currently approved, but the CDC has released a "best practice" document to guide PCR use. DFA testing is no longer recommended for diagnosis! An elevated WBC count with an absolute lymphocytosis is suggestive in a clinical setting of paroxysmal cough in infants and children but is not often seen in adolescents.

Infants < 6 months of age with underlying medical conditions commonly require hospitalization.

Treat infants and children > 1 month of age with azithromycin, erythromycin, or clarithromycin. Give TMP/SMX for those who are macrolide-allergic. For infants < 1 month of age, azithromycin is recommended—because of the increased association of erythromycin use and infantile hypertrophic pyloric stenosis. (This is a 2012 Red Book recommendation, but azithromycin is not FDA-approved in children < 6 months of age.)

Chemoprophylaxis (same medications as for treatment) is recommended for all household and day care contacts. Booster dosages of pertussis vaccine should be given if they are due, and especially adolescents 11–18 years of age need to be immunized with Tdap.

Moraxella catarrhalis

Moraxella catarrhalis (formerly *Branhamella catarrhalis* [formerly *Neisseria catarrhalis*]) is a gram-negative diplococcus that causes respiratory infections. It is the 3rd most common cause of otitis media and sinusitis in children (behind *S. pneumoniae* and non-typeable *H. influenzae*). Rarely, it can cause bacteremia or bronchopulmonary infections, particularly in immunocompromised children or children with chronic lung disease.

Almost 100% of *Moraxella* strains produce β-lactamase. Amoxicillin-clavulanic acid, cefuroxime, cefprozil, cefpodoxime, azithromycin, and TMP/SMX are all generally effective agents (and fluoroquinolones in adults).

Pseudomonas aeruginosa

Pseudomonas aeruginosa is a small gram-negative rod with a single flagellum. *Pseudomonas* is commonly found in cystic fibrosis (see Respiratory Disorders, Book 4). Consider *Pseudomonas aeruginosa* if there is a history of nail-puncture wounds (especially if through a tennis shoe), osteomyelitis and endocarditis in IV drug abusers, bacteremia in burn patients, and chronic otitis externa (can be especially severe in diabetics). You might see ecthyma gangrenosum (a round, indurated, black lesion with central ulceration) with pseudomonal bacteremia—especially in neutropenic patients who are also at risk for typhilitis and perirectal cellulitis from *Pseudomonas*. In normal hosts, *Pseudomonas* is the cause of "hot tub rash," which people get from improperly chlorinated hot tubs. (This is usually self-limited.)

Treatment is with broad-spectrum PCNs, such as piperacillin-tazobactam and ticarcillin-clavulanic acid, or cephalosporins, such as ceftazidime and cefepime, or aminoglycosides. Quinolones are also effective, as are imipenem and meropenem. [Know: Never use ceftriaxone for *Pseudomonas* infection.]

Burkholderia cepacia and B. pseudomallei

B. cepacia and *B. pseudomallei* used to be known as *Pseudomonas* species. *B. cepacia* is common in cystic fibrosis and chronic granulomatous disease, is very difficult to treat, and has a poor prognosis. *B. pseudomallei* is a common infection in children in Southeast Asia (known as melioidosis) and can result in localized infection or septicemia. Treatment is even more difficult than for *Pseudomonas aeruginosa*; both are resistant to aminoglycosides! Meropenem, ceftazidime, quinolones, doxycycline, chloramphenicol, and trimethoprim/sulfamethoxazole may be helpful.

Salmonella

Salmonella are gram-negative bacilli that are generally motile. Non-typhoidal *Salmonella* is a fairly common cause of diarrhea and rarely causes bacteremia, meningitis (with brain abscess formation), and bone infections (very common cause of osteomyelitis in sickle

Quick Quiz

- What is the treatment for uncomplicated gonococcal ophthalmia in the newborn?

- True or false? Most *Moraxella* produce β-lactamase.

- A child steps on a nail through his tennis shoe. What organisms would you be concerned about if he developed an osteomyelitis in the foot?

- Iguana = what organism?

- Which group of patients should you treat for *Salmonella* gastroenteritis?

- In what settings do many *Shigella* infections occur?

- Which requires many fewer organisms for transmission: *Shigella* or *Salmonella*?

- What laboratory finding is common in *Shigella* infections?

cell patients). Young infants are at higher risk of invasive disease. (Common risk factor = bottles prepared in same sink that family uses to wash raw chicken.)

Because the bacteria are not host-adapted, like *S.* serotype Typhi (formerly known as *S. typhi)*, they can be found in many different non-human host animals. Recent foodborne outbreaks include: frozen foods (especially chicken), milk, eggs, produce, and peanut butter. Baby chicks, iguanas, frogs, turtles, and other exotic pets also may be sources of infections. Treatment increases the risk of developing a carrier state—it does not decrease symptoms and can prolong fecal excretion; so, for uncomplicated gastroenteritis, do not give antibiotics!

However, give antibiotic therapy for *Salmonella* diarrhea in children < 3 months of age and older children with immunocompromising diseases (e.g., HIV, agammaglobulinemia, malignancy, Crohn's). Invasive infections should be treated with a 3rd generation cephalosporin until susceptibilities are available.

Salmonella serotype Typhi is, unlike most *Salmonella*, non-motile and encapsulated. It causes typhoid fever, usually from contaminated food, milk, or water. Adults are more likely to be carriers because *S.* serotype Typhi tends to seed in gallstones. (Did "typhoid Mary" have gallstones?) The infection tends to cause leukopenia. The classic "rose spots" form on the trunk about a week after the fever starts; these look like small, 2–3-mm angiomas. Blood (60% sensitive), bone marrow (90% sensitive), or bile culture is diagnostic of *S.* serotype Typhi. (Organisms are frequently absent from the stool.)

Typhoid vaccine is recommended for individuals (> 2 years old) traveling to the Indian subcontinent, Latin America, Asia, the Middle East, and Africa.

Treatment of typhoid fever: Options include 3rd generation cephalosporins, ampicillin, TMP/SMX, quinolones, and chloramphenicol, depending on susceptibilities. (Resistance is increasing worldwide!) Carriers without gallbladder disease or stones can typically be cleared with 4 weeks of ciprofloxacin or norfloxacin. High-dose IV ampicillin can be used if fluoroquinolone therapy is not well tolerated.

Shigella

Shigella sonnei is the most common serotype in the U.S., with *S. flexneri* 2nd in frequency. Highest incidences occur in day care centers, among people living in crowded conditions or institutions, and among people living on Native American reservations. Children ages 1–4 years have the highest incidence, with a peak between July and October. Outbreaks also occur due to contaminated pools and lakes. Houseflies are recognized as vectors (transport infected feces). Foodborne outbreaks, especially from fresh fruits and vegetables, also occur.

Person-to-person transmission of *Shigella* plays a key role (unlike *Salmonella* infection). *Shigella* can infect with only 10–100 organisms vs. the thousands to millions for *Salmonella*!

Incubation is most often 24–48 hours. Most children's infection begins with fever, malaise, poor appetite, vomiting, and/or headache. Diarrhea is typically watery and can progress to dysentery within hours or days: frequent small stools with mucus or blood accompanied by lower abdominal cramps and tenesmus.

A classic *Shigella* scenario is when an infant presents with fever and new-onset seizures, and while you are performing the lumbar puncture, the baby has a large, bloody stool.

Complications include rectal prolapse (5–8%), pseudomembranous colitis, and HUS. Peripheral WBCs are usually elevated; bandemia is very common. Seizures occur with increased frequency of *Shigella* infection in young children. Reactive arthritis can occur, especially in patients with HLA-B27.

Once *Shigella* is identified in a day care attendee or household, all other symptomatic individuals in these environments should be cultured for *Shigella* as well. Anyone found to have *Shigella* cannot return to day care until the diarrhea has stopped > 24 hours and stool cultures test negative.

Most clinical infections with *S. sonnei* are self-limited. Treat children with severe disease or underlying conditions with ceftriaxone, ciprofloxacin (if older than 18 years), or azithromycin. Antibiotics shorten disease course and limit spread to others (opposite of *Salmonella*). Oral cephalosporins are not useful. TMP/SMX and ampicillin were once the drugs of choice, but resistance is increasing (50% in 2009).

E. coli

E. coli is a gram-negative, lactose-fermenting, motile rod belonging to the *Enterobacteriaceae* family. *E. coli* is a common cause of UTI. It also is a cause of meningitis in the neonate.

There are > 200 different serotypes, with 5 phenotypes causing diarrhea:

1) Enteropathogenic *E. coli* (**EPEC**) causes acute and chronic diarrhea in infants.

2) Enterotoxigenic *E. coli* (**ETEC**) causes watery diarrhea in infants and "traveler's diarrhea."

3) Enteroinvasive *E. coli* (**EIEC**) causes diarrhea and fever.

4) Enterohemorrhagic *E. coli* (**EHEC**) and also now known as **STEC** (Shiga toxin-producing *E. coli*) is responsible for hemorrhagic colitis and hemolytic uremic syndrome. No antibiotics (see below).

5) Enteroaggregative *E. coli* (**EAEC**) causes persistent diarrhea in children in developing countries and in travelers.

Do not give antimotility agents to children with inflammatory or bloody diarrhea! Treatment is generally supportive care only (orally-administered electrolyte-containing solution should be adequate to prevent dehydration). For severe watery diarrhea or traveler's diarrhea, use azithromycin or a fluoroquinolone. Most experts advise against prescribing antimicrobial therapy for children with STEC.

Enterohemorrhagic (EHEC, STEC) results from outbreaks of *E. coli* O157:H7. Foodborne infections are becoming more frequent—especially in the U.S. The incidence of *E. coli* O157:H7 infection is more common than *Shigella*! Dairy cattle appear to be a major reservoir; the disease is linked to eating undercooked beef and unpasteurized milk or apple juice. Outbreaks at petting zoos have also been reported.

This *E. coli* produces a Shiga toxin (STX), which may cause bloody diarrhea, hemorrhagic colitis, hemolytic uremic syndrome (HUS), and can simulate TTP.

HUS classically has the triad of:

1) Kidney failure
2) Thrombocytopenia with purpura
3) Hemolytic anemia

E. coli culture medium requires sorbitol-enhanced agar.

Do not treat with antibiotics! An initial study showed that treating patients infected with O157:H7 strains increased the risk of HUS—however, meta-analysis failed to confirm this. But most experts would not treat children with O157:H7 because no benefits have been proven and adverse events may occur.

Children may not return to day care until the diarrhea has resolved and they have had 2 negative stool cultures after diarrhea resolution.

Non-O157 STEC strains are also associated with outbreaks and HUS. A 2011 outbreak of O104:H4 associated with contaminated sprouts occurred in Germany.

Haemophilus influenzae

Overview

Haemophilus influenzae is a small, "pleomorphic," gram-negative coccobacillus. *H. influenzae* type b (Hib) used to be the most common cause of meningitis, bacteremia, pneumonia, epiglottitis, and septic arthritis in children. However, the introduction of the *H. influenzae* vaccine quickly reduced the incidence of encapsulated *H. influenzae* type b (the etiology of severe invasive disease) to the point where it has become almost nonexistent in some centers. Unimmunized children < 4 years of age are at increased risk of invasive Hib disease.

Risk factors for invasive disease include sickle cell disease, asplenia, HIV, malignancies, and primary immunodeficiencies. Hib was also more common in boys; African-American, Alaska Native, Apache, and Navajo children; child care attendees; and children living in crowded conditions.

Today, non-typeable strains are still responsible for a large number of mucosal infections, including conjunctivitis, otitis media, sinusitis, and bronchitis.

In newborns, incidence of non-typeable *H. influenzae* has increased for bacteremia and meningitis. Most of the organisms are picked up from the mother when traversing the birth canal. Around 80% of cases occur in the 1st day of life. *In utero*, infection also occurs. Because of this increased incidence, some centers have added a 3rd generation cephalosporin to standard ampicillin and gentamicin in the newborn, particularly if meningitis is suspected.

Vaccine use has also resulted in "herd immunity," whereby those not vaccinated have some protection because of the reduced incidence of nasopharyngeal carriage for pathogenic strains. Many of these infections are more historical, but you still need to know them for the exams!

Meningitis

Symptoms are nonspecific for *H. influenzae* meningitis. Peak age is < 1 year. Around 1/3 of children have seizures with *H. influenzae* meningitis. Petechial rash also occurs, as in meningococcal infection. Other sites of infection are common, including septic arthritis or buccal cellulitis. Common complications include subdural empyema, brain infarcts, cerebritis, ventriculitis, brain abscess, and hydrocephalus. Mortality is ~ 5%. Long-term sequelae occur in 15–30% of survivors, with sensorineural hearing loss (6–15%) the most common. Other sequelae include language disorder, intellectual disabilities, and developmental disorders.

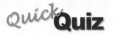

Quick Quiz

- Name the diseases with which *E. coli* O157:H7 is associated.
- What food products are associated with *E. coli* O157:H7?
- At what age are newborns at greatest risk for serious disseminated disease from non-typeable *H. influenzae*?
- What is the most common long-term sequela of *H. influenzae* meningitis?
- Know the treatment for *H. influenzae* meningitis.
- How is the epiglottis described in acute epiglottitis?
- Historically, what was buccal cellulitis associated with?
- What is the most common cause of bacteremic periorbital cellulitis?
- What is a common cause of periorbital cellulitis if a bug bite or scratch was the inciting injury?
- True or false? You should treat all occult bacteremias due to *H. influenzae* with parenteral antibiotics.
- What is the drug of choice for otitis media? What if you suspect or find a β-lactamase–producing *H. influenzae*?

Prior to or concurrent with the initiation of antibiotics (ceftriaxone or cefotaxime), use dexamethasone 0.6 mg/kg/day divided q 6 hours x 2 days to decrease the incidence of hearing loss and neurologic sequelae.

Epiglottitis

Epiglottitis occurs primarily in children age 2–7 years with an abrupt onset of high fever, dysphagia, and drooling. The epiglottis is described as "cherry red." These kids have the "I'm going to die" look with the classic "tripod" position: trunk leaning forward, neck hyperextended, and chin thrust forward. Do not try to examine the oropharynx of an uncooperative child with possible epiglottitis without the presence of an adequate airway or anesthesiologist/ENT in the operating room. For children in whom the diagnosis is certain—based on presentation and clinical examination—intraoral examination is likely unnecessary. In those for whom the diagnosis is unclear, many experts advocate the use of a tongue depressor in a cooperative child. You must view individual factors for each case. (More in Respiratory Disorders, Book 4.) Bacterial tracheitis due to *S. aureus* is now more common than epiglottitis in the U.S.

Septic Arthritis / Osteomyelitis

Before the Hib vaccine was available, *H. influenzae* was the most common cause of septic arthritis in children < 2 years of age. Septic arthritis of the hip and shoulder requires surgical drainage.

Buccal Cellulitis

Buccal cellulitis previously was virtually always caused by *H. influenzae* infection, but now the vaccine has all but prevented this infection from occurring. If present, the child is almost always bacteremic with *H. influenzae*. Buccal cellulitis is palpable on both sides of the cheek and is purplish in color; these children are very toxic in appearance.

Periorbital Cellulitis

Periorbital or preseptal cellulitis also used to be commonly due to *H. influenzae*. Today, pneumococcus is the most common etiology for bacteremic periorbital cellulitis. A significant portion of cases of preseptal cellulitis is related to minor trauma of the eyelids or insect bites and is due to *S. aureus* or a group A *Streptococcus*.

Occult Bacteremia

Occult bacteremia with *H. influenzae* is very different from occult bacteremia with pneumococcus. Pneumococcal "occult" bacteremia tends to spontaneously resolve without therapy, while bacteremia with *H. influenzae* results in 30–50% developing meningitis or other deep, focal infection from occult bacteremia!

Pneumonia, Otitis Media, Sinusitis

Pneumonia from *H. influenzae* used to cause ~ 1/3 of bacterial pneumonia in the pre-Hib vaccine era. Today, it is rare. Most cases have pleural effusion; blood cultures are positive in 90%.

Treat invasive *H. influenzae* with a 3rd generation cephalosporin—either ceftriaxone or cefotaxime. You can use cefuroxime (2nd generation) for non-meningitis infection but with caution, because it does not cross the blood-brain barrier well. Treat uncomplicated Hib meningitis with IV therapy for at least 10 days; septic arthritis requires 14–21 days. Those with osteomyelitis, pericarditis, or empyema are generally treated for 4–6 weeks IV, followed by oral therapy. Occult Hib infection requires therapy to prevent focal infection from developing.

For noninvasive disease, such as otitis media and sinusitis, amoxicillin is the drug of choice. If amoxicillin fails, use agents active against β-lactamase-producing strains, including amoxicillin-clavulanic acid, TMP/SMX, azithromycin, clarithromycin, cefuroxime axetil, cefixime, or cefpodoxime.

Chemoprophylaxis is important for those exposed to invasive strains of *H. influenzae*. The rules guiding who gets prophylaxis are quite complicated, and you may have to re-read the guidelines several times to make sense of it. In general, for the exam, you'll give prophylaxis. Give rifampin 20 mg/kg (max 600 mg) q day x 4 days to household contacts and day care attendees (although, hopefully, most of them are immunized).

Classically, though, look for the following scenarios on an exam:

• Give prophylaxis to all household members if the household has:
  ◦ at least 1 contact < 4 years of age who is incompletely immunized or
  ◦ an immunocompromised individual in the household.
• Give prophylaxis to preschool and child care center contacts when the child care center has had at least 2 patients with invasive Hib disease within 60 days.

Yersinia

Yersinia pestis

Yersinia pestis is a gram-negative coccobacillus that causes plague. Reservoir is wild rodents. It is transmitted by fleas or direct contact, such as skinning animals, and has high mortality.

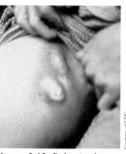
Image 5-12: Bubonic plague
Courtesy of CDC

The **bubonic** type causes large, localized lymphadenopathy ("buboes") that suppurate (Image 5-12). If not treated, it can lead to the **septicemic** form characterized by hypotension, respiratory distress, organ failure, and death. The bubonic type also may lead to a **pneumonic** form that is rapidly transmitted to bystanders by coughing. (Bioterrorism has brought some attention to this organism on exams.)

Note: Plague and tularemia present similarly (adenopathy after hunting, etc.), except that the geographic locations are different—desert Southwest for plague vs. Arkansas, Missouri, and Oklahoma for tularemia.

Diagnose plague by culture (blood, lymph node aspirate, sputum) or by serology.

Treat plague with gentamicin or streptomycin. 2nd line choices: tetracycline, doxycycline, TMP/SMX, or quinolones.

Yersinia enterocolitica

Yersinia enterocolitica is a small, gram-negative coccobacillus. It produces entero- and endotoxin. Most humans become infected from ingesting contaminated food, milk, or water. Pigs are commonly infected; so those who handle pork products, especially chitterlings, are at increased risk. A fairly common scenario is for a grandparent to prepare chitterlings, or handle raw pork, and then feed or handle the baby without washing the hands well—resulting in the infant becoming colonized and then infected. Contaminated blood transfusions have also been implicated in transfusion-related sepsis. *Yersinia* is found in ~ 1% of diarrheal illnesses.

Older children and adolescents present with the "pseudo-appendicitis syndrome," which can be due to *Yersinia pseudotuberculosis* or *Y. enterocolitica*. This presents clinically just like appendicitis.

Adults are more likely to get the reactive arthritis (especially with HLA-B27) and erythema nodosum associated with *Yersinia* infection.

Bacteremia occurs in the very young (< 1 year of age) and in those with iron overloads (especially children who are transfusion-dependent with sickle cell disease, beta-thalassemia, aplastic anemia, etc.).

Treat patients with bacteremia (and non-GI disease) and immunocompromised hosts with TMP/SMX, aminoglycosides, 3rd generation cephalosporins, tetracycline, or quinolones.

Legionella pneumophila

The *Legionellae* family comprises many species—of which *Legionella pneumophila* causes 80–90% of human *Legionellae* infections. *Legionellae* infections are rare in children. *Legionellae* are aerobic, gram-negative bacilli that require a particular media (enriched, buffered, charcoal yeast extract) to grow.

L. pneumophilia is found in water, and modes of transmission are multiple—with aspiration the most likely.

L. pneumophila infection (legionellosis) causes legions of problems. Multisystem disease is the clue! Patients with "Legionnaires' disease" often have diarrhea, CNS symptoms (H/A, delirium, and confusion), and renal disease in addition to the pneumonia (mild to severe). Presentation is similar to, and often confused with, *Mycoplasma pneumoniae*. Like *M. pneumoniae*, the CXR looks much worse than the exam indicates. It can also cause "Pontiac fever," which is a milder multisystem flu-like illness without pneumonia.

Treat moderate infections with azithromycin or quinolones.

Klebsiella

Klebsiella is a rare cause of pneumonia, bacteremia, and meningitis in children. It also can cause UTIs but is much less common than *E. coli*. It can be an important cause of neonatal septicemia. Most *Klebsiella* organisms are uniformly resistant to ampicillin. Resistance to the cephalosporins is increasing due to AmpC beta-lactamases and extended-spectrum beta-lactamases ([ESBL] the drug of choice for an ESBL-producing *Klebsiella* is meropenem), and some *Klebsiella* isolates are even carbapenem-resistant.

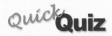

Quick Quiz

- A day care center in a commune (that does not allow immunizations) has 2 cases of *H. influenzae* meningitis. What should the other children in the day care center receive?
- How is *Yersinia pestis* transmitted?
- How is plague diagnosed? Treated?
- What organism is associated with "pseudoappendicitis syndrome" in older children and adolescents?
- For which type of atypical pneumonia is multisystem disease a diagnostic clue?
- What is a common atypical presentation of cat-scratch disease?

Brucella

Brucellosis is a zoonosis caused by an aerobic gram-negative bacillus that, worldwide, is most commonly *B. melitensis* (goats, sheep, and camels). Other strains: *Brucella abortus* (cattle), *B. suis* (pigs), and *B. canis* (dogs).

It is often transmitted to humans via unpasteurized milk or cheese, by inhalation (work-related), or by handling carcasses. It affects the heart (especially suspect in culture-negative endocarditis), lungs, GI tract, GU (orchitis, abortion), and endocrine glands (thyroiditis, adrenal insufficiency, SIADH). Osteoarticular disease, especially sacroiliitis, is relatively common! Granulomatous hepatitis can also occur.

Check for brucellosis in a fever of unknown origin (FUO) workup! Confirming the diagnosis is difficult. Cultures may take up to 4 weeks to grow (newer BACTEC™ systems can detect *Brucella* species in 5–7 days). In some types, you can do serotyping. (Look for increasing specific IgM titers.)

Treatment requires combination therapy:

- Doxycycline x minimum of 6 weeks + aminoglycoside x 2 weeks or
- Doxycycline + rifampin x at least 6 weeks

Quinolones are not appropriate 1st line single agents—but can be given in combination with doxycycline or rifampin.

For children < 8 years, most recommend TMP/SMX for 4–6 weeks + rifampin. Add gentamicin for serious or complicated infections.

Relapses generally are associated with premature discontinuation of therapy or monotherapy (and not resistance).

Francisella tularensis

Francisella tularensis is a small, gram-negative pleomorphic bacillus that causes tularemia ("rabbit fever"). It is found in many animals and is especially prevalent in Arkansas, Missouri, and Oklahoma. It is transmitted by ticks and blood-sucking flies; the organism may also be ingested or inhaled. Typically, patients with tularemia present with a sudden onset of fever, chills, myalgias, and arthralgias, followed by an irregular ulcer at the site of inoculation. Known as the "ulceroglandular form," it may persist for months. Regional lymphadenopathy develops, and these nodes may necrose and suppurate. Other forms include:

- Glandular (without the ulcer)
- Oculoglandular (conjunctivitis and preauricular lymphadenopathy)
- Oropharyngeal (acute pharyngitis)
- Vesicular skin lesions
- Pneumonic (pneumonia and hilar adenopathy—from inhalation of aerosolized organisms [not common but could be used for bioterrorism])
- Typhoidal (high fever, hepatosplenomegaly)

Base diagnosis of tularemia on the typical clinical syndrome, and confirm with serologic testing for *Francisella tularensis*. Differentials include plague, which occurs mostly in the Desert Southwest.

Treat with gentamicin or streptomycin x 10 days. Alternative agents include ciprofloxacin and doxycycline. Relapse tends to occur more commonly with tetracyclines, so treat for 14 days.

Bartonella

Bartonella henselae causes cat-scratch disease (CSD) or, in the immunocompromised patient, bacillary angiomatosis.

Cat-scratch disease is characterized by > 3 weeks of chronic, tender, regional lymphadenopathy, a history of cat (especially kitten) contact or scratch, and a primary skin lesion, which appears as a small, nondescript pink papule (~ 60% have the skin lesion) (Image 5-13). Most common involved lymph nodes are cervical, axillary, inguinal, and epitrochlear. Dog contact may be responsible in some cases.

Humans become infected through inoculation of the bacteria through a scratch or bite from an infected cat or by hands contaminated with infected flea feces touching an open wound or eye. The enlarged node (Image 5-14) spontaneously resolves in 4–6 weeks, but 25% will suppurate. The oculoglandular syndrome of Parinaud's is one of the more common atypical presentations. This occurs when the patient is scratched or inoculated around the eye, gets conjunctivitis, and develops an ipsilateral preauricular lymphadenitis. Less common manifestations of CSD (about 25% of cases) include systemic disease with hepatosplenic granulomas,

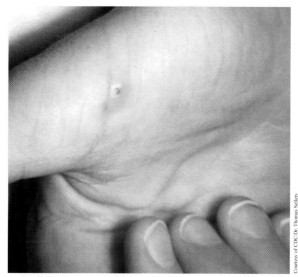

Image 5-13: Cat-scratch disease, 1° lesion

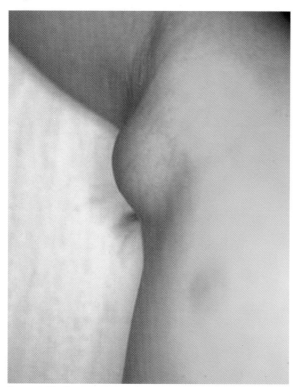

Image 5-14: Cat-scratch disease, adenopathy

neuroretinitis, encephalopathy, aseptic meningitis, osteomyelitis, endocarditis, and FUO.

Diagnosis is usually clinical; however, use of PCR and serum antibodies is available. Recovery of the organism in culture is rarely achieved. Do not incise and drain because a persistent sinus tract infection will likely develop. Node biopsy may be required in atypical cases to confirm the diagnosis, and bacilli may be demonstrated by Warthin-Starry silver stain, although not specific for *B. henselae*. Histologic findings on lymph node would typically show necrotizing granulomas.

Treatment of localized CSD is aimed at symptom relief since the disease usually resolves in 2–4 months. Painful suppurative nodes can be relieved by needle aspiration, but incision and drainage should be avoided. Some experts recommend treating with a 5-day course of oral azithromycin early on, prior to development of lymph node suppuration, to speed recovery. Antibiotics may hasten recovery in acutely or severely ill patients with systemic symptoms, especially those with hepatosplenic involvement or painful adenitis, and is recommended for all immunocompromised people. Additional agents include TMP/SMX, fluoroquinolones, rifampin, and gentamicin.

Bacillary angiomatosis occurs mainly in HIV-infected adults. The skin lesions of bacillary angiomatosis are identical to "verruga peruana." Treatment: azithromycin or doxycycline +/– rifampin for months.

Pasteurella

Pasteurella multocida is best known for causing infection in cat or dog bites—it classically causes rapidly progressing cellulitis within 24 hours of the bite, often accompanied by fever and regional lymphadenopathy. It is the most common cause of infection in cat bites with *Staphylococcus aureus* being #2. Local complications can include septic arthritis, osteomyelitis, and tenosynovitis. The drug of choice for isolated *Pasteurella* infection is penicillin, but commonly in cat and dog bites, amoxicillin-clavulanate is used because of mixed flora. In penicillin-allergic children, trimethoprim/sulfamethoxazole plus clindamycin are the drugs of choice for bite wounds. Treat all cat bites (tend to be deep puncture wounds) and only those dog bites that are infected or are deep wounds.

Kingella

Kingella kingae causes osteomyelitis and suppurative arthritis in children under the age of 5 years. Osteomyelitis most commonly occurs in the distal femur and suppurative arthritis most commonly involves the knee, and next most often, the hip and ankle. *K. kingae* can also cause endocarditis (one of the HACEK organisms), diskitis, and meningitis. Penicillin is the treatment of choice (if beta-lactamase negative); most strains are susceptible to ampicillin-sulbactam, TMP/SMX, aminoglycosides, and fluoroquinolones.

Campylobacter

Campylobacter produces fever and diarrheal gastroenteritis. Stools can be bloody. Children can present with febrile seizures, and abdominal pain can mimic appendicitis or intussusception. It is the most common cause of Guillain-Barré syndrome (more in Neurology, Book 3) and can also be associated with reactive arthritis (arthritis, urethritis, bilateral conjunctivitis). Chicken and turkey are common sources, and carcasses are generally contaminated. Puppies and kittens typically

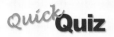

Quiz

- What antibiotics may be useful in cat-scratch disease?
- What do you suspect in a neonate with *Citrobacter* growing in the CSF?
- Where does the rash occur with RMSF?
- What is the drug of choice to treat RMSF?

harbor the infection. Cultures require an incubation temperature of 42°–43° C (107.6°–109.4° F). Azithromycin or erythromycin is the preferred drug and eradicates the organism from stool in 2–3 days. Fluoroquinolones (e.g., ciprofloxacin) can be effective, but resistance is common and these antibiotics are not FDA-approved for kids < 18 years of age for this indication.

Helicobacter pylori

Helicobacter pylori is a gram-negative, spiral, flagellated bacillus. It causes gastritis and peptic ulcer disease and is a risk factor for adenocarcinoma of the stomach. Infection is frequently acquired in childhood; most individuals remain asymptomatic for life. More in Gastroenterology & Nutrition, Book 4.

Citrobacter

Citrobacter is rare. However, if the exam mentions a neonate with *Citrobacter* growing in a blood or CSF culture, immediately get a CT/MRI of the head to look for brain abscess!

Enterobacter sakazakii and *Serratia marcescens* also cause brain abscesses in neonates!

RICKETTSIAE

Rickettsia

Rickettsia rickettsii, a gram-negative coccobacillus, causes Rocky Mountain spotted fever (RMSF)—[Know!] This disease has a 3% mortality. Classic signs and symptoms include a rash, fever, headache, arthralgias (but not overt arthritis), and a history of recent exposure to ticks. The peak incidence is in children ages 5–9 years. It is common in the Carolinas, Georgia, Virginia, Missouri, Tennessee, Arkansas, and Oklahoma. The rash occurs on the distal extremities (Image 5-15). It progresses from maculopapular to petechial to purpura. Most infected persons get the rash—but few get all of the classic signs/symptoms. Patients may also present with diarrhea and abdominal pain. Hyponatremia and thrombocytopenia are helpful lab clues.

Other rickettsial infections include *R. typhi* (endemic typhus), *R. prowazekii* (epidemic typhus), *R. akari* (rickettsialpox), *R. conorii* (Mediterranean spotted fever), and *Coxiella burnetii* (Q fever).

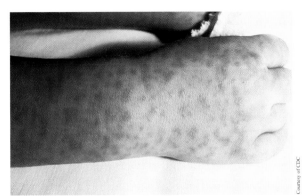

Image 5-15: Rocky Mountain spotted fever (RMSF)

[Know:] Q fever is a zoonosis that is transmitted to humans mainly by inhalation of the aerosol released from the infected animal. Q fever is seen in abattoir (slaughterhouse) workers and in people exposed to an infected animal's products of conception during birthing. Buzzwords: Cattle or Cats or Conception = *Coxiella* (Q fever).

Diagnose by serology (IFA usually) or by staining tissue specimens (biopsy) obtained from the site of the rash—the staining method is very specific, but not very sensitive—and do this before you give antibiotics.

Treat all *Rickettsia* infections with doxycycline, which is the drug of choice for all ages (even those < 8 years of age) because of its clinical superiority to other agents. Chloramphenicol is essentially no longer available in the U.S. as an oral agent.

Ehrlichia / Anaplasma

Ehrlichia (ehrlichiosis) and *Anaplasma* (anaplasmosis) infections have been called "Rocky Mountain spotless fever." There are 2 forms of the disease:

1) Human monocytic ehrlichiosis (HME, due to *E. chaffeensis*)
2) Human granulocytic anaplasmosis (HGA, due to *Anaplasma phagocytophilum*)

The organisms are small, gram-negative, and obligately intracellular. HME is mainly prevalent in Texas, Oklahoma, Missouri, and Arkansas; HGA predominates in the Northeast and Midwest. There is frequently a

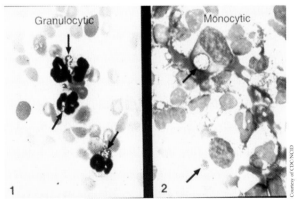

Image 5-16: Morulae seen in ehrlichiosis

rash in children. The organism affects the monocytes or neutrophils, and patients typically present with the viral picture of fever, headache, and leukopenia. They may also have thrombocytopenia and elevated liver transaminases. Think of this in an exam presentation of pancytopenia and tick bite! Diagnosis is usually by serologic testing, but the organism can be isolated in culture from blood/CSF, by PCR, or by detection of a cytoplasmic cluster of organisms (morulae) in the WBCs (Image 5-16).

Treat ehrlichiosis with doxycycline.

Note: There are reports of dual infection with *Ehrlichia* + *Babesia microti* (an intraRBC protozoan parasite) and *Ehrlichia* + *Borrelia burgdorferi* (Lyme) in the endemic Northeast areas.

GRAM-VARIABLE

Gardnerella vaginalis (previously called *Haemophilus vaginalis*) is **g**ram-**v**ariable. Treat with metronidazole. It is associated with a vaginosis.

ANAEROBES

Anaerobes are listed briefly in the ABP content outline. For the most part, anaerobic infection is mainly a concern with oral, pulmonary or intraabdominal abscesses (*Bacteroides, Prevotella*). Treatment of dental infections typically includes penicillin; clindamycin is active against almost all oral and lung anaerobic organisms and is the drug of choice by some experts, especially for severe lung infection. *Bacteroides* species of the GI tract are predictably susceptible to metronidazole.

Fusobacterium is an anaerobe that causes Lemierre disease, which is more common in adolescents and young adults and results in internal jugular vein thrombophlebitis or thrombosis with signs of septic lung emboli. Initially there is fever and sore throat that progresses to severe neck pain (angina) with associated unilateral neck swelling, trismus, and dysphagia. Metronidazole is recommended by many, but combination therapy with ceftriaxone/cefotaxime is common to cover for coinfection with aerobic oral and respiratory pathogens.

ACID-FAST

Overview

All *Mycobacteria* are acid-fast (red on a green background). *M. avium complex* (MAC) and *M. scrofulaceum* cause lymphadenitis in immunocompetent children (Image 5-17). Treat by excising the nodes! Do not incise the node—it will cause a chronic draining lesion! The nodes are usually painless.

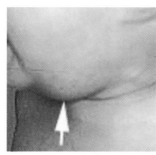
Image 5-17: Lymphadenitis

M. leprae causes leprosy. Transmission is probably via person-to-person respiratory droplets. Diagnose with histopathology and Fite stains of skin or nerve biopsy.

M. marinum is the "fish-tank bacillus." It causes non-healing skin ulceration in people working around fish tanks. It often causes strings of lesions along the lymphatic channels. Treat *M. marinum* with ethambutol + rifampin or clarithromycin + rifampin.

M. bovis is associated with fresh cow's milk and especially in San Diego, California, where 3–11% of tuberculosis cases were due to *M. bovis*!

M. abscessus and MAC are associated with pulmonary infections in children with cystic fibrosis.

M. chelonae and *M. fortuitum* are associated with catheter-associated infections. *M. fortuitum* is also associated with osteomyelitis in children who have puncture wounds contaminated with soil!

M. tuberculosis—we will cover this in detail next.

Disseminated infections with nontuberculous mycobacteria occur in children with impaired cell-mediated immunity, especially in children with primary immunodeficiencies such as interleukin-12 deficiency, NF-kappa-B essential modulator (NEMO) mutations, and interferon-gamma receptor defects. Children who have undergone stem cell transplants or have advanced HIV are also at risk.

Mycobacterium tuberculosis

Overview

TB is a favorite exam topic! Tuberculosis infection occurs when aerosolized, contaminated droplets (coughed up by a person with the disease or the "source case") are inhaled by another and the droplet or droplet nucleus reaches an alveolus.

Note: Children < 10 years of age commonly don't spread the organism by the respiratory route, and most children get their tuberculosis infection from an adult. So if you are asked about the likelihood of spread from a 4-year-old to another 4-year-old in day care, the answer is "very unlikely." Usually an adult is responsible for spread if an outbreak occurs in a day care facility.

TB infection is almost always a latent infection—called latent tuberculosis infection (LTBI). We no longer give "prophylaxis" after a diagnosis of LTBI, but rather "treat" the LTBI.

TB disease may occur days to years after initial infection, if at all. Of those infected, 90% remain disease-free. The risk of conversion is 5% within 2 years (these individuals are said to develop rapidly progressive or primary disease) and another 5% thereafter (reactivation disease). Reactivation disease is more likely to occur in children and adults with immunosuppressive conditions—such as HIV and AIDS, end-stage renal disease, diabetes, malignancies, corticosteroid use, and use of TNF-alpha inhibitors. HIV patients have a 40% risk of conversion.

- With what signs/symptoms do most children with tuberculosis present?
- How may tuberculous pericarditis present?
- How common is tuberculous meningitis, and what age group is most commonly affected?
- What will the serum sodium likely be (high, low, or normal) in a patient with symptomatic tuberculous meningitis?
- How will an older adolescent with pulmonary tuberculosis present?
- Who should be screened for tuberculosis?

Non-latent primary TB infection (i.e., occurring with the initial tuberculosis exposure followed immediately by pulmonary disease)—seen in adolescent and adult HIV patients—is primarily a lower lobe disease (reflecting normally increased airflow to the lower lobes); while reactivation TB disease (again, pulmonary disease occurring months to years after the initial exposure) is primarily an upper lobe/apical disease.

Report all persons with current TB disease or suspected current TB disease to the state or local health department.

Presentations in Children / Adolescents / Adults

Many children with tuberculosis infection have no signs or symptoms at any time! Infants and adolescents are more likely to have symptoms. Infants are most likely to have nonproductive cough, mild dyspnea, and wheezing, especially at night. CXR will show hilar lymphadenopathy—this is your clue on the examination! Frequently, the lymph node swelling compresses bronchial structures and results in air trapping, hyperinflation, and lobar emphysema.

Children with pulmonary tuberculosis frequently have a local, asymptomatic pleural effusion. However, pleural effusions are infrequent in children < 6 years. Pleural effusions associated with *M. tuberculosis* have a lymphocyte count of 1,000–6,000/mm³, a low-glucose, elevated protein, and elevated LDH. Pleural fluid is usually acid-fast bacilli (AFB) smear-negative, but a pleural biopsy increases the yield. Tuberculous pericarditis occurs in 4/1,000 children infected with tuberculosis and may present as a rub or distant heart sounds. Fluid is typically negative for the organism and may be bloody.

Meningitis is the most serious TB complication in children and occurs in 3/1,000 untreated patients. It most commonly occurs in children ages 6 months to 4 years. (It can occur in children < 3 months if the infant's mother had disseminated tuberculosis with placental involvement.) A caseous lesion generally forms in the cerebral cortex or meninges during the occult lymphohematogenous dissemination of the initial infection. This caseous lesion enlarges and forms what is known as a "rich focus" and seeds the subarachnoid space. It also can cause a communicating hydrocephalus. SIADH with resultant hyponatremia is common. CSF protein is typically significantly elevated, and CSF glucose is typically low; the CSF WBC count is usually mild-to-moderately elevated with lymphocyte predominance.

A tuberculoma is another serious complication in children and presents clinically as a brain tumor. Tuberculomas are rare in the U.S. but make up 40% of brain tumors in developing areas of the world. In children, the lesions are infratentorial, near the cerebellum. Headache, seizures, and fever are the most common symptoms. Tuberculomas are rare, but if they occur, they frequently—and paradoxically—do so after the patient has started anti-tuberculosis medications!

The most common extrapulmonary manifestation in children is lymph node involvement. The most common sites are the anterior or posterior cervical triangles; submandibular and supraclavicular node involvement also occurs. Involvement is usually unilateral, but bilateral disease occurs in 1/4 of patients.

Common presenting signs of TB disease in adolescents and adults include fever, weakness, night sweats, and weight loss. Look out for these presenting symptoms in your patients! They'll be coughing all over the kids who are asymptomatic, and you'll have to know to check them for tuberculosis! Symptoms of pulmonary TB disease in adolescents and adults are cough, pleuritic chest pain, and hemoptysis. The chest x-ray may show an upper lobe infiltrate and hilar lymphadenopathy. The hilar adenopathy is usually out of proportion to the size of the infiltrate. Acid-fast stains of the sputum may show "red snappers," and you can also send sputum for PCR and culture. In older adolescents and adults, most TB disease is pulmonary; 15% is extrapulmonary. Image 5-18 shows a cavitary apical lesion.

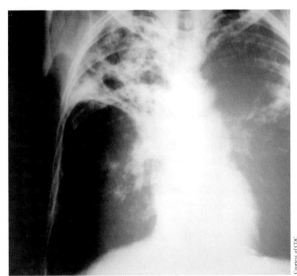

Image 5-18: TB with cavitary apical lesion

Screening for Latent TB Infection (LTBI)

Who gets screened? High-risk groups including:

- HIV or high risk for HIV
- Close contacts of those with TB disease
- IV drug abusers
- The homeless
- Migrant workers
- Residents of long-term care facilities (nursing homes and prisons)
- Patients who are about to start or are receiving long-term steroids or TNF-alpha antagonists
- Children traveling to or immigrating from countries (international adoptees!) with endemic infection
- Children with radiographic or clinical features suggestive of disease

How are they screened for TB? 2 methods:

1) The tuberculin skin test (TST; also called purified protein derivative, PPD) is the most widely used and is preferred for children < 5 years of age.

2) Immunologic-based blood tests called interferon-gamma release assays (IGRA) are preferred in children > 5 years who have received the Bacille Calmette-Guérin (BCG) vaccine or in children > 5 years who are unlikely to return for TST reading. Data are not available for IGRA use in children < 5 years.

So on an exam, if they ask you about an asymptomatic child who has received BCG vaccine and who has a positive TST but a negative IGRA, then the diagnosis of latent TB is unlikely.

For people easily lost to follow-up, such as in some jails and homeless shelters, screen for actual disease (chest x-ray and sputum for AFB).

Note: Tuberculin skin tests are positive in most infected people, but 10% of children will be initially anergic then eventually react, suggesting that tuberculosis itself may contribute to the anergy. The TST is contraindicated only if there has been a necrotic skin reaction to previous tests. You can give the TST if the child has had the BCG vaccine (used in some non-U.S. countries as a TB vaccine). All current guidelines recommend that you "ignore" the history of BCG vaccine and follow the same cutoffs as listed for everyone else!

The standard Mantoux skin test is an intradermal injection of 0.1 mL (5 tuberculin units) of purified protein derivative (PPD) tuberculin in the forearm. Evaluate the injection site after 48–72 hours. The reading is based on the diameter of the indurated/swollen area—not the red area—measured perpendicularly to the long axis of the forearm.

The current recommendations from the CDC as to what constitutes a positive reading (listed below) take into account the degree of clinical suspicion of LTBI. The following list shows how a particular diameter of induration may be a positive test in 1 group but negative in another. All the following are considered positive skin tests:

- **5 mm** is positive for those in the high-risk group:
  - Those with CXR findings or clinical evidence consistent with TB disease
  - Those with HIV or major, cell-mediated dysfunction
  - Anyone with fibrotic changes on CXR, consistent with prior TB
  - Close contacts with a documented case
  - Patients with organ transplants and other immuno-suppressed patients (who are receiving the equivalent of ≥ 15 mg/day of prednisone for ≥ 1 month)

- **10 mm** is positive for those in the moderate-risk group:
  - Homeless persons
  - Recent travel or birth in a high-prevalence region of the world
  - IV drug abusers who are HIV-negative
  - Prisoners
  - Health care workers!
  - Nursing home patients and staff
  - Diabetics, chronic renal failure patients
  - Persons undergoing immunosuppressive therapy (equivalent of < 15 mg/day prednisone)
  - Children < 4 years of age

- **15 mm** is positive for those in the low-risk group (≥ 4 years without risk factors). This includes most people in the community.

A shortcut to remember cutoffs for positive TSTs:

- HIV+, abnormal chest x-ray, close contacts, severely immunocompromised = 5 mm
- No risk factors and ≥ 4 years of age = 15 mm
- All the rest = 10 mm

False-negative skin tests—consider:

1) Too recent an exposure: It takes up to 10 weeks for the TST test to turn positive after exposure; so if a recently exposed patient has a negative skin test, recheck 10–12 weeks after exposure. Children < 4 years of age who have been exposed to TB are at high risk for disseminated disease, so start therapy for LTBI while you wait to repeat the TST at 10–12 weeks.

   or

2) Anergy: The CDC used to recommend that all HIV patients and other patients suspected of being anergic have 2 additional skin tests simultaneously with the TST—mumps and *Candida*. This is no longer recommended. Even so, do remember that anergy can cause a false-negative TST.

- For what age are interferon-gamma release assays (IGRA) recommended?
- How do you interpret a TST in a child who has received BCG vaccine?
- What groups are considered high-risk, moderate-risk, and low-risk for tuberculosis?
- What are the "cut-offs" for a positive TST in the groups listed in the previous question?
- A child has a positive TST. What is the workup if he is asymptomatic?
- If a child with a positive TST has no disease present after his workup (LTBI), what is the necessary treatment?

Treatment of LTBI

This section is summarized in Table 5-3.

Who gets treated for LTBI?

What do you do if the patient has a positive skin test? [Know!] A positive skin test indicates that the patient has, or has had, LTBI, but not necessarily active disease. If the patient has had no previous TB workup, do a workup for active disease: clinical evaluation, a chest x-ray, and a sputum (if old enough) or morning gastric aspirate for acid-fast bacilli (AFB) smear, PCR, and culture (x3).

If disease is present, treat for tuberculosis as discussed next.

If no disease is present, treat all previously untreated persons with positive TSTs; this includes the 80-year-old and the 1-year-old, HIV-positive and HIV-negative, and recent or old seroconverters. (Simple, huh?)

What about negative TSTs? Treat all immunocompromised (e.g., HIV infection) and children < 4 years of age with negative TSTs who are close contacts to patients with active TB disease; then recheck with another TST. For older children and adolescents, repeat TST in 8–10 weeks. If the repeat TST is positive, continue for 9 months. If the repeat TST is negative, stop. That's it!

How Do You Treat LTBI?

Treatment of LTBI: Give isoniazid ([INH] 10–15 mg/kg/day, max 300 mg/day) to eradicate the TB infection before it can develop into the disease. Again, the risk of conversion is 5% within 2 years for "normal" persons and ~ 40% within several months for those with HIV. Optimal duration of INH treatment of LTBI is 9 months.

Table 5-3: Treatment of Latent Tuberculosis Infection	
Positive TST Determination Based on Preexisting Conditions in Infants, Children, and Adolescents	
Certain groups are at high risk of developing TB disease once infected. These people are candidates for treatment regardless of their age—after ensuring active infection is not present. The current optimum treatment regimen for all patients is 9 months of daily INH. See text for treatment of drug-resistant organisms. Treat **all** of the following (**all** ages!):	
TST Result (Induration)	**In Children with the Following Conditions**
≥ 5 mm is positive in these high-risk groups	In close contact with known or suspected contagious cases of tuberculosis disease Suspected to have tuberculosis disease: • Findings on chest radiograph consistent with active or previously active tuberculosis • Clinical evidence of tuberculosis disease Receiving immunosuppressive therapy or with immunosuppressive conditions, including HIV infection
≥ 10 mm is positive in these moderate-risk groups	At increased risk of disseminated disease: • Those < 4 years of age • Those with other medical conditions, including Hodgkin disease, lymphoma, diabetes mellitus, chronic renal failure, or malnutrition With increased exposure to tuberculosis disease: • Those born, or whose parents were born, in high-prevalence regions of the world • Those frequently exposed to adults who are HIV-infected, homeless, users of illicit drugs, residents of nursing homes, incarcerated or institutionalized, or migrant farm workers • Those who travel to high-prevalence regions of the world
≥ 15 mm is positive in this low-risk group	≥ 4 years of age without any risk factors
TST negative but high risk	High-risk contacts of active cases

For patients with known exposure to INH-resistant organisms or with history of INH intolerance, give rifampin for 6 months instead.

In 2011, the CDC recommended an alternative therapy for LTBI of a weekly (x 12-weeks) dose of INH + rifapentine, given through directly observed therapy (DOT), for individuals 12 years of age and older. This regimen was equally effective compared with the 9 months of self-administered INH therapy in a large clinical trial.

Treatment of Tuberculosis

Treatment: The emergence of multidrug-resistant (MDR) strains has changed the treatment of TB disease. We will first define the 4-drug and 3-drug regimens. [Know!]

The 4-drug regimen consists of:

1) Rifampin
2) Isoniazid (INH)
3) Pyrazinamide (PZA)
4) Either ethambutol (oral preferred) or streptomycin (injection)

The 3-drug regimen consists of the first 3 drugs (rifampin, INH, and PZA). To remember: **RIP**; Rest In Peace for the TB patient who doesn't get **r**ifampin, **I**NH, and **PZA**.

In the U.S., initially treat all patients with TB disease for 2 months with 4-drug therapy—unless criteria for 3-drug therapy are met (see below). After the first 2 months, give INH and rifampin for an additional 4 months (as long as MDR TB is not suspected or susceptibilities are known). Give HIV-infected patients on protease inhibitors rifabutin instead of rifampin. Duration of therapy (6 months total) for HIV-infected patients is the same for those on a rifabutin regimen.

Give drugs daily for the first 2 months, then 2–3x per week thereafter, although this is fairly flexible.

All patients must be observed taking the medication unless you can absolutely assure compliance. Treatment is the same for extrapulmonary TB (except for CNS disease).

When can 3 drugs be used? Only if there is a slight chance of drug-resistant infection. All of the following criteria must be met:

• Child resides in an area with low rates of INH resistance
• No known exposure to a patient with a drug-resistant infection
• Source case has no risk factors for resistant disease

Vitamin B_6 (pyridoxine) is also given to some with INH-containing regimens to prevent peripheral neuropathy and mild central nervous system effects. Give to exclusively breastfed infants, children on milk- or meat-deficient diets, those with nutritional deficiencies, symptomatic HIV-infected children, and pregnant adolescents.

Some other scenarios:

• If the patient cannot take PZA, give INH and rifampin for a total of 9 months.
• If the TB is resistant to INH only, stop INH and give the other 3 drugs for 6 months (total).
• Multidrug-resistant TB (i.e., to at least INH and rifampin) is difficult, and treatment is based on susceptibilities; 4 drugs are used for 12–24 months of therapy.

Side effects: Rifampin, INH, and PZA are all hepatotoxic.

Rifampin causes orange discoloration of all secretions and urine. It also can make oral contraceptives ineffective by speeding up their metabolism!

INH: In all patients on INH, regardless of age, monitor monthly only for signs/symptoms of liver toxicity. Laboratory testing is indicated only if signs or symptoms develop!

Ethambutol is not hepatotoxic, but it can cause a decrease in visual acuity. Often, decreased color perception is the 1st sign of this deterioration. It is usually reversible if you discontinue the drug quickly. Patients should have an ophthalmologic exam before treatment and periodic checks thereafter (Snellen chart, gross confrontation eye exam, and question the patient). Any inflammatory disease of the eyes is at least a relative contraindication for ethambutol.

Streptomycin is an older aminoglycoside. It tends to cause vertigo and ataxia in children. Ototoxicity and nephrotoxicity are less common in children than in adults.

Nocardia

Nocardia asteroides is only weakly acid-fast (easily missed). Its shape is beaded, branching, and filamentous. It commonly starts as a lung infection—occasionally causing a thin-walled cavitary lesion. It can cause focal brain abscesses and a neutrophilic chronic meningitis. (Most chronic meningitides are lymphocytic.) Nodular skin lesions are common. It is hard to isolate.

Usual treatment is with high-dose sulfonamides or TMP/SMX. In severely ill patients, add combinations of drugs, including amikacin + ceftriaxone or amikacin + imipenem. Minocycline and linezolid are alternate choices for those sulfa-allergic.

OTHER ORGANISMS

Actinomyces is a microaerophilic/facultative anaerobic organism that causes an infection in which there are growing, characteristically yellow, "sulfur" granules that are actually clusters of organisms. The usual presentation of actinomycosis is cervicofacial involvement caused by a dental infection (Image 5-19). Thoracic

Quick Quiz

- What is the treatment of active TB disease?

- Which children should receive pyridoxine with INH therapy?

- True or false? You should routinely monitor laboratory in patients on anti-tuberculosis medications.

- What is the concern of ethambutol use?

- A draining lesion of the face has sulfur granules noted on microscopy. What is the likely etiology?

- What organism causes pneumonia and splenomegaly and is associated with having parrot exposure?

- What organism is common as an etiology for pneumonia in adolescents?

- True or false? Antibiotic ointment in infants' eyes at birth prevents *Chlamydia* infection.

- An infant presents at 6 weeks of age with a "staccato cough," no fever, and CXR consistent with pneumonia. What organism should you suspect?

- Swimming in a pond with an infected dog could predispose a child to what infection?

disease occurs after aspiration, and abdominal disease occurs after penetrating trauma or intestinal perforation.

Actinomyces is a cause of pelvic inflammatory disease (PID) when there is an intrauterine device (IUD) in place. The organism can also be associated with appendicitis. It occasionally causes a chronic neutrophilic meningitis (as do *Nocardia* and fungi).

Treat with PCN or ampicillin. 2nd choice includes clindamycin, doxycycline, or tetracycline.

Image 5-19: Actinomycosis

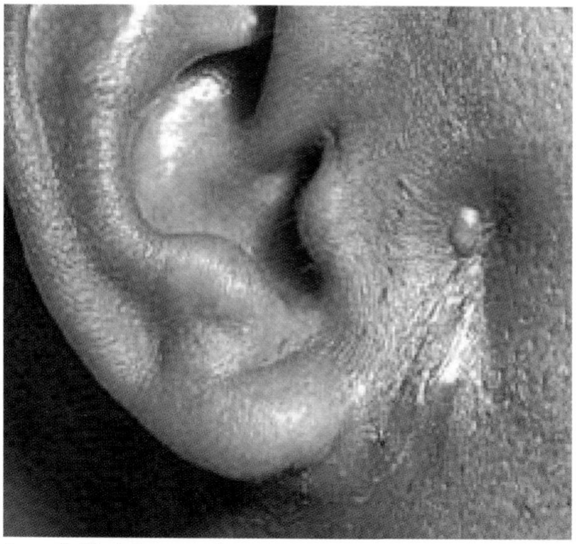

Chlamydiae are obligate intracellular parasites. *Chlamydophila psittaci* (formerly *Chlamydia psittaci*), *Chlamydia trachomatis*, and *Chlamydophila pneumoniae* (formerly *Chlamydia pneumoniae* and TWAR) are pathogenic in humans.

C. psittaci is found in psittacine and other birds and causes psittacosis (pneumonia and splenomegaly). Again, with any pneumonia associated with poultry, especially with splenomegaly, strongly suspect *C. psittaci*. (Differential: *Histoplasma* also causes pneumonia and splenomegaly; it is associated with bird and bat droppings.) Onset of psittacosis: myalgias, rigors, headache, and high fever—to 105° F.

C. pneumoniae causes community-acquired pneumonia in children > 5 years of age and adolescents. (It is not associated with bird exposure; rather, person-to-person spread.) Bronchospasm is particularly prominent in respiratory infection caused by *C. pneumoniae*.

C. trachomatis causes the GU infections and trachoma. Trachoma is a chronic external eye infection causing cataracts—but not glaucoma. It causes a chronic follicular keratoconjunctivitis with neovascularization and is found especially in Asia and Africa. ~ 5% of pregnant women have *Chlamydia trachomatis* in their genital tracts; antibiotic ointment in infants' eyes at birth does not prevent *Chlamydia* conjunctivitis but does prevent gonorrheal eye infection.

The same *C. trachomatis* can cause neonatal pneumonia! Chlamydial pneumonia is a common infection in the first 4 months of life; 10–20% of newborns will develop infection if born through an infected birth canal. Most infants do well with an afebrile pneumonia and a persistent staccato cough. Lymphogranuloma venereum is an STD caused by the same *C. trachomatis*, but it is a different biovar (serovars L1, L2, and L3).

Treat chlamydial organisms with macrolides or tetracyclines.

SPIROCHETES

SYPHILIS

Syphilis is caused by *Treponema pallidum*. It is covered in Adolescent Health and Gynecology, Book 1.

LEPTOSPIROSIS

Leptospirosis is a spirochetal disease transferred by contact with infected animals or contaminated water. It is considered to be the most widespread zoonosis in the world. Clue: Look for contact with dog or rat urine (e.g., a kid who swims in a pond with dogs). It causes a wide range of symptoms, from myalgias, fever, and headache, with or without aseptic meningitis, to Weil disease—severe hepatitis with renal failure and hemorrhagic complications (renal or hepatic symptoms may predominate). Conjunctival suffusion without purulent discharge and myalgias of the calf and lumbar regions are distinct clinical findings. Pulmonary symptoms are also common. The hepatitis is characterized by the bilirubin disproportionately elevated compared to the liver enzymes. The variety of presenting symptoms makes for a high incidence of initial misdiagnoses. Many patients also have a biphasic illness (2 phases separated by 3–4 days of no fever).

Diagnosis: Blood cultures may be positive in the initial septicemic phase (days 4–7), while urine cultures will be positive thereafter; but isolation of *Leptospira* organisms is very difficult. Serology and PCR are probably more useful in real-world settings.

Treat with PCN, ceftriaxone, or doxycycline.

LYME DISEASE

Borrelia burgdorferi causes Lyme disease. Transmission occurs by the *Ixodes scapularis* (previously *Ixodes dammini*) tick in the eastern U.S. and the *Ixodes pacificus* tick in the California area. (The protozoa *Babesia* is also transmitted by *Ixodes scapularis*.) 95% of cases occur in 13 states: Minnesota, Wisconsin, Vermont, New Hampshire, Maine, Massachusetts, Connecticut, New York, New Jersey, Pennsylvania, Delaware, Maryland, and Virginia. Reported cases are about 30,000/year. It is estimated that only 1 in 10 cases are reported! (Image 5-20)

Rarely, Lyme disease can cross the placenta and cause fetal infection and death.

For the most part, ticks (usually *I. scapularis*) transmit Lyme disease during the nymph stage, probably because nymphs are more likely to feed on a person and are rarely noticed because of their small size (< 2 mm!). Thus, the nymphs typically have ample time to feed and transmit the infection; ticks are most likely to transmit infection after ~ 2 or more days of feeding. If a person reports a tick on him/herself for a few hours the previous day, provide reassurance that no treatment is necessary.

Diagnosis is clinical: Erythema migrans is the pathognomonic skin lesion of the early localized disease (Stage I); it starts at the site of the bite and is a slowly spreading, irregular erythematous lesion with either a bull's eye or a clear center (Image 5-21). Other early symptoms include myalgias, arthralgias, fever, HA, and lymphadenopathy. Then, weeks to months later, early disseminated (Stage II) disease occurs with recurring

erythema migrans (usually multiple lesions), neurologic problems (lymphocytic meningitis and/or neuritis), and heart problems (myocarditis, which may cause a rapidly alternating 1st, 2nd, or 3rd degree AV block). The neuritis often presents as a peripheral neuropathy, a cranial nerve palsy, or both; consider it in a patient with a suggestive history and Bell's palsy, foot drop, or both. Months to years later, late disseminated disease (Stage III) occurs, most commonly with arthritis (oligo- or migratory—small or large joints—generally large), but there can also be chronic neurologic syndromes. A definite diagnosis may be difficult to establish. Serology is negative in 90% of early localized disease, so base the diagnosis on clinical findings.

Should you check Lyme serology on a patient with erythema migrans. No! Just treat! Again, erythema migrans is pathognomonic for the disease.

A 2-step approach is recommended for the serologic diagnosis of Lyme disease. A positive EIA or IFA should be followed by a Western immunoblot. Treat only patients with positive results on both tests.

Treat early disease and isolated Bell's palsy with oral doxycycline 100 mg bid, or amoxicillin (for children < 8 years of age) for 14–21 days. Initially, treat Lyme arthritis with oral agents, as described above but for 28 days; then re-treat with the same oral agent—or ceftriaxone—if there is no response. Nonresponders frequently are HLA-DR4 allele-positive. Treat cardiac and neurologic sequelae with ceftriaxone 75–100 mg/kg/day (maximum 2 grams) or PCN G 300,000 U/kg/day divided q 4 hours (maximum daily dose 20 million U) IV x 21 days. No prophylaxis is indicated; i.e., do not give medications prior to camping out or to "defend against" tick bites.

At one time, there was a recombinant outer-surface protein (OspA) Lyme disease vaccine (LYMErix™), but it was pulled from the market.

Note: If on the exam, they present a patient with fatigue, joint stiffness (not arthritis), muscular aches, and/or tenderness: Do not check Lyme titers and do not treat for Lyme based on these nonspecific findings!

Other *Borrelia* infections are *B. recurrentis* and *B. vincentii*, which cause relapsing fever (in this, spirochetes are seen in the blood smears) and Vincent angina.

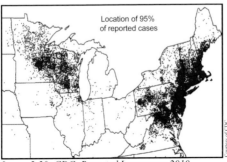

Image 5-20: CDC: Reported Lyme cases 2010

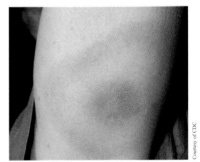

Image 5-21: Erythema migrans

Quick Quiz

- How do you diagnose leptospirosis in the first 4–7 days of infection? In the 2nd week of infection?

- A child visits a "Lyme-prone" area for several hours. On return from his visit, a tick is noted. The tick was likely attached for between 2 and 3 hours. What is the appropriate therapy (if any) for this child?

- Describe erythema migrans.

- A child presents with isolated Bell's palsy and lives in rural Connecticut. What diagnosis should you consider?

- In a patient with erythema migrans, should you check Lyme serology to confirm your diagnosis?

- What are the treatments for Lyme disease at its various stages? Especially know the different therapies that depend on if the child presents with isolated erythema migrans, heart block, Bell's palsy, meningitis, or arthritis.

- A 15-year-old adolescent in an endemic area for Lyme presents with chronic fatigue as a presenting (and only) symptom. Physical examination is normal. Is it appropriate to check Lyme titers?

- Describe the classic *Candida* diaper rash.

FUNGI

OVERVIEW

Fungi are roughly divided into 2 morphologic types: yeasts and molds. There is also a dimorphic type that changes from a yeast to a mold and vice-versa, depending on temperature. The dimorphs are the type most likely to cause systemic disease in the immunocompetent host. The dimorphic fungi are also more limited in the environment. The infecting form of fungi is usually spores (molds), which convert to yeasts in a moist environment at body temperature. The *Deuteromycetes* are a class of fungus that contains the yeasts *Candida* and *Cryptococcus*, the molds that cause skin and nail disease (dermatophytes), and the dimorphic fungi: *Histoplasma*, *Coccidioides*, and *Blastomyces*. *Mucor* is of the class *Phycomycetes* (nonseptate hyphae), and *Aspergillus* is of the genus *Ascomycetes*.

CANDIDA

Note

Candida albicans is a common infection in pediatrics, especially in newborns. It can cause problems ranging from simple superficial infection of the skin to life-threatening meningitis or sepsis.

Skin Infections

Cutaneous Candidiasis

Superficial skin infection is benign and tends to occur in locations of wet, macerated skin, such as the perineum in infants or diabetics and intertriginous areas of obese children/adolescents. In infants, the peak age is 2–4 months; ~ 10% will be affected. *Candida* diaper rash has a classic presentation: a bright red, fiery rash with sharp borders and pinpoint, "satellite" papules and pustules. If you scrape one of the pustules and examine it under a microscope with KOH, you will see the classic pseudohyphae of *Candida*. Treatment: Keep the area dry and use topical antifungals (usually nystatin).

Nail infection is fairly common in thumb suckers and appears as dry, heaped-up, gray granulomatous tissue around and on top of the nail.

Chronic mucocutaneous candidiasis (CMCC) is associated with a T-cell problem in which the T cell does not recognize *Candida*. It generally starts in those < 2 years of age. Patients present with a bad chronic oral and facial rash, alopecia, nail disease, and, occasionally, esophageal stricture. It is associated with a spectrum of immunodeficiencies, endocrinopathies, and autoimmune disorders. CMCC is a prominent feature of autoimmune polyendocrinopathy-candidiasis-ectodermal dystrophy (APECED; in which there can be hypoparathyroidism, Addison disease, DM, hypothyroidism, and/or vitiligo). These patients respond well to fluconazole.

GI Tract Candidiasis

Oropharyngeal candidiasis, or "thrush," is one of the most common presentations of *Candida* infection in infants < 5 months of age. After 5 months of age, it is seen in children who are receiving antibiotics, are immunocompromised (think about HIV or SCID), or are debilitated and malnourished. The lesions are classically described as "pearly white plaques" on the mucosal surface of the oropharynx. Removing the plaques results in pinpoint bleeding. Use topical therapy with nystatin or clotrimazole troches in the immunocompetent and fluconazole in the immunocompromised. (Grandparents still like Gentian violet—"because you can see it is working," especially when it gets all over the drooling child's clothes.)

Esophagitis occurs in immunocompromised patients. They complain of pain with swallowing. Most start with fluconazole and, if no response, proceed to esophagoscopy with washings or biopsy, if indicated. *Candida* also can spread to the rest of the GI tract in the immunocompromised.

GU Infections

Cystitis

Candida infections of the urinary tract are common in immunocompromised children and especially in those with an indwelling urinary catheter. DM and antibiotics are also risk factors. Urine smear and culture will diagnose the infection readily. Most give fluconazole but for some, removal of the catheter may be the only treatment required.

Candiduria also may indicate obstructive uropathy or "fungus balls" of the kidneys/ureters. (Look for this on ultrasound.)

Vaginitis

Candida vaginitis occurs in adolescent women with increased frequency in those on birth control pills, antibiotics, or who are pregnant. White vaginal discharge (pH < 4.9) and pruritus are common. Numerous topical agents are available; a single, 150-mg fluconazole dose successfully treats the infection.

Candida Sepsis

Treat *Candida* fungemia aggressively and never ignore a positive blood culture with *Candida* as a "contaminant." Take special care to examine the skin and the eyes because discrete lesions may occur at both sites. Retinal lesions present as white, cotton-like chorioretinitis (everyone with candidemia needs an eye exam!). Hepatosplenic or renal candidiasis is also seen. CT is helpful and may show hypodense abscesses.

If a catheter is involved in the infection, you must remove it.

CNS involvement is usually secondary to dissemination from the blood stream—and rarely primary.

Candidemia can result in 3 deadly syndromes:

1) **Septic peripheral thrombophlebitis**.
2) **Septic thrombosis of the great central veins** (especially with central venous catheters).
3) **Hepatosplenic candidiasis** (mentioned above): This should be considered in recovering leukemia patients who present with fever and have negative cultures. CT scan shows focal areas of involvement in the liver/spleen.

Treat all of these by first removing any infected catheter. Amphotericin B is preferred for neonates; they should be treated for 3 weeks when systemic candidiasis is present. In non-neutropenic children, fluconazole or an echinocandin (caspofungin, micafungin, or anidulafungin) is the recommended treatment and should be continued for 2 weeks after *Candida* is cleared. In critically ill neutropenic patients, use an echinocandin or lipid amphotericin B. In addition, resect any suppurative peripheral vein. Suspect septic thrombosis of great central veins if there is edema of the upper body and/or candidemia persists > 2 days after removal of the catheter. Resistance to antifungal medications is uncommon, but amphotericin B resistance has been reported in *C. lusitaniae*, *C. krusei*, and *C. glabrata*; and fluconazole resistance in *C. krusei* and *C. glabrata*.

CRYPTOCOCCUS

Cryptococcus neoformans typically causes minimally symptomatic, self-limited infections. Patients may have a low-grade fever, cough, and a pulmonary infiltrate—all of which resolve. It is not associated with any particular geographical location. Although it is found in old pigeon droppings, most patients have no recollection of being in contact with any. Cryptococcal pneumonia may form cavitary lesions and peripheral "cannon ball" skin lesions.

Dissemination is more likely in T-cell–deficient patients (AIDS, corticosteroid therapy, Hodgkin disease, ALL, diabetes, immunodeficiencies like idiopathic CD4 lymphopenia, and post-organ transplant). These patients are especially likely to get cryptococcal meningoencephalitis—the most common presentation of severe cryptococcal infection.

Confirm presence of the organism with a CSF cryptococcal antigen test (preferred) or a CSF India ink test, which is positive when you see the large "halo" due to the thick capsule around the organism. Definitive diagnosis is made by culturing the organism.

Treat cryptococcal meningitis with amphotericin B and 5-flucytosine (5-FC). You can treat less severely ill patients with fluconazole. HIV-infected patients and others chronically immunosuppressed require fluconazole for life after their initial therapy. Recurrent severe headaches and signs of increased intracranial pressure may be treated with repeated large volume lumbar punctures.

Of note, *C. gattii*, which is associated with trees and soil, has recently emerged as an outbreak-associated pathogen in the Pacific Northwest U.S., as well as Canada. It causes disease in immunocompetent and immunocompromised adolescents and adults, but rarely causes disease in children.

COCCIDIOIDES, HISTOPLASMA, BLASTOMYCES

Coccidioides, *Histoplasma*, and *Blastomyces* are dimorphs that can cause severe disease, especially in immunocompromised patients.

The spores of *Coccidioides immitis* are found in the soil of the arid Southwest U.S. and northern Mexico (often called "valley fever"—think of San Joaquin Valley or Death Valley). Once inhaled, it converts to a yeast that, days to weeks later, causes a self-limited, flu-like illness with arthralgias, erythema multiforme, and/or erythema nodosum. It often has a sarcoid-like presentation. Disease often results in a pulmonary "coin lesion." In immunocompromised patients, the disease is usually more severe (see AIDS-related infections). Think of this disease in a patient from Arizona or California with a flu-like illness!

Diagnosis can be established using serologic, histopathologic (spherules in tissues), or culture techniques.

Quick **Quiz**

- A child presents with *Candida albicans* fungemia and central venous line infection. True or false? It is appropriate to try and "treat through the line" in hopes of "clearing the line" and saving it for later use.

- What geographic locations are risk factors for *Coccidioides*? *Histoplasma*? *Blastomyces*?

- What children are at highest risk for developing aspergillosis?

- What disease entity is *Malassezia furfur* associated with in adolescents? In infants?

- In infants with *Malassezia furfur*, what type of hyperalimentations were they likely receiving?

For disseminated infections or CNS infections, fluconazole is the drug of choice. If the infection does not respond to fluconazole, consider amphotericin B.

Histoplasma is confined to the Mississippi and Ohio River valleys and is especially prevalent in bat and bird droppings. Do not confuse *Histoplasma* with the "valley fever" described above. Most infections are asymptomatic, and past infection can cause an incidental calcified granuloma on CXR. Histoplasmosis can present with interstitial pneumonia, palate ulcers, and splenomegaly. 1/3 of patients have anemia, neutropenia, or pancytopenia. The pneumonia and splenomegaly are similar to that seen in *C. psittaci* infection. *Histoplasma* occasionally causes a cavitary pneumonia similar to that seen in TB.

Diagnosis can be made by culturing the organism, by detection of the histoplasma antigen in urine, serum, or CSF, or by serology. Acute pulmonary disease generally does not require therapy.

Treat chronic or severe acute disease with itraconazole and disseminated disease with amphotericin B, followed by itraconazole.

Blastomyces causes an illness similar to *Histoplasma* and *Coccidioides*. It is seen in Arkansas and Wisconsin hunters and loggers. (An outbreak occurred in some kids who visited a Wisconsin lodge and messed around with a beaver dam.) On the exams, if you see the words "beaver dam," think blastomycosis! In addition, *Blastomyces* disseminate to the skin, causing crusted lesions. Bone lesions also are commonly seen in blastomycosis. Treat with itraconazole or amphotericin B in severely affected patients.

ASPERGILLOSIS

Aspergillus species are molds that grow on decaying vegetation and in soil. Aspergillosis manifests as invasive, noninvasive, chronic, or allergic disease dependent upon the immune status of the host. Transmission occurs by inhalation of conidia (spores) from the environment, construction sites, soil, and water supplies (showerheads).

Invasive aspergillosis occurs almost exclusively in immunocompromised patients with prolonged neutropenia due to chemotherapy, graft-versus-host disease, or impaired phagocytic function (chronic granulomatous disease, corticosteroids, immunosuppressive therapy). Children at highest risk for this infection are new onset or relapse of hematologic malignancy or stem cell transplant patients. The 2 most common causes of invasive disease are Aspergillus *fumigatus* and Aspergillus *flavus*. Invasive infection involves pulmonary, sinus, cerebral, or cutaneous sites. The hallmark of invasive aspergillosis is angioinvasion with resulting thrombosis and dissemination to other organs.

Isolation of *Aspergillus* species from lung, sinus, and skin biopsy specimens from Sabouraud dextrose agar is required for definitive diagnosis. Seeing branched and septate hyphae on KOH stain from similar specimens is suggestive. A positive enzyme immunosorbent assay (serum galactomannan) can be used in both adults and children to support a diagnosis of invasive disease. Voriconazole is the drug of choice for invasive disease. Use amphotericin B in neonates.

DERMATOPHYTES

Dermatophytes are the skin and hair fungi. Treat ringworm (*Tinea corporis*) with topical clotrimazole, miconazole, or terbinafine (> 12 years). If these are not successful, oral griseofulvin is recommended. Never use amphotericin B. These organisms are discussed further in Dermatology, Book 2.

MALASSEZIA FURFUR

Malassezia furfur is responsible for 2 disease types in children. 1st, it causes a superficial dermatosis called pityriasis (a.k.a. tinea) versicolor. The lesions are hypo- or hyperpigmented patches that scale. Heat, moisture, and occlusive clothing make it worse. It is very common in adolescents. Look for "spaghetti and meatballs" on a skin scraping. Treat with topical 2.5% selenium sulfide or oral ketoconazole/itraconazole/fluconazole. (Note that the most common cause of pityriasis versicolor is *M. globosa*.)

The 2nd disease type is a serious infection which occurs in NICU babies who are receiving IV lipids and TPN. These infants have fever, bilateral interstitial pulmonary infiltrates, increased WBC count, and thrombocytopenia. Clue: If the lab tells you the organism required an olive oil overlay to grow, it's *Malassezia furfur*!

Treat by removing the catheter, stopping the lipid infusion, and starting amphotericin B.

SPOROTRICHOSIS

Sporotrichosis is caused by *Sporothrix schenckii*—a dimorphic fungus associated with plants. Cases have occurred in children on farms, especially if they deal with hay bales or straw. Gardeners tend to get it, often after being pricked by a rose thorn.

Sporotrichosis can be a chronic problem. The disseminated type is more common in immunodeficient gardeners. (Warn your post-transplant rose gardeners!) Remember: *Mycobacterium marinum* can cause similar lesions over lymphatic channels—but exposure is from fish tanks!

Of the 4 types of clinical presentations, the cutaneous and the lymphangitic (nodules form on the skin over lymph channels) types are treated with itraconazole (an alternative treatment includes saturated solution of potassium iodide), while the pulmonary and disseminated types are treated with amphotericin B followed by itraconazole.

ZYGOMYCOSIS (MUCORMYCOSIS)

Mucor, *Rhizopus*, and *Cunninghamella* organisms can cause zygomycosis. Risk factors include trauma, diabetes mellitus, immunosuppression (hematological malignancies, organ transplantation, AIDS), and deferoxamine therapy. There are rhinocerebral, pulmonary, cutaneo-articular, and disseminated forms of zygomycosis. The infection usually starts after inhalation of the spores or inoculation of the skin due to trauma. Pulmonary mucormycosis affects immunocompromised patients, causing pulmonary infarcts. In diabetics, sinusitis is more common. Rhinocerebral mucormycosis starts as a black necrotic spot in the nose or paranasal sinuses and extends intracranially; it has a poor prognosis.

Treat with amphotericin B and surgical debridement. Posaconazole is an effective agent but with limited data in children. [Know:] Both *Aspergillus* and *Mucor* can cause a necrotizing, cavitating pneumonia.

PNEUMOCYSTIS JIROVECI

Pneumocystis pneumonia (PCP) is a potentially life-threatening opportunistic infection that occurs in immunocompromised individuals and is due to *Pneumocystis jiroveci* (species that infects humans). It was formerly called *Pneumocystis carinii* (species that infects rats). *P. jiroveci* is classified as a fungus on the basis of DNA analysis but is resistant to most antifungal agents. It does retain some morphologic and biologic similarities to protozoa, including some susceptibility to antiprotozoal agents.

HIV-infected patients with low CD4 counts are at the highest risk of *Pneumocystis* pneumonia; this is covered in the HIV section page 5-58. Others at risk include hematopoietic stem cell and solid organ transplant recipients, those with cancer (especially hematologic malignancies like leukemia or lymphoma), and those receiving glucocorticoids, chemotherapeutic agents, and other immunosuppressive drugs.

The most significant of these risk factors for PCP in patients without HIV are steroid use and defects in cell-mediated immunity.

In patients without HIV infection, PCP typically presents as fulminant respiratory failure with fever, dry cough, and hypoxia.

CXR shows diffuse, bilateral, interstitial infiltrates. More unusual x-ray patterns include lobar infiltrates and solitary or multiple pulmonary nodules, which may become cavitary.

Diagnosis can be made by demonstration of organisms in lung or respiratory tract secretions. Least invasive methods to obtain specimens include bronchoscopy with bronchoalveolar lavage, induction of sputum in older children/adolescents, and deep endotracheal aspiration as compared to open lung biopsy, which is the most sensitive method. Methenamine silver, toluidine blue O, calcofluor white, and fluorescein-conjugated mono-clonal antibody are the most useful stains to identify the thick-walled cysts of *P. jiroveci*. PCR assays for *P. jiroveci* are experimental and not approved by the FDA.

Treatment: The drug of choice is IV TMP/SMX x 21 days. Use IV pentamidine if the patient cannot tolerate TMP/SMX or if they have not responded to TMP/

Table 5-4: Classification of Parasites		
Protozoa (replicate within the body) (no eosinophilia)	Sporozoa	*Toxoplasma gondii, Cryptosporidium, Isospora belli, Cyclospora, Plasmodium, and Babesia*
	Ameba	*Entamoeba histolytica*
	Flagellates	*Giardia lamblia*—GI; *Trichomonas vaginalis*—GU; *Trypanosoma, Leishmania*—blood
Helminths (do not replicate within the body—except *Strongyloides*) (+ eosinophilia)	Nemathelminthes (= nematodes) (= roundworms)	Pinworms, hookworms, whipworms (*Trichuris trichiura*), *Trichinella, Strongyloides, Ascaris*
	Platyhelminthes	Cestodes (tapeworms), trematodes (flukes)

Quick**Quiz**

- Cutaneous sporotrichosis can be treated with which 2 agents?
- At which stage of pregnancy is the mother more likely to transmit toxoplasmosis to her fetus?
- At which stage of pregnancy is the infection more likely to cause serious sequelae?
- What are the classic physical findings in congenital toxoplasmosis? What is the CT scan of the head likely to show?
- What pharmaceutical agents are used to treat a fetus with congenital toxoplasmosis?

SMX after 5–7 days. For moderate-to-severe PCP (PaO$_2$ of < 70 mmHg), add corticosteroids. Atovaquone is approved for mild-to-moderate PCP in adults, but experience in children is limited.

PCP prophylaxis

For HIV-exposed or infected children: see HIV (page 5-58).

Prophylaxis is recommended for children who have received hematopoietic stem cell transplants (HSCT), all HSCT recipients with hematologic malignancies (leukemia/lymphoma), and HSCT recipients receiving intense conditioning regimens or graft manipulation. Prophylaxis should be initiated at engraftment and administered for 6 months. It should be continued longer in all children receiving immunosuppressive therapy (prednisone or cyclosporine) or in those with graft-versus-host disease.

Recommended drug regimens include TMP/SMX, aerosolized pentamidine, daily oral dapsone, and IV pentamidine.

PARASITES

PROTOZOA

Overview of Protozoa

There are 2 main types of parasites—**protozoan** and **helminthic** organisms (Table 5-4).

The protozoa are single-celled and can replicate within the body, so it takes only a small number of organisms to cause infection. Protozoa do not cause eosinophilia.

The 3 types of common clinically relevant protozoa are:

Sporozoa: *Toxoplasma gondii*, *Cryptosporidium*, *Isospora belli*, *Cyclospora*, *Plasmodium*, and *Babesia*

Ameba: *Entamoeba histolytica*

Flagellates: *Giardia lamblia*, *Trichomonas vaginalis*, *Trypanosoma*, and *Leishmania*

Protozoa Type I: Sporozoa

Toxoplasma gondii

Toxoplasma gondii is the protozoan that causes toxoplasmosis. Cats are the definitive host because all of the oocysts (infectious form) that eventually infect humans are shed in cat feces. It is common: 10–30% of U.S. adults have had it, and, in France, prevalence rates are > 85%. Diagnose active infection by finding an elevated IgM antibody.

There are 4 types of toxoplasmosis: toxoplasmosis in the immunocompetent host, during pregnancy, in the immunocompromised, and ocular toxoplasmosis.

Toxoplasmosis in the Immunocompetent

Toxoplasmosis in the immunocompetent is most often asymptomatic but may cause a "mono"-like illness with nontender lymphadenopathy, night sweats, and atypical lymphs. It is self-limited.

Toxoplasmosis During Pregnancy

Toxoplasmosis during pregnancy can be very problematic. This type is serious in the immunocompetent only if acquired during pregnancy, when it causes congenital toxoplasmosis (causing intellectual disabilities and necrotizing chorioretinitis in the fetus). The fetus is more likely to have a congenital infection if the disease is acquired later in pregnancy (25%: 1st trimester; 54%: 2nd trimester; 65%: 3rd trimester; but in contrast, the severity of clinical disease is inversely related to gestational age, so those infected later in pregnancy are usually asymptomatic).

For severe congenital infection in a newborn, be on the lookout on the exam for an infant with the following findings:

- Microcephaly
- Hydrocephalus
- Hepatosplenomegaly
- Maculopapular rash or thrombocytopenic purpura
- Chorioretinitis
- Cerebral calcifications, which can be fairly widespread in the brain parenchyma with toxoplasmosis! Note: If calcifications "**CircuMV**ent" the ventricles [periventricular], the cause is almost always CMV and not toxoplasmosis!

Treatment of the mother can begin during pregnancy if the diagnosis is made. If the infection occurs in weeks 7–34 of gestation, you could give spiramycin (though not licensed in the U.S., it is available as an investigational drug) 1 gram q 8 hours for up to 18 weeks of gestation. If fetal infection is excluded, spiramycin is continued until term; if you confirm infection of the fetus, switch therapy to pyrimethamine, sulfadiazine, and leucovorin. For maternal infections after 34-weeks gestation, the 3-drug regimen can be used.

For congenital infections, treat the fetus *in utero* as discussed above. After delivery, continue treating the infant even if there are no clinical signs/symptoms. Once you completely evaluate the healthy newborn and you rule out infection, therapy can stop. The congenitally infected child must receive 12 months of therapy.

Treat toxo during pregnancy with a pyrimethamine, sulfadiazine, and leucovorin (which is folinic acid, not folic acid). If neutropenia occurs, increase the leucovorin dose. It is important to monitor CBC in these infants. At the end of 12 months, repeat eye exams at 3 and 6 months out to check for new chorioretinitis lesions. How to prevent this? Make sure pregnant women do not eat rare or undercooked meat—and have them avoid cat litter duties in the house. Pregnant gardeners should always wear gloves and wash their hands well because cats frequently defecate in garden soil areas as well.

Toxoplasmosis in the Immunocompromised

Toxoplasmosis in immunocompromised patients tends to cause CNS infection and multiple mass lesions caused by a reactivation of a latent infection. Patients with AIDS remain on therapy for life. Treat with pyrimethamine, sulfadiazine, and leucovorin.

Ocular Toxoplasmosis

Finally, localized ocular toxoplasmosis causes retinal lesions that look like yellow-white cotton patches and also causes irregular scarring and pigmentation (disseminated candidiasis produces white, cotton-wool patches). Treat with pyrimethamine, sulfadiazine, leucovorin, and corticosteroids until the infection has resolved.

Cryptosporidium

Cryptosporidium is a protozoan that causes infection, especially in the immunocompromised (especially in HIV and hyper-IgM syndrome) but also in the immunocompetent. The oocytes are passed in animal and human feces (vs. just cats in toxo). Symptoms in immunocompetent patients usually consist of a watery diarrhea that is self-limited, lasting 1–2 weeks. In the immunosuppressed, it can persist indefinitely and is refractory to medications. Immunocompetent patients often require no therapy. Nitazoxanide (Alinia®) is the drug of choice. Alternative therapy includes paromomycin + azithromycin. Diagnose by acid-fast stains (small and round). This organism causes major metropolitan (Wisconsin) outbreaks of diarrhea due to contaminated city water as well as water park and swimming pool outbreaks; be aware of this for the exams!

Isospora belli

Isospora belli is another acid-fast protozoan that, in patients with AIDS, causes a watery diarrhea identical to *Cryptosporidium*. On the acid-fast stain, it is large and oval, whereas *Cryptosporidium* is small and round. Treat with TMP/SMX.

Cyclospora

Cyclospora is a newly described acid-fast, intestinal protozoan parasite that causes diarrhea in immunocompromised and immunocompetent patients. Usual source is imported fruits and vegetables from developing countries. Outbreaks have occurred due to raspberries, basil, lettuce, snow peas, and contaminated water. Systemic symptoms (e.g., malaise, myalgia, low-grade fever, fatigue) are commonly seen with *Cyclospora* infection. Treat with TMP/SMX.

Malaria

Plasmodium is a protozoan that causes malaria. It affects the RBCs and is transmitted via the *Anopheles* mosquito. There are 4 major types: *P. vivax*, *P. ovale*, *P. malariae*, and *P. falciparum*. (*P. knowlesi* can also infect humans and is associated with severe disease.) Patients who are asplenic have more severe cases of malaria. Travelers with fever, upon returning from a malarial endemic area, should have thick and thin smears of their peripheral blood to test for malaria. Do the thick smears in case they have low numbers of parasites and thin smears in order to determine the malarial species.

P. falciparum is the worst type of malaria and can cause cerebral malaria (seizures, stupor, coma, etc.), hypoglycemia, renal failure, respiratory failure, metabolic acidosis, severe anemia, and shock. It is the cause of virtually all of the fatal infections. It also has widespread chloroquine resistance. Most cases of *P. falciparum* are acquired in mid-Africa.

The blood smear in *P. falciparum* shows "banana gametocytes" (Image 5-22). Often you see > 1 infected RBC on the slide and even multiple parasitized RBCs. This greatly contrasts with the other forms of malaria in which the parasitized RBCs are often hard to find. Finding a banana gametocyte on the peripheral blood smear is diagnostic for *P. falciparum*. Even though *P. falciparum* causes the highest levels of parasitemia, the schizonts are not seen on peripheral smear. If you see schizonts, the patient has one of the other types.

Non-falciparum: The Duffy RBC antigen is the site of attachment for *P. vivax*. Syndromes associated with *P. vivax* and *P. ovale* include anemia, hypersplenism, and relapsing disease (up to 3–5 years later, secondary to the latent hepatic stages—hypnozoites). Any type of malaria can cause nephritis from immune complex deposition, but *P. malariae* is most commonly associated with

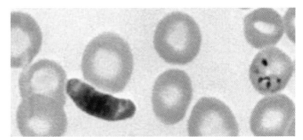

Image 5-22: P. falciparum, "banana gametocytes"

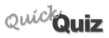

Quick Quiz

- What drug is used to treat *Isospora belli* infection?

- What is the food associated with *Cyclospora* infection?

- If you see "banana gametocytes" on a peripheral smear, what type of malaria does the patient have?

- Which type of malaria is more commonly associated with nephrotic syndrome?

- What type of anemia must you screen for before treating someone with primaquine for malaria?

- What drug must be taken after chloroquine for successful treatment of *P. vivax* and *P. ovale*?

nephrotic syndrome. Antibody production causes a decrease in parasitemia, but not in the number of intracellular parasites!

Treatment (Table 5-5): Use chloroquine for infections of *P. vivax*, *P. ovale*, and *P. malariae*. Recent reports of *P. vivax* resistance have occurred in Papua New Guinea, Indonesia, and in parts of Asia and South America. Primaquine is adjunctive medication for infections with *P. vivax* and *P. ovale* to eradicate hypnozoites in the liver. Remember: Hypnozoites are the malarial forms responsible for relapse! Chloroquine-sensitive *P. falciparum* is treated with chloroquine, of course. For *P. falciparum* that is likely to be chloroquine-resistant, see Table 5-5. Another option is mefloquine (Lariam®). Mefloquine is effective against the chloroquine-resistant

and the pyrimethamine/sulfadoxine-resistant *P. falciparum*. It is also effective against the chloroquine-sensitive *Plasmodia*.

Remember: The use of pyrimethamine/sulfadoxine (Fansidar®) is rarely associated with the risk of severe Stevens-Johnson syndrome (which is due to the sulfa)! Also remember: Primaquine induces hemolytic anemia in G6PD-deficient persons, so you must screen for G6PD deficiency before prescribing it.

For malaria prophylaxis, use chloroquine if there is no chloroquine-resistant *P. falciparum* present in the region in question. Start it 1–2 weeks before arrival to the endemic area and continue for 4–6 weeks after leaving the area. Use mefloquine, doxycycline, or atovaquone/proguanil (Malarone®) for prophylaxis in chloroquine-resistant regions. Primaquine can be given the last 2 weeks of a prophylaxis period with either chloroquine or mefloquine and after travel to regions where there is *P. vivax* or *P. ovale*. [Know:] The main causes of malaria in the U.S. are either not taking prophylaxis before traveling to endemic regions or stopping prophylaxis too soon after returning from endemic areas!

A fixed combination of atovaquone and proguanil (Malarone®) is approved for the prophylaxis and treatment of uncomplicated *P. falciparum* malaria. For prophylaxis, the advantage is that it can be started just prior to leaving and stopped soon after return; it also has fewer side effects. The disadvantage is that it must be taken daily.

Encourage the use of DEET and picaridin-containing insect repellants—and mosquito netting impregnated with permethrin. DEET is not recommended by the AAP for children < 2 months of age.

Table 5-5: Treatment and Prophylaxis of Malaria		
Type of Malaria	**Treatment**	**Prophylaxis**
Non-falciparum malaria	Chloroquine and primaquine	Chloroquine 500 mg (300 mg base) weekly. Give daily in endemic areas.
P. falciparum Chloroquine-sensitive	Chloroquine Atovaquone/proguanil	Choose any 1 of the following: Chloroquine Atovaquone/proguanil Mefloquine Doxycycline
P. falciparum Chloroquine-resistant Not very ill	Atovaquone/proguanil or Quinine sulfate PO plus either pyrimethamine + sulfadoxine, doxycycline, or clindamycin or Mefloquine	Mefloquine: 1 dose weekly, including 1 week before and 4 weeks after or Atovaquone/proguanil: 1 dose daily, including 1–2 days before and 7 days after or Doxycycline: 100 mg 1–2 days before travel and continued 4 weeks after return
P. falciparum Chloroquine-resistant Very ill	Artemisinin derivative (best choice) or IV quinidine gluconate +/– IV clindamycin	

Babesia

Babesia microti is an intra-RBC protozoan parasite that causes babesiosis. This disease is a febrile, hemolytic anemia seen especially in debilitated elderly patients and patients who are asplenic. The organism is transmitted via the *Ixodes* tick from rodents (as is the spirochete *Borrelia*, which causes Lyme disease). It is mostly seen in the Northeast U.S.—usually in summer or early autumn.

Symptoms, which may persist for months, include fever, profuse sweats, myalgias, and shaking chills. Hemoglobinuria is a predominant sign. Patients often are emotionally labile. Because of the symptoms and the parasitized RBCs, it may be misdiagnosed as malaria.

B. microti is distinguished from *Plasmodium* by the classic intra-RBC tetrad appearing as a "Maltese cross" (Image 5-23), but more often looks like 4 dots in a square shape (the malaria parasites have a ring form).

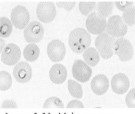
Image 5-23: Maltese cross

Mild babesiosis infections are generally self-limited. Treat moderate infections with clindamycin + quinine or atovaquone + azithromycin. If severe, do an exchange transfusion, then give antibiotics. Again, patients who are asplenic have more severe disease.

Protozoa Type II: Ameba

Human amebiasis is caused by the protozoa *Entamoeba histolytica*. Transmission is fecal-oral and can be food- or waterborne. In the U.S., the usual population groups in which it is found are the institutionalized, immigrants, and gay/bisexual men.

For intestinal disease, diagnose by examining the stool with an O+P. However, the aspirate of an amebic liver abscess often shows no ameba or PMNs—diagnose with serology!

For asymptomatic infection, a luminal agent is fine: diloxanide furoate (available only from the CDC), paromomycin, or iodoquinol. Follow-up stool studies are recommended because no regimen is 100% effective.

For liver abscesses or invasive colitis, metronidazole is the treatment of choice (alternatives: tinidazole, nitazoxanide); follow with a luminal agent (iodoquinol or paromomycin). Even large amebic abscesses respond very quickly.

Protozoa Type III: Flagellates

Organisms

The flagellates: *Giardia lamblia*, *Trichomonas vaginalis*, *Trypanosoma*, *Leishmania*.

Giardia lamblia

Giardia is the most common disease-causing parasite in the U.S. It also is the most frequently identified diarrheal agent in waterborne-associated infections. *Giardia* infections are found in campers, travelers, children in day care, gay men, and in patients with IgA deficiency and/or hypogammaglobulinemia. It infects the duodenum. (Remember: *Shigella* is also found among day care kids and gay/bisexual men.) 75% of infected persons are asymptomatic. Acute symptoms include a watery, smelly diarrhea and flatulence. Chronic giardiasis causes flatulence, sulfuric belching, soft stools, and frequent weight loss.

Diagnose with microscopic examination of fresh stool samples x 3 or *Giardia* antigen test on 1 stool. For chronic giardiasis, a string test may be required: Have the patient swallow a capsule on a string, leave it for several hours, then retrieve it and check for trophozoites. This is rarely done today.

Nitazoxanide (Alinia®) is an anti-*Giardia* medication available in a suspension form. Tinidazole has the advantage of being a single-dose tablet available for children ≥ 3 years of age. Metronidazole is also frequently used. The dose for metronidazole is 5 mg/kg tid x 7 days or a maximum of 250 mg tid x 7 days. The 2012 Red Book lists tinidazole, metronidazole, or nitazoxanide as the drugs of choice. If relapse occurs, repeat treatment with the same drug. Relapse is common in immunocompromised patients and may require more aggressive therapy.

Trichomonas vaginalis

Trichomonas vaginalis causes an STD. Treat with metronidazole. See more in Adolescent Health and Gynecology, Book 1.

Trypanosomiasis

Trypanosoma causes trypanosomiasis. There are 2 main types. The African disease is sleeping sickness. It is caused by *Trypanosoma brucei* and is transmitted via the tsetse fly.

The American illness, Chagas disease, is caused by *T. cruzi*; it is found in Central/South America and Mexico, and is transmitted by the triatomine insects ("kissing bugs"). The acute phase is usually asymptomatic or mild, nonspecific symptoms. The chronic form can cause problems with the heart (from heart block to CHF), the GI system (especially achalasia, megaesophagus, and megacolon), and occasionally the CNS. Be suspicious of trypanosomiasis in child from Mexico or Central/South America who presents with unilateral firm edema of the eyelids (Romaña sign, Image 5-24) followed by fever, generalized lymphadenopathy, and malaise (acute phase). Myocarditis can follow. The heart failure and cardiomyopathy may occur years later after the initial infection.

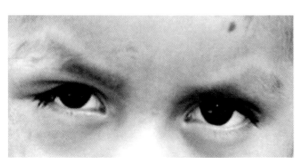

Quick Quiz

- How is *Babesia* infection distinguished from malaria?

- Do you diagnose an amebic liver abscess with stool studies or serology?

- What is the most common cause of diarrhea due to parasites in the U.S.?

- How do you treat *Giardia* in a child who cannot swallow pills?

- A child presents from South America with heart block and CHF. What parasitic infection is a possible etiology?

- True or false? Most helminth (worm) infections cause a peripheral eosinophilia.

- What is the largest roundworm that infects humans in the U.S.?

All patients with Chagas disease should be treated; benznidazole and nifurtimox are the only drugs with proven efficacy.

Leishmaniasis

There are 3 major clinical syndromes associated with leishmaniasis:

1) **Cutaneous**: An erythematous papule at the site of the sand fly bite slowly enlarges and becomes ulcerative. After weeks to years, lesions scar (flat, atrophic, "cigarette paper" scar). Caused by: *L. braziliensis, L. panamensis*, and *L. guyanensis*. Location: Western Hemisphere.

2) **Mucosal** (a.k.a. **espundia**): Granulomatous inflammation presents on the nose and lips. Same organisms and locations that cause the cutaneous form. May occur years to months after cutaneous lesions heal.

3) **Visceral** (a.k.a. **kala-azar**): Fever, anorexia, weight loss, hepatosplenomegaly, pancytopenia, thrombocytopenia, peripheral lymphadenopathy. Caused by: *L. donovani* and *L. infantum*. Location: Eastern Hemisphere.

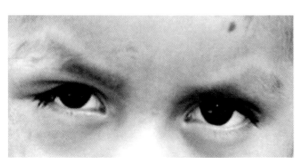

Image 5-24: Romaña sign in trypanosomiasis

Amphotericin B is the only treatment approved by the FDA. Sodium stibogluconate (pentavalent antimony) is available as an investigational drug but is associated with increased toxicity.

HELMINTHIC ORGANISMS

Overview

The helminthic organisms are the other major type of parasite. [Remember: 1) protozoan and 2) helminthic organisms.] They are multicellular worms that, in general, do not replicate in the body—but do cause eosinophilia.

The 2 types of helminthic organisms are:

1) Nemathelminthes: the nematodes or roundworms, which include pinworms, hookworms, whipworms (*Trichuris trichiura*), *Trichinella, Strongyloides*, and *Ascaris*.

2) Platyhelminthes: cestodes (tapeworms) and trematodes (flukes).

Nematodes (Roundworm)

Ascaris lumbricoides

Ascaris lumbricoides is the largest intestinal roundworm that infects humans. Worms are 20–40 cm long. The female lays 200,000 eggs daily. Eggs then pass in the host's feces and become infective in the environment—only after the 1st stage larva molts within the egg. Children often infect themselves and others while playing in the same areas where they poop. Mature worms set up shop in the jejunum, where they lay their eggs.

The larval form has a complex migration pattern in humans and must cross from the duodenum into the mesenteric lymphatics, to the portal circulation, and then reach the pulmonary vascular bed. There, they cut through the alveolar wall, go up the respiratory tree to the epiglottis, and are finally swallowed. During this period of going through the lungs, patients frequently have cough, fever, and rales. Hemoptysis can occur. A key to look for is "shifting" infiltrates or atelectasis

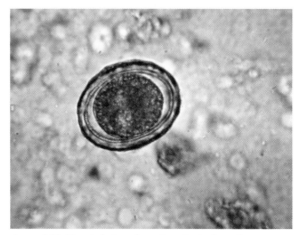

Image 5-25: Nematode (roundworm) egg in stool sample

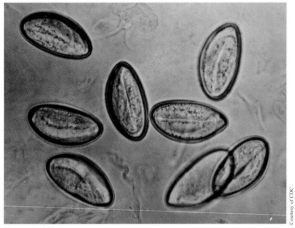

Image 5-26: Pinworm eggs

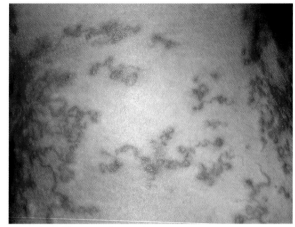

Image 5-27: Cutaneous larva migrans

occurring with Löffler syndrome (which usually also has a high eosinophil count).

Diagnose by finding the eggs or worms in the stool. (See Image 5-25 of the fertilized egg.) Mebendazole, albendazole, or ivermectin are the drugs of choice; however, mebendazole is no longer available in the U.S.

Pinworms (*Enterobius vermicularis*)

Pinworm infection is ubiquitous. It occurs when eggs (Image 5-26) are ingested by oral contact with contaminated hands, toys, or other fomites. Some feel that "slumber parties" are the pinworm's heaven (all those kids jumping around on the bed, the eggs flying up in the air—aerosolized and easily ingested). The eggs hatch in the duodenum, then travel to the cecum, where they have worm sex. The pregnant female worm travels to the large bowel and out the anus at night, leaving a trail of eggs on the surface of the skin. The female worms are 8–13 mm long. The prime time for the worms to exit the rectum is "10–11 p.m." Know that reinfection is common, as is autoinoculation. "Pruritus ani" occurs with pinworms quite commonly. Diagnose by visualization of worms in the perianal region or use the clear adhesive tape test for eggs.

Treat pinworms with pyrantel pamoate or albendazole (not FDA-approved for this use). Both are given as a single dose and then repeated in 2 weeks. Again, mebendazole is no longer available in the U.S. Also, treat all family members. Be sure to launder the sheets and bedclothes, but don't shake those dirty sheets too much!

Hookworm (*Necator americanus*)

Hookworm infection in the U.S. is due mainly to *Necator americanus,* which causes anemia, weakness, and fatigue. (It also can cause cutaneous larva migrans, Image 5-27). Know that children with hookworms may have failure to thrive! "Catch-up" growth usually occurs when the worms are killed. Treat with albendazole, mebendazole, or pyrantel pamoate.

Whipworm (*Trichuris trichiura*)

Whipworm infection (trichuriasis) is due to infection of the large intestine with *Trichuris trichiura*. Infection is most predominant in the southern U.S. and occurs by ingesting eggs.

If only a few worms are present, the infection is asymptomatic. If more worms are present, look for fever, abdominal pain, weight loss, and itching. Heavy infestations can cause diarrhea, blood-streaked stools, and rectal prolapse.

Diagnose whipworm by finding the eggs in the stool. Treat with albendazole or ivermectin x 3 days (not approved by the FDA to treat trichuriasis).

Mebendazole is the drug of choice but is no longer available in the U.S. But for the exam, if mebendazole is given as a choice, pick it!

Trichinosis (*Trichinella spiralis*)

Trichinella spiralis larvae, which are usually found in pork (but also found in venison, horse, bear, boar, seal, walrus), cause trichinosis. In the U.S., there were 66 cases documented between 2002 and 2007—commonly from undercooked wild meat, especially bear meat. Human infection is much more common in other parts of the world.

Symptoms are determined by where the worm is. After ingestion, the eggs hatch and the larvae invade the duodenum, which can cause abdominal pain, nausea, and vomiting. From here, they go into the blood stream and reach muscle tissue, which can cause muscle pain. Calcifications occur in skeletal muscle. If they reach the heart, myocarditis can occur. Ocular involvement is common, as is eosinophilia. Chemosis and periorbital edema suggest the diagnosis, which is confirmed by finding rising serologic titers or muscle biopsy.

Treat with mebendazole or albendazole. Corticosteroids are useful in severe disease (especially CNS and myocardial disease) and also help alleviate symptoms.

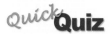

Quick Quiz

- Know everything there is to know about pinworms. Diagnosis? Treatment?
- What time of day do most pinworms emerge from the anus? (Just kidding.)
- What is the only worm to replicate in humans?
- What causes visceral larva migrans?
- In a child with a history of pica, pneumonia, and eosinophilia, what should you think about?
- What is cysticercosis? How does it present?

Filariasis (*Wuchereria bancrofti*)

The mosquito transmits *Wuchereria bancrofti*. It is one of the causes of lymphatic filariasis (lymphatic blockage) and 2° elephantiasis! It may take thousands of bites by infected mosquitoes to inoculate enough of the organism to cause this. Remember: With the exception of *Strongyloides*, helminthic organisms do not multiply in the human body. Diagnose by presence of microfilariae in the blood.

Treat with diethylcarbamazine citrate (DEC) in combination with albendazole or ivermectin in a single dose.

Strongyloides stercoralis

Strongyloides stercoralis infection is common in certain areas of the U.S. and is very common in South America and Southeast Asia. Highly endemic areas exist in Southeast Asia and South America, where up to 60% of the population is infected. In the U.S., studies found infection rates of 3% among Kentucky school children and 6% at the Tennessee VA hospital.

It is (virtually) the only helminthic organism that replicates in the body. With this autoinfection, the infection can persist for decades. (Strong!)

Symptoms are usually GI, but there can be pulmonary symptoms during the infective part of the larvae's lifecycle. Patients often have larva currens, a serpiginous rash with erythematous tracks. Eosinophilia commonly is present.

In immunosuppressed patients, potentially fatal, disseminated strongyloidiasis may occur—some call it "hyperinfection"—presenting with abdominal pain and distension, neuro and pulmonary symptoms, and shock.

Diagnose with serial stool samples for larvae—not eggs. Treat with ivermectin.

Toxocariasis (*Toxocara canis* and *T. cati*)

Toxocara canis (and sometimes *Toxocara cati*) causes visceral larva migrans. Older children may get retinal involvement alone (ocular larva migrans). The normal host for *Toxocara canis* is dogs, and it is transmitted to humans by ingesting soil contaminated with dog excreta.

In humans, the larvae do not develop into adult worms but rather migrate through the host tissue—eliciting eosinophilia. Look for this in a child with fever, hepatosplenomegaly, "migratory pneumonia," hypergammaglobulinemia, and eosinophilia! In the U.S., *Toxocara* seropositivity is 20% in kindergarten children and 2% in the general population; especially consider on the exams in a 1–4-year-old with a history of pica (e.g., eating dirt).

Hypereosinophilia and hypergammaglobulinemia associated with increased titers of isohemagglutinin to the A and B blood group are presumptive evidence of infection. Serum *Toxocara* antibodies are available but can't distinguish between current or past infection.

Either observe (most will get better) or treat with albendazole.

Platyhelminthes (Cestodes and Trematodes)

Platyhelminthes include **cestodes** (tapeworms) and **trematodes** (flukes).

Cestodes are the flatworms (tapeworms). The pork tapeworm, *Taenia solium*, has 2 clinical entities:

1) If the cysticerci are ingested, taeniasis develops. (A tapeworm grows in the intestines.)
2) If an egg-contaminated food (from animal or human feces) is ingested, the patient will develop cysticercosis. The eggs hatch and the oncospheres go into the blood and, most significantly, cause cysticerci in the CNS and eyes. These cysts do nothing until the organism dies. In the brain (neurocysticercosis), the resulting inflammation usually causes seizures as the 1st symptom. Especially consider cysticercosis in a patient with new-onset seizures who is an immigrant from Mexico, Central or South America, or who is from a household with an immigrant from these areas. Characteristically, head CT initially shows single or multiple cysts, which then progress to calcified granuloma.

T. saginata is the most common tapeworm in humans and is a beef tapeworm.

T. asiatica is found in parts of Asia and is a pig tapeworm.

Praziquantel or niclosamide is the usual treatment for all intestinal tapeworms. Use albendazole (1st choice) or praziquantel along with corticosteroids for neurocysticercosis. Note: If ocular or spinal cysts are present, do not treat—this causes irreparable damage!

Trematodes are the flukes:

- *Clonorchis sinensis* is the Chinese liver fluke. It is endemic in the Far East. Infection is caused by eating raw fish and is often associated with biliary obstruction.
- *Schistosoma haematobium* infects the bladder, causing urinary symptoms (hematuria!). Risk factors include swimming in infested endemic waters. Infected children have an increased risk of bladder cancer as adults.
- *Schistosoma mansoni* is a fluke found in Africa, the Middle East, and South America.
- *Schistosoma japonicum* is found in Asia.

Schistosoma causes acute schistosomiasis (Katayama fever) ~ 2 months after inoculation. This infection presents with fever, lymphadenopathy, diarrhea, hepatosplenomegaly, and marked eosinophilia. The most serious complication of schistosomiasis is cirrhosis with esophageal varices. Schistosomiasis does not cause the other stigmata seen with alcoholic cirrhosis (spiders, gynecomastia, or ascites).

Finding the eggs in the stool makes the diagnosis.

Give praziquantel for 1 day (!) for any *Schistosoma* and most other fluke infections. Repeat therapy in 1–2 months because therapy does not kill developing worms.

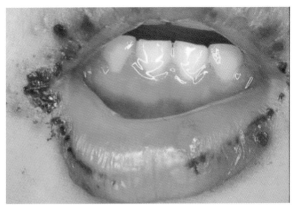

Image 5-28: HSV-1 infection

VIRUSES

HERPES SIMPLEX VIRUS

Herpes Viruses

The herpes viruses are double-stranded DNA viruses that include the herpes simplex viruses (HSV-1 and HSV-2), CMV, Epstein-Barr, human herpesviruses (HHV 6, 7, and 8), and varicella-zoster viruses.

HSV-1

HSV-1 causes orofacial infections in ~ 40% of the population. By the later adult years, 70–90% of individuals are infected with HSV-1. In the primary infection, the vesicular lesions and ulcers are usually localized to the oral mucosa, lips, and surrounding skin, whereas in recurrent infections, ulcers are typically on the outer lip (Image 5-28). Peak incidence of initial infection occurs at 1–5 years of age.

Herpetic whitlow refers to an HSV infection of the fingers (Image 5-29). It is painful and may be confused with a bacterial infection. Do not surgically open these infections because the infection may worsen and spread. Herpes gladiatorum occurs in wrestlers and herpes rugbiaforum (or scrum pox) in rugby players and occurs in abraded skin that has contact with oral secretions infected with HSV.

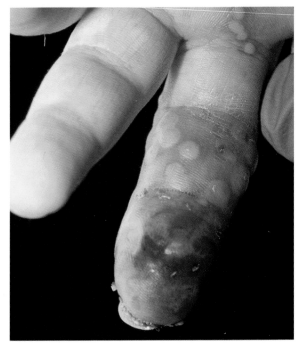

Image 5-29: Herpetic whitlow

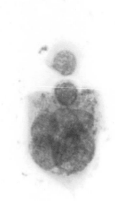

Image 5-30: Giant cell on Tzanck test

Quick Quiz

- Which fluke infects the bladder?

- In a patient with herpetic whitlow, do you need to consult a surgeon for I & D?

- If a skin lesion is HSV, what will the Tzanck smear show?

- What is the concern with HSV near the eye?

- A pregnant woman has herpetic-like lesions in her vaginal area at the time of delivery. True or false? A C-section is recommended.

- A pregnant woman has recurrent herpes 4 weeks before delivery. At the time of delivery, she has no symptoms and no signs of lesions. True or false? She should have a C-section just in case she is shedding.

- Which infant is more likely to be infected with HSV—one born to a mother with her 1st episode of HSV at delivery or an infant born to a mother with her 20th episode of HSV?

- True or false? The majority of women who deliver an infant with HSV infection have a prior history of HSV.

- Where do the lesions of neonatal HSV tend to occur?

Tzanck test is done by scraping down to the bottom cellular layer of a vesicle, placing the material on a slide, then staining with either Giemsa or Wright. The test is no longer recommended but commonly appears on exams. In herpes simplex and varicella (including zoster), it shows multinucleated giant cells (Image 5-30). Herpes direct fluorescent antibody testing (DFA), PCR, and glycoprotein G-based type-specific assays are now more commonly used and are much more sensitive and specific. However, culture remains a very reliable and fast way to diagnose infection, especially in those with lesions or skin, eye, mucosa (SEM) disease.

It is possible to autoinoculate the virus; thus, the infection can spread from the lips (or other areas) to the eyes of a patient. Recurrent HSV-1 eye infection resulting in a keratitis is the most common infectious cause of blindness in industrialized nations. It presents with characteristic dendritic, branched, fluorescent-staining corneal ulcers.

HSV-2

HSV-2 causes "genital herpes." Actually, it causes ~ 75% of HSV genital infections—the rest are due to Type 1. Note that the prevalence of HSV-2 is 25%, and, of those, only 25% have symptoms! In 10% of patients, the initial occurrence of HSV-2 is associated with only a herpetic exudative pharyngitis. New data suggest that asymptomatic shedding of virus spreads many HSV infections.

Neonatal HSV

Most cases of neonatal HSV are from intrapartum contact, so a C-section is recommended if the mother has symptoms or signs of genital herpes, or its prodrome, at the time of delivery. (Otherwise, vaginal delivery is fine.) The risk for transmission to the neonate is high (25–60%) among women who get their 1st episode of genital herpes (primary infection) near the time of delivery and low (~ 2%) among women with a history of recurrent herpes. However, 60–80% of women who deliver infants with neonatal HSV have no prior history of HSV!

Serology that can distinguish type-specific HSV antibodies are more reliable now so that the type of maternal infection can be determined and thus guide in the management of infants born to women with active genital HSV lesions. The AAP has now published an algorithm for the evaluation of asymptomatic HSV disease in neonates following vaginal or C-section delivery to women with active genital HSV lesions, using a combination of viral and serologic tests. The guidelines do not address how to manage asymptomatic neonates born to women with a history of genital herpes but no active lesions at delivery.

Neonatal HSV can manifest in 3 clinical syndromes:

- ~ 45% of infections are localized to the SEM (skin, eyes, mouth); presents in the 1st or 2nd week of life
- 30% to the CNS only; typically presents in the 2nd or 3rd week of life
- 25% disseminated (including liver, lung, and CNS involvement); usually presents in the 1st or 2nd week of life

HSV infection in the neonate is often severe, with high mortality and severe CNS sequelae even with appropriate antiviral therapy.

Think about HSV in neonates with skin lesions, conjunctivitis, fever, seizures, or sepsis/shock! Workup includes:

- HSV culture of the mouth, nasopharynx, conjunctivae, and anus
- HSV culture and PCR of skin lesions and CSF
- Whole blood sample for HSV PCR and liver enzymes

Skin lesions start as macules and quickly become vesicular on a red base. The lesions commonly occur at sites of trauma, such as fetal scalp monitor sites or eye margins. Never overlook HSV as a possibility in a neonate with a vesicular-looking lesion! Conjunctivitis, keratitis, or chorioretinitis may occur with the eye. SEM disease does well if the diagnosis is made quickly and acyclovir is given early. It is common for skin lesions to recur during the next several years.

Treat neonatal HSV with IV acyclovir for 14 days for SEM disease, and a minimum of 21–28 days for both CNS infections (treat until HSV CSF PCR is negative) and disseminated infections. After completing the course of IV acyclovir, it is now recommended that neonates with HSV continue oral acyclovir suppressive therapy x 6 months to prevent HSV skin reoccurrences. This is associated with improved neurodevelopmental outcome in babies with CNS disease and in infants with SEM disease.

HSV in Older Children

Encephalitis is the predominant cause of HSV-related mortality in older children. (The most commonly identified etiologies of encephalitis are arboviruses, but the majority of encephalitis etiologies are still not identified.)

Patients with herpes encephalitis usually present with constitutional symptoms, altered mental status, and may have focal neurologic signs. Because it has a predilection for the temporal lobe, patients may have temporal lobe seizure symptoms (e.g., abnormal behavior, smells burning rubber). > 60% are left with neurologic sequelae!

HSV PCR, EEG, and MRI are all sensitive for diagnosis. Bloody CSF is not pathognomonic for HSV encephalitis, but CSF pleocytosis with a predominance of lymphocytes and some erythrocytes is typically seen.

HSV is one of the many causes of erythema multiforme. (See Dermatology, Book 2.)

Treatment of HSV in children and adolescents: Use acyclovir for all the types of herpes infections. Give IV in immunosuppressed patients, but be careful—it can cause acute renal insufficiency, although rarely in children.

For genital herpes, give acyclovir or one of its analogs (famciclovir, valacyclovir) orally. Acyclovir (or famciclovir, or valacyclovir) can also be given to suppress chronic infection or as a treatment for acute recurrence. Use foscarnet to treat HSV that is resistant to acyclovir. Ganciclovir is not helpful for resistant HSV because it is also inactivated by the same mechanism.

VARICELLA
Overview

Varicella-zoster virus (VZV) causes chicken pox (Image 5-31) and herpes zoster (shingles, Image 5-32). The incubation period is 10–21 days (up to 28 days if varicella zoster immune globulin [VARIZIG®] or IVIG has been given). Children present with low-grade fever, headache, and malaise, followed in 24–48 hours with the vesicular exanthem, described as "dew drops on a rose petal." It appears most commonly on the trunk and extremities, but the face and scalp can be involved as well. The vesicles appear in crops for 3–5 days and are worse in areas of eczema or trauma. (Patients usually have 250–500 lesions total.) Eventually, the vesicles become cloudy with cellular debris and finally involute and crust over. Itching is the most common complaint. Healing tends to occur in 7–10 days without scar formation.

Patients are contagious from 1–2 days prior to onset of rash until all lesions are crusted over. Children may return to school or day care when the lesions are crusted over. Those exposed while hospitalized should be placed in a negative-pressure isolation room from days 8 to 21 *after* exposure (up to 28 days if given VARIZIG). For most children, varicella is a benign illness. More severe disease occurs in infants, adolescents, and adults compared to children. Suspect bacterial infection if fever occurs after the initial 48 hours or if there is progression of redness or tenderness around lesions that are crusting over. Other things to look for: mental status changes, hemorrhagic lesions, or significant abdominal pain or vomiting.

Children immunized with vaccine can still get disease, but generally it is mild with few lesions (< 50).

Complications of Varicella

The most common complication is secondary bacterial infection. Most commonly, *Streptococcus pyogenes* and *Staphylococcus aureus* are involved. Infection can range from simple impetigo to necrotizing fasciitis. Also, deep tissue abscesses, bone infections, or severe lymphadenitis may occur.

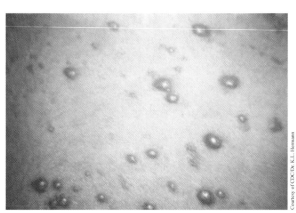

Image 5-31: Chicken pox

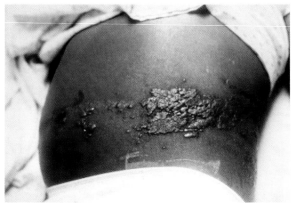

Image 5-32: Shingles

Quick Quiz

- How long should you treat an infant with acyclovir that has HSV localized to SEM? CNS encephalitis? Disseminated disease?

- A college student presents with abnormal behavior, focal seizures, and signs of encephalitis. What radiologic test will best diagnose this if HSV is the etiology? What empiric therapy should you start while awaiting test results?

- What is the incubation period for chicken pox?

- When may a child with chicken pox return to day care or school?

- A child with cystic fibrosis is in the hospital for a "tune-up." He was exposed to a child with chicken pox 5 days before admission. The CF child has not received the varicella vaccine and has not had chicken pox. When should this child be placed in isolation, and when may he be removed from isolation if he is still hospitalized?

- What is the most common complication of chicken pox?

- What is the most common CNS complication of chicken pox?

- Which patients are more likely to get chicken pox pneumonia?

Hepatitis, with mild liver enzyme elevations, is common in varicella. More extensive hepatitis is rare, but can occur. Reye syndrome has been associated with aspirin use and varicella infection.

Children have pneumonitis in ~ 10% of cases; it is usually mild. Adults and adolescents are more likely to have severe disease. Progression to pneumonia is more likely in these older age groups.

Thrombocytopenia can occur and result in bleeding problems.

The most common CNS complication is transient cerebellar ataxia and encephalitis. Cerebellar ataxia is self-limited and may occur before or after the onset of the exanthem. Encephalitis can be quite severe in some patients. Other, rarer CNS complications include aseptic meningitis, transverse myelitis, and Guillain-Barré syndrome.

Immunocompromised Patients

Children with defects in the ability to mount an antigen-specific T-cell immune response are at risk for progressive, disseminated varicella infection. These include patients:

- With lymphoproliferative malignancies, stem cell or solid organ transplant recipients, severe combined immunodeficiency, short-limbed dwarfism, Wiskott-Aldrich syndrome, and ataxia-telangiectasia.
- With HIV and AIDS. These patients are also at risk for recurrent disease; shingles also is very common.
- Receiving chronic steroids, or even receiving a temporary dose of steroids (even for asthma) during the varicella incubation period.

Disseminated varicella begins with severe abdominal pain or back pain before the appearance of the rash. Fever is very high, may reach 104° to 106° F, and persists for several days. Liver involvement, pneumonitis, low platelet counts, coagulopathy, encephalitis, and renal dysfunction may all occur. Mortality is high. Also, infectiousness is longer in these individuals.

Pregnancy

Symptoms of chicken pox may be severe in adolescents, adults, and especially in pregnant women. Pneumonia is more likely to occur in these older patients. Besides increased severity and pneumonia in the mother, if she is infected between 8- and 20-weeks gestation, her newborn is more likely to have birth defects. These defects can include classic cicatricial skin scarring and limb atrophy, microcephaly, cortical atrophy, seizures, chorioretinitis, and neurologic defects. Maternal zoster does not carry this risk.

Current recommendation for pregnant patients exposed to chicken pox: Give zoster immunoglobulin (VARIZIG) within 10 days of exposure. If VARIZIG is not available, give IVIG. Do not give varicella virus vaccine (VARIVAX®) to pregnant patients because it is a live vaccine.

Infants born to mothers who develop varicella < 5 days before delivery, or < 48 hours after delivery, are at risk of severe neonatal varicella because they are likely to have acquired significant virus in the absence of transplacental varicella antibody. Mothers who develop varicella > 4 days prior to delivery make varicella-specific IgG in sufficient time to permit placental transfer of antibody. This will generally prevent severe disease but may not protect newborns against infection. Infants whose mothers have varicella at any stage of pregnancy, or infants who acquire varicella during the first few months of life (especially < 6 months of age), may manifest zoster early in life. Give infected term infants IV acyclovir. Most authorities recommend treating adults/adolescents with oral acyclovir 20 mg/kg/dose every 6 hours for 5 days (maximum: 800 mg/dose) if they present within the first 24 hours of the exanthem. Also, if the case is the 2nd or later in the household, many will treat that child presumptively with acyclovir (because the disease is usually more severe than in the primary case in the household). Give immunocompromised patients IV acyclovir. (Toxicity: acute renal insufficiency, but again, very rare in children.) Avoid aspirin because of Reye syndrome risk.

VARIZIG® (Varicella Zoster Immune Globulin)

Consider VARIZIG for significantly exposed, susceptible (without evidence of immunity) children at risk for severe disease.

Susceptible patients include:

- Immunocompromised children
- Pregnant women
- Newborns whose mothers had varicella < 5 days before or < 48 hours after delivery
- Hospitalized premature infants ≥ 28-weeks gestation born to varicella antibody-negative mothers or no reliable history of varicella
- Hospitalized premature infants < 28-weeks gestation or ≤ 1,000 grams (regardless of mothers' varicella status)

Note: If the mother has zoster, then neither VARIZIG nor IVIG is given to the newborn.

What is significant exposure?

- Active case residing in the same household
- Active case sharing the same hospital room
- Visit by person deemed contagious
- Face-to-face indoor play with an active case (5 minutes to 1 hour)
- Intimate contact with a person with active zoster

In 2012, the FDA extended the period you could give VARIZIG to within 10 days after significant exposure. Be aware that VARIZIG may not prevent infection and may prolong the incubation period up to 28 days. Do not give as a treatment to those with active infection. If VARIZIG is not readily available, IVIG can be given or, alternatively, a course of acyclovir can be given.

If these children (exposed and susceptible) have not received VARIZIG by day 7, consider a course of acyclovir.

You can also give varicella vaccine to someone (> 12 months of age) without immunity to varicella, ideally within 3 days but up to 5 days after exposure to try to prevent varicella infection.

Infection Control

[Know.] Children with varicella are excluded from school until the lesions are crusted. Those exposed are potentially contagious from day 10 after exposure to the end of the incubation period (21 days). Therefore, any child admitted to the hospital with a history of exposure must be in a negative-pressure isolation room with airborne precautions during the incubation period—specifically from days 8-21 after exposure.

In the hospital setting, a child with varicella is considered infectious and remains in isolation until all lesions are crusted over (or at least a minimum of 5 days if crusting occurs earlier).

Zoster (Shingles)

Herpes zoster (shingles) is caused by reactivation of the varicella-zoster virus. Varicella vaccine virus can also cause zoster in immunocompetent children, but it is usually mild. A Tzanck smear shows multinucleated giant cells, which are pathognomonic for herpes viruses. A varicella virus direct fluorescent antibody (DFA) is diagnostic. Postherpetic neuralgia is more likely with increasing age in adults > 60. Shingles recurs in < 5% of immunocompetent patients. If a young child develops shingles, the 1st question to ask is when did they have chicken pox—commonly it was when they were a young infant (< 6 months of age).

Most commonly, zoster affects 1 or 2 adjacent dermatomes with thoracic, cranial nerve, and lumbosacral areas most frequently involved. The lesions increase in number over 3–5 days and crust over by 2 weeks.

Prednisone, previously used with acyclovir, prolongs the course of herpes zoster in immunosuppressed patients. Immunosuppressed patients often get severe cases of shingles. Although it was previously thought that prednisone decreases the incidence of postherpetic neuralgia in the immunocompetent, well-designed studies have shown no benefit.

To treat zoster, use high-dose oral acyclovir; although it shortens the course of acute illness a little, it does not decrease the incidence of postherpetic neuralgia. Only famciclovir and valacyclovir are shown to decrease the incidence of postherpetic neuralgia. Valacyclovir is an L-valyl ester of acyclovir, has 3–5x greater bioavailability than acyclovir, and is almost completely converted to acyclovir after oral administration. For pain control, tricyclics, gabapentin, and lidocaine patches have some efficacy. Narcotics are effective and underused in this instance! Amitriptyline may be helpful for treatment of postherpetic neuralgia.

A zoster vaccine for adults (Zostavax®) has been licensed by the FDA in the U.S. for people ≥ 50 years of age, and currently is recommended by the CDC to give to healthy people ≥ 60 years of age for prevention of herpes zoster.

If a patient presents with back pain and you think it is a herpes zoster prodrome, what should you do? Answer: Nothing, except follow closely. Do not begin the acyclovir or its analogs until you see vesicles.

Quick Quiz

- Which antiinflammatory drug should be avoided in chicken pox?

- Who should be considered for VARIZIG® therapy after exposure to chicken pox? In particular, which term newborns should be considered for VARIZIG?

- True or false? If you have a mother with herpes zoster, you give VARIZIG to her newborn.

- How long after exposure to varicella can you give VARIZIG to a susceptible person to protect them?

- Where does herpes zoster tend to occur?

- How is CMV transmitted?

- Describe the clinical findings in an infant with severe congenital CMV infection.

- What is the greatest concern regarding infants born with asymptomatic CMV infection?

- True or false? The hearing loss associated with congenital CMV is conductive.

- What would a CT scan look like in an infant with congenital CMV?

CYTOMEGALOVIRUS (CMV)

Overview

Cytomegalovirus (CMV) is a DNA virus that has been designated as human herpesvirus 5 (HHV-5). CMV infection is usually asymptomatic and is fairly common. Prevalence rates depend on geography and socioeconomic status. In developing countries, 100% will have seroprevalence by their early 20s. By contrast, only 50% of the middle-upper socioeconomic population in the U.S. has anti-CMV antibodies by the age of 35.

CMV is transmitted through contact with infected urine, respiratory secretions, or blood. It can also be transmitted with organ or hematopoietic stem cell transplantation. Approximately 1% of all newborns are congenitally infected with CMV. (CMV is the most common congenital infection.) Most of these infections are clinically silent and occur in mothers with existing immunity; however, clinically significant infections can occur. Breastfeeding is also a common method of transmission.

If the infant is not infected congenitally or in the perinatal period, the infant is likely to be infected in day care. Day care center prevalence rates approach 80%!

Congenital CMV Infection

Whether or not an infant will be infected depends largely on if the mother has IgG antibodies to CMV. Infants who are exposed *in utero* when the moms have a primary infection with CMV are at a high risk of congenital infection, and 5–20% of babies born to mothers with primary infection are symptomatic at birth.

There is some confusion about infection rate if an infant is exposed *in utero* when mom is reinfected with a new strain or has reactivation of existing CMV. Previously, it was taught that the chance of infection in these infants is much lower, ~ 1%. There are new data showing that infants born to women who are reinfected with a new strain during pregnancy are equally likely to be infected as infants born to moms with primary infection. Distinctly different conclusions! Obviously, we need more time for this to be sorted out.

The most severe form of congenital CMV infection is cytomegalic inclusion disease. It presents with the following findings:

- IUGR
- Hepatosplenomegaly
- Jaundice
- Thrombocytopenia
- "Blueberry muffin" baby (petechiae/purpura as in congenital rubella syndrome)
- Microcephaly
- Cerebral atrophy
- Chorioretinitis
- Sensorineural hearing loss
- Periventricular intracerebral calcifications ("**CircuMV**ent the ventricles")

Some infants are born asymptomatic at birth but can have subtle findings, including growth retardation. Some neurological lesions may not occur for years! The greatest concern is that 15–20% of these children will have sensorineural hearing loss.

Diagnosis of congenital CMV requires isolation of the virus from urine, stool, respiratory tract secretions, or CSF obtained within 2–4 weeks of birth.

Data for neonates with symptomatic CMV disease involving the CNS suggest a benefit from 6 weeks of IV ganciclovir for decreasing hearing loss and potentially improving neurologic outcome at 1–2 years of age. Valganciclovir (an oral analog of ganciclovir) achieves the same ganciclovir exposure as the IV form.

Even so, at this time, routine use of ganciclovir is not recommended by the AAP or the Red Book Committee due to possible antiviral toxicities (mainly neutropenia). If IV ganciclovir or PO valganciclovir is used, the use should be limited to those infants with congenital CMV with CNS disease or intractable thrombocytopenia, and started within the 1st month of life. Oral valganciclovir (Valcyte®) is being evaluated in a clinical trial conducted by the National Institute of Allergy and Infectious Diseases Collaborative Antiviral Study Group comparing 6 weeks to 6 months of treatment in infants with symptomatic congenital CMV infection.

Perinatal CMV

Most perinatal CMV infections are asymptomatic and have no long-term risk of neurologic disease or hearing loss. Some infants (especially preterm) may present with lymphadenopathy, hepatitis, or pneumonitis, but these also do not predispose to future hearing loss.

Mononucleosis-like Syndrome (Heterophile-Negative)

This tends to occur in adolescents with fever and malaise, mild hepatitis, and the presence of atypical lymphocytes. Ampicillin/amoxicillin can cause a rash with this form. Diagnosis is usually through serology (+ CMV IgM).

Immunocompromised Hosts with CMV Infection

CMV is a very common infection in patients with decreased cellular immunity (post-transplant and AIDS). 75% of seronegative transplant recipients get CMV if the donor is seropositive. With a post-transplant systemic CMV infection, the patient can have concurrent "-itises," which may include encephalitis, hepatitis, retinitis, colitis, pneumonitis, and adrenalitis (causing adrenal insufficiency). These are especially common and more severe if the recipient is seronegative prior to the transplant.

CMV is a common cause of eye problems in adult and adolescent AIDS patients with low CD4 count. CMV can cause chorioretinitis, pneumonitis, esophagitis, and colitis. The CMV retinitis is distinctive; it has both retinal blanching and hemorrhage. Diagnosis is confirmed if CMV is cultured from the buffy coat smear. Diagnose CMV pneumonitis in transplant patients by finding inclusion bodies on the biopsy specimen or a BAL (bronchoalveolar lavage) with a postive CMV PCR. Finding CMV antigenemia or a positive-serum CMV PCR may be helpful also.

Treat CMV chorioretinitis (usually in AIDS patients) with ganciclovir, foscarnet, or a combination of both. Also, intraocular ganciclovir-release devices (with oral ganciclovir) have been effective. Cidofovir is also approved. However, all of these agents have only a suppressive effect and must be given until the CD4+ T-lymphocyte count increases to > 200.

Major toxicities of ganciclovir include granulocytopenia (30%!) and low platelets. The major toxicity of foscarnet is reversible renal failure; it also causes hypocalcemia, hypomagnesemia, and hyperphosphatemia (patients may present with seizures). Because they are only suppressive, these drugs do not cure the symptoms; once they are stopped, the disease resumes.

EBV (EPSTEIN-BARR VIRUS)

Epstein-Barr virus (a DNA virus) causes infectious mononucleosis. Incubation period is 1–2 months. Most (> 90%) IM patients have pharyngitis or tonsillitis, fever, lymphadenopathy, and abnormal liver function. Lymphocytosis is common with > 10% atypical lymphocytes: enlarged with abundant cytoplasm, vacuoles, and indentations of the cell membrane. 50% have splenomegaly. Patients commonly develop a macular rash if given ampicillin. Heterophil antibody titers (monospot) decrease within 6 months, but the EBV IgG antibodies are present for years. The atypical lymphs are T cells. Recurrence is unusual but possible—typically with high titers of antibody to EBV early antigen (> 1:5,000).

Children < 4 years of age rarely have the "classic" symptoms. Most are subclinical but can present with rashes and hepatosplenomegaly. Otitis media, FTT, abdominal pain, and recurrent pharyngitis are common in young children. Prolonged fever may be the only manifestation. The monospot test is rarely positive in a child < 2 years of age and has ~ 50% sensitivity in children 2–4 years of age.

EBV-specific antibodies are a pain to learn, but please do so for exams. Here is a simplified version:

If the IgM-VCA is +, the patient has acute primary EBV or a very recent-past EBV infection.

EBNA (EB nuclear antigen) positivity means the patient is convalescent or post-EBV. So again, if IgM-VCA is positive and EBNA is negative, your patient should have acute primary EBV infection, and this is not reactivation.

IgG-VCA doesn't help you at all. It is positive before the patient has symptoms and remains so for life. It will be positive if the patient is in convalescence—or had EBV years ago.

Anti-early antigen (anti-EA) isn't much help either. It can be positive in acute-primary, recent-past, chronic, reactivation, or in EBV malignancies. It should go away in convalescent or post-EBV infection. So someone convalescing should have only a +IgG-VCA (or maybe an EBNA).

Thus, the only really helpful test findings are an isolated +IgM-VCA (which means acute-primary or recent past infection) or an isolated +IgG-VCA (which generally means an infection in the past).

There are no antivirals effective for infectious mononucleosis. Corticosteroids are used sometimes for severe life-threatening complications—especially airway obstruction, neurologic complications, severe hepatitis, myocarditis, or hemolytic anemia. Give corticosteroids to only a minority of patients with EBV. Affected persons should avoid contact sports and other activities during the time of splenomegaly (usually 1–3 months).

EBV causes oral hairy leukoplakia; this mucocutaneous lesion may be seen as an early manifestation of HIV disease. High-dose acyclovir may offer some benefit

Quick Quiz

- What infection does CMV produce in adolescents?
- What clinical manifestations can CMV infection cause in immunocompromised patients? (transplants, HIV)
- What is the primary toxicity of ganciclovir?
- What is the characteristic WBC finding in patients with EBV infection?
- How do children < 4 years of age present with EBV?
- How sensitive is the monospot test for detecting acute EBV infection in a child 3 years of age?
- Which EBV antibody tests are positive in an acute infection?
- Describe the infection associated with HHV-6 infection.

in treatment of oral hairy leukoplakia. Chronic fatigue has no proven association with EB virus. EBV is associated with X-linked lymphoproliferative syndrome, post-transplant lymphoproliferative syndrome, Burkitt lymphoma, and nasopharyngeal carcinoma.

A patient with mononucleosis symptoms and who is heterophile-negative usually has CMV.

HUMAN HERPESVIRUS 6

Human herpesvirus 6 (HHV-6) is a DNA virus. Nearly all children < 3 years of age have been infected with HHV-6. Children can be asymptomatic, have fatal disseminated disease (extremely rare), or anything in between. Most commonly, HHV-6 causes exanthem subitum (roseola or "sixth disease"). It presents as fever for 3–5 days, followed by the abrupt cessation of fever and the appearance of a macular-to-maculopapular rash (Image 5-33). Seizures are not uncommon during the febrile stage. Don't be fooled on an examination by an 8-month-old with fever for 3 days who is placed on amoxicillin and then has a "drug reaction." The answer is more than likely exanthem subitum!

CNS disease is usually mild, but HHV-6 likely accounts for a large percentage of febrile seizures occurring in children < 2 years of age. Severe CNS disease can occur in immunocompromised patients, especially bone marrow transplant patients.

HUMAN HERPESVIRUS 7 AND 8

HHV-7 and HHV-8 were "discovered" in the 1990s. HHV-7 is associated with roseola infantum (see above), and HHV-8 is associated with Kaposi sarcoma in AIDS and other immunocompromised patients.

RUBELLA (GERMAN MEASLES)

Rubella is "German measles" (ssRNA virus). In March 2005, the CDC declared that rubella had been eliminated from the U.S. There were 117 cases in 1989, 100 in 2001, and only 10 in 2004. Of the 67 rubella cases reported from 2005 through 2011, a total of 28 (42%) cases were known importations. We will review this because it continues to be endemic in many areas of the world.

Rubella is spread by person-to-person transmission of infected droplets. Patients are infectious a few days before the rash and a few days into the rash. It peaks in the late winter and spring. Congenitally acquired infection is chronic, but postnatal infection is not.

Clinically, rubella presents with adenopathy, rash, and low-grade fever.

The usual incubation period is 14–21 days. The tender adenopathy begins 1st and is generally postauricular (Image 5-34), occipital, and posterior cervical. Older children and adolescents complain of malaise, headache, sore throat, and mild coryza during a 1- to 5-day prodrome before the rash develops.

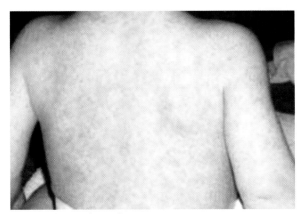

Image 5-33: Exanthem subitum

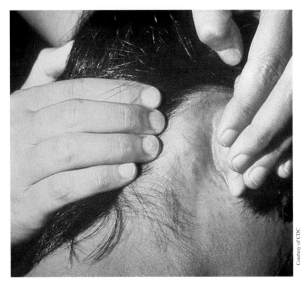

Image 5-34: Rubella infection with postauricular adenopathy

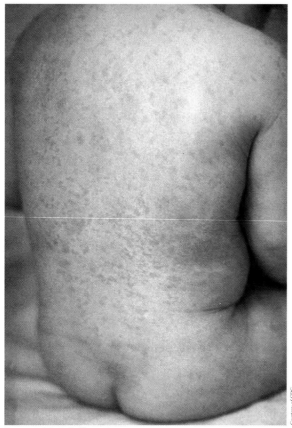

Image 5-35: Rubella rash

The rash changes appearance throughout its course. It may be a "quick blush" but typically persists for 2–3 days. Most commonly, it begins as macules on the face that spread quickly to the neck, trunk, arms, and finally, the legs (Image 5-35). Usually, the rash is gone from the face by the time it has reached the legs.

Rubella also has an enanthem called Forchheimer spots. These are pinpoint or slightly larger red spots on the soft palate and may occur during the late prodrome or at the beginning of the rash appearance. They are not specific for rubella, however, and can appear with other viral exanthems.

Fever is common but can be absent in some cases. Women tend to have polyarthralgia/arthritis, but this is rare in children. CNS involvement is less common than in measles.

Congenital rubella occurs when the mother is infected during pregnancy. The trimester the infection occurs has important prognostic predictors:

- 1st trimester: 90% fetal infection risk with almost all having defects—cardiac, cataracts, and glaucoma common; hearing loss and neurologic manifestations.
- 2nd trimester: 54% infection risk with defects during the initial 2nd trimester falling to 25% near the end of the 2nd trimester; some risk of hearing or neurologic manifestations.
- Last weeks of gestation: Infection risk is 60–100%, but infection is generally non-teratogenic.

The difficulty is that infants with congenital rubella may present with multiple anomalies, be stillborn, or have no abnormalities at all.

The most severe syndrome manifestations include:

- Thrombocytopenic purpura, "blueberry muffin" lesions, which are reddish-purple macular lesions and the most common manifestation of congenital rubella (Image 5-36). This is extramedullary hematopoiesis. (These blueberry muffin lesions also may appear in congenital CMV infection.)
- Radiolucencies in the metaphyseal long bones.
- Hepatosplenomegaly.
- Hepatitis.
- Hemolytic anemia.
- Bulging anterior fontanelle.
- CSF pleocytosis.
- Congenital heart disease: Most common is PDA with or without pulmonary artery stenosis; ASD and VSD.
- Sensorineural deafness (due to damage to the organ of Corti); this may be the only manifestation if infection occurs after the first 8 weeks of pregnancy.
- Cataracts with microphthalmia (Image 5-37).
- Congenital glaucoma.
- Retinopathy with patchy deep pigmentation.
- Intellectual disability.

A rare complication is progressive rubella panencephalitis, which is a severe, progressive neurologic deterioration that begins in the 2nd decade. It presents with mental

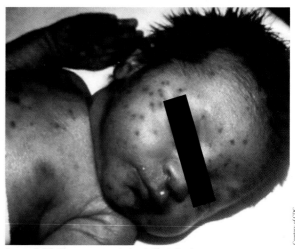

Image 5-36: Severe congenital rubella infection

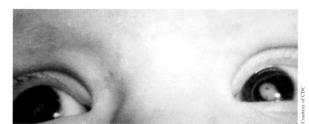

Image 5-37: Cataracts from congenital rubella

- Describe a typical 10-year-old with rubella.

- Describe the differences in outcome in infants with congenital rubella depending on the trimester their mothers acquired rubella.

- Describe a newborn with severe congenital rubella infection.

- What type of muffin do you think about when you see the rash of congenital rubella? What causes it?

- What are the "3 Cs" associated with measles?

- Characterize the presentation for rubeola infection. Differentiate rubeola from rubella infection.

- What are the oral spots called in rubella? In rubeola?

deterioration, myoclonus, ataxia, and seizures, with progression to death in several years.

Children with a history of congenital rubella have a much higher risk of IDDM! By age 10, the risk is nearly 4x greater; by adulthood it is 10–20x greater.

Increased risk of thyroiditis has also been described.

Mortality is highest in the first 6 months of life. In those infants with congenital rubella and neonatal thrombocytopenic purpura, the mortality rate is ~ 40%. Most children die from sepsis or congestive heart failure.

RUBEOLA (MEASLES)

Rubeola is "measles" (Image 5-38). Measles is one of the most highly communicable of all infectious diseases! It is spread via respiratory droplets, or less commonly by airborne spread. Unfortunately, measles still occurs rather commonly in mini-outbreaks with the most recent occurring in 2011—most occur because of an infected traveler coming to the U.S. and then exposing under-immunized or nonimmunized individuals. College outbreaks are common as well. Symptoms start ~ 10 days after the initial exposure. Symptoms at the onset: the "3 Cs"—cough, coryza, and conjunctivitis (with photophobia). The conjunctivitis causes edema of the lids, and the child has increased tearing. Vitamin A deficiency (prevalent in developing countries) results in more severe disease—including eye disease, with corneal ulcers and loss of vision.

Children also have malaise and fever. Koplik spots (whitish spots on an erythematous base) appear on the buccal mucosa 2–3 days before the onset of the skin rash and are considered pathognomonic. The Koplik spots are usually gone by 24 hours after the skin rash appears (Image 5-39).

The skin rash starts at the hairline and spreads downward. It lasts ~ 5 days and then resolves, also from the hairline downward. Lymphadenopathy and splenomegaly are common. Occasionally diarrhea, vomiting, and abdominal pain occur. Immunocompromised patients might not develop the characteristic rash.

Complications of the CNS are common; 10% of children develop a CSF pleocytosis, and 50% have EEG changes! Encephalomyelitis occurs in 0.1% (1/1,000) of cases and presents with seizures, altered mental status, and coma. Mortality approaches 10–25%—with motor, mental cognition, or behavioral problems developing in 20–50% of the survivors.

Subacute sclerosing panencephalitis (SSPE) is a rare degenerative CNS disease, classically characterized by behavior and intellectual decline, that occurs 7–10 years after an infection with wild-type measles. Think about SSPE in a 10-year-old child who was adopted at age 3 from a country in which measles vaccination is not routine.

Measles also can reactivate tuberculosis.

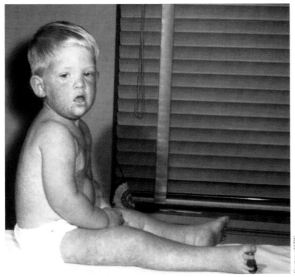

Image 5-38: Rubeola (measles)

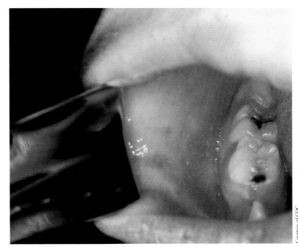

Image 5-39: Measles, Koplik spots

Gestational measles can induce premature delivery, stillbirth, or abortion but does not cause a congenital syndrome of malformations, as is seen with rubella.

Treatment with vitamin A can be helpful in reducing eye abnormalities and pneumonia, especially in individuals at risk for vitamin A deficiency.

Measles vaccine, if given within 72 hours of measles exposure, will provide protection in some cases and is the intervention preferred for measles outbreaks that occur in schools and day cares. During a measles outbreak, MMR vaccine can be given to children as young as 6–11 months old (instead of the usual 12 months). Doses given prior to the 1st birthday should not count toward the recommended 2-dose series of MMR.

Immunoglobulin (IG) can prevent or modify measles from developing in a susceptible at-risk child, but you must give it within 6 days of exposure. IG is recommended for susceptible household members or other close contacts of patients with measles, especially for those < 1 year of age, pregnant, immunocompromised, or those in whom measles vaccine is contraindicated.

No specific antiviral therapy is available. While not approved by the FDA for the treatment of measles, ribavirin has been given to severely affected and immunocompromised children with measles.

RETROVIRUS

Retroviruses—RNA viruses. HTLV-1 causes T-cell leukemia. HTLV-2 causes a rare T-cell variant of hairy cell leukemia. HIV-1 (previously called HTLV-3) causes AIDS. HIV-2, found in West Africa and parts of the U.S., is a virus that causes an illness indistinguishable from AIDS (more on HIV later in this section).

RESPIRATORY VIRUSES

Rhinoviruses

Rhinoviruses are a common cause of URI, usually during the autumn. They are RNA viruses that replicate best at cooler body temperatures (93°–95° F), such as in the nasal mucosa. The numerous serotypes are responsible for the "common cold." Controlled trials have yet to prove that vitamins, minerals (including zinc, except in 1 adult study), or herbal remedies (e.g., echinacea) are effective for reducing the duration of the typical cold.

Adenovirus

Adenovirus is a common cause of respiratory tract infection. It is a DNA virus with 51 serotypes recognized in humans. Most children are infected early with serotypes 1, 2, and 5; serotypes 3, 7, and 21 are less common but important causes of respiratory infection.

Respiratory manifestations: Infants present with coryza, conjunctivitis, otitis media, and pharyngitis, generally due to serotypes 1, 2, and 5. In infants with serotypes 3, 7, and 21, more severe infection is likely, with progressive, severe bronchiolitis, pneumonia, and long-term sequelae. Serotype 14 can cause severe disease in all age groups. Adenovirus can also cause a pertussis-like syndrome.

Pharyngoconjunctival fever: This syndrome is frequently due to adenovirus 3 and presents with fever, pharyngitis, conjunctivitis, rhinitis, and cervical adenitis. It occurs most commonly in the summer and is transmitted while swimming—frequently causing epidemics in summer camp settings.

Epidemic keratoconjunctivitis: This occurs with conjunctivitis, corneal involvement, and preauricular lymph node enlargement. It too is seen more commonly in the summer and is associated with swimming.

Diarrhea: Adenoviruses 40 and 41 are common causes of infant diarrhea. ELISA or electron microscopy can detect the virus in stool. Some adenoviruses have been implicated in the diagnosis of intussusception.

Acute hemorrhagic cystitis: Adenovirus types 11 and 21 are associated with acute hemorrhagic cystitis. The hematuria can last for several days or up to 2 weeks. Initially, it can be confused with post-streptococcal glomerulonephritis.

Meningoencephalitis: This can occur on occasion with adenovirus infection, particularly in the immunocompromised and in patients with AIDS.

Treatment for all of the above is symptomatic. Antivirals are not helpful routinely. Cidofovir is used in immunocompromised patients or immunocompetent patients with severe, pulmonary or disseminated disease.

Because of the common association between adenovirus and "close quarters" in adults, military recruits are given the live, oral vaccine; however, the vaccine is effective only for serotypes 4 and 7.

Health care workers with adenoviral conjunctivitis should avoid direct patient care x 14 days from the onset of illness.

Coronavirus and SARS-CoV

Coronavirus is an enveloped RNA virus. It is responsible for 3–5% of "common colds." It is more likely to be the etiology of the cold during the winter months.

Severe acute respiratory syndrome (SARS) has now emerged as a concern and is due to SARS-associated coronavirus (SARS-CoV). In 2003, there were > 8,000 cases worldwide and > 800 deaths. Be concerned about someone on the exam who presents with recent travel to Asia (or an epidemic area like Toronto) and who has early "flu-like" symptoms—but quickly progresses to severe respiratory distress. However, an elderly person is more likely to be severely affected.

In 2012, a novel coronavirus was reported and termed Middle East respiratory syndrome coronavirus (MERS-CoV). This has been limited to the Middle East and a

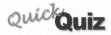
Quiz

- True or false? Rubeola can cause a "congenital rubeola syndrome."
- What vitamin deficiency worsens rubeola? In what way?
- What can be given within 6 days of exposure to prevent or modify rubeola in a susceptible immunocompromised child?
- Describe the eye diseases associated with adenovirus infection.
- Which virus can cause acute hemorrhagic cystitis?
- Is there a vaccine available for adenovirus, and to whom do you give it?
- What causes SARS?
- Describe the symptoms of influenza.
- What 2 bacteria are likely to cause pneumonia in a patient with a preceding influenza infection?

few in travelers returning from the Middle East. As of Sept 20, 2013, there were a total of 130 laboratory confirmed cases.

RSV (Respiratory Syncytial Virus)

Respiratory syncytial virus (RSV) infections occur yearly, during the autumn and winter. RSV infections are more severe in the infant, occasionally resulting in pneumonia. Only 1% of affected infants are hospitalized. Diagnose RSV by doing an ELISA test or PCR on nasal secretions. RSV is discussed in more detail in Respiratory Disorders, Book 4.

Parainfluenza Virus

Parainfluenza virus is discussed in Respiratory Disorders, Book 4.

Human Metapneumovirus

Human metapneumovirus was discovered in 2001 and is one of the leading causes of bronchiolitis in infants and also causes pneumonia, asthma exacerbations, croup, and URIs with concomitant acute otitis media in children. Rapid diagnostic immunofluorescent assays, or PCR, can be used to confirm infection.

Influenza Virus

Influenza is still a major cause of death in the U.S. and can be quite severe in adult populations, particularly those > 55 years old or in young children and children with chronic medical conditions such as underlying lung or CNS disease. Vaccination decreases mortality!

There are 3 types of influenza viruses: **influenza A**, **B**, and **C**. Influenza A and B cause the yearly epidemics of respiratory illnesses. Type A is widely distributed in animals, especially horses, hogs/pigs, and chickens/birds. Influenza C causes very mild, if any, symptoms.

Virus is spread by hand-to-nose droplets of respiratory secretions or small-droplet aerosol.

"Antigenic shift" refers to major changes in the viral hemagglutinin (HA) or neuraminidase (NA) on the outer surface—this occurred with the 2009 H1N1 influenza outbreak! These "shifts" occur only in influenza A and result in a new virus, to which humans or other animals have no natural immunity. These shifts resulted in the "pandemics" of the last century and are among the concerns with the "bird flu" scare of this century. "Antigenic drift" refers to minor changes in the virus and occurs with both influenza A and B.

Influenza causes fever, chills, headache, and myalgias after 1–3 days of incubation. After 24 hours, rhinitis and lower respiratory symptoms develop. Tracheobronchitis is the most common manifestation of lower respiratory tract infection.

Most children recover without complication. However, 3 types of pneumonia are possible:

1) Viral bronchopneumonia: usually occurs between days 3 and 5 of illness.

2) Secondary bacterial pneumonia: typically occurs 5–7 days into the illness. Common bacteria include *S. pneumoniae* and *S. aureus*.

3) Diffuse viral hemorrhagic alveolitis.

Other manifestations can include nausea, vomiting, diarrhea, otitis media, and acute myositis characterized by calf tenderness and refusal to walk. Severe disease, including myocarditis and CNS disease/encephalitis, can also occur.

Diagnose by isolating the virus or by an EIA-based antigen detection assay or PCR.

Treatment of Influenza

Treatment of influenza typically involves 2 types of antivirals:

1) Oseltamivir (Tamiflu®—oral) and zanamivir (Relenza®—powder for inhalation) were the 1st of the neuraminidase inhibitors, a newer class of treatment for influenza A and B (FDA-approved in 1999). Zanamivir is contraindicated in children with chronic lung disease or asthma.

2) Amantadine and rimantadine are older drugs that block the uncoating of influenza A viruses only (so neither has activity against influenza B).

In 2012–2013, circulating influenza A strains (H3N2 and 2009 H1N1) were both resistant to amantadine and rimantadine. Fortunately, both were susceptible to the neuraminidase inhibitors—making oseltamivir and zanamivir the drugs of choice for all types of influenza in the 2012–2013 season.

Treating influenza patients within 48 hours of the onset of symptoms yields the best chance at decreasing the length and severity of illness. However, you should treat all hospitalized or high-risk children—no matter how long they have had symptoms.

The "bird flu" (H5N1—now H7N1) continues to lurk as a potential cause of the next pandemic.

Infection control for alternate H1N1 or potential bird flu:

• Single room with negative pressure.
• Use gloves, gowns, eyewear, and fit-tested N95 respirator when in the room. (Note: Regular droplet precautions/respiratory mask are OK for seasonal influenza, but guidelines for pandemic influenza specifically call for the respirator because of current lack of knowledge of how this particular virus is transmitted.)
• Patients are infectious 1 day before symptoms develop until a minimum of 7 days after they first have symptoms.
• Control measures: influenza vaccine.

All people ≥ 6 months of age should receive the influenza vaccine annually. It is especially important for people at greater risk of severe complications of influenza such as those with:

• Asthma or other chronic pulmonary disease (cystic fibrosis)
• Hemodynamically significant cardiac disease
• Immunosuppressive therapy
• HIV infection
• Sickle cell anemia and other hemoglobinopathies
• Patients on long-term aspirin therapy (rheumatoid arthritis, Kawasaki disease due to risk of Reye syndrome)
• Chronic renal disease
• Chronic metabolic disease (diabetes mellitus)
• Any condition that can compromise respiratory function (spinal cord disorders, neuromuscular disorders, seizures)
• Pregnancy

Influenza Vaccination

There are 2 types of influenza vaccines available: the trivalent inactivated influenza vaccine (TIV) and the live-attenuated influenza vaccine (LAIV). Both vaccines contain 3 virus strains (one each: A [H3N2], A [H1N1], and B). Quadrivalent influenza vaccines (QIV) with 2 A strains and 2 B strains were added to the choices for the 2013–2014 influenza season.

Why the QIV? Each year the public health authorities have chosen between the 2 main strains of influenza B that cause illness. And they guess right about half the time. The QIV contains both B strains and should overcome this issue. Both TIV and QIV (along with the LAIV) were available for the 2013-2014 season.

Thimerisol is used only in the multidose vials of influenza vaccine. Single-dose units do not contain thimerisol.

TIV is licensed for use in people ≥ 6 months of age. LAIV is licensed for healthy people age 2–49 years of age and is given via intranasal spray. LAIV should not be given to:

• Pregnant women
• People with asthma or children < 5 years of age with recurrent wheezing
• Anyone < 2 years or ≥ 50 years
• Immunosuppressed patients

Remember, TIV and QIV contain only killed, noninfectious viruses and therefore cannot cause active infection.

For children < 9 years of age who have never been vaccinated, give 2 doses of vaccine, 1 month apart, to achieve adequate antibody levels. Thereafter, they receive 1 annual vaccine. If they miss the 2nd dose the 1st year, they get 2 doses with the next flu season and then go to once annually. Vaccine efficacy is not established for children < 6 months of age.

Both TIV and LAIV vaccines are produced in eggs, but data have shown that TIV is well tolerated in recipients who have allergy to egg. The data is not sufficient to use LAIV in people allergic to egg. Mild reactions to eggs are defined as hives alone, while severe reactions include anaphylaxis. If your patient has severe allergy to egg, consult an allergist; otherwise, it's OK to give TIV vaccine without referring to an allergist.

ENTEROVIRUS

Overview

The enterovirus group includes:

1) Coxsackievirus A
2) Coxsackievirus B
3) Echovirus
4) Poliovirus

Poliovirus is considered below as a separate entity.

It turns out that there is a large amount of overlap in the biology of the viruses and they have also been classified by serotype EV-1, EV-2, … EV-71, etc., based on antibody tests. Newer isolates go simply by their serotype (e.g., EV-71).

Enteroviruses occur year-round but have increased infection rates between May and October in warmer climates. Transmission is by the fecal-oral and person-to-person routes.

Infection is most common in children < 4 years of age and in lower socioeconomic groups.

- What are the contraindications for giving live-attenuated influenza vaccine?
- Can the flu shot (TIV or QIV) cause influenza?
- An 8-year-old is to receive her 1st influenza vaccine this year. How should this be administered?
- Is it safe to give flu vaccine to someone with egg allergy? When do you refer to an allergist?
- What causes hand-foot-and-mouth disease?
- What virus can cause an acute hemorrhagic conjunctivitis?

Clinically, enteroviruses can present in multiple ways. In particular, be most familiar with EV-71, which can cause hand-foot-and-mouth disease, herpangina, severe neurologic disease, brainstem encephalomyelitis, paralytic disease, pulmonary edema/hemorrhage, and cardiopulmonary collapse.

Diagnosis of all enterovirus disease has been aided by PCR technology. Sensitivity and specificity approach 95% for many of the enteroviruses. Finding the virus in CSF or blood suggests an active infection.

No FDA-approved therapy is available at this time, but many experts recommend IVIG. Pleconaril was being evaluated for use in neonates in the past, but is not commercially available.

Congenital and Neonatal Infections

Group B coxsackievirus can cause serious and fatal disseminated disease in newborns. It can be transplacentally transmitted as well. It can cause hepatitis, myocarditis, meningoencephalitis, and adrenal cortex failure. Illness onset is abrupt. Hepatic necrosis is common.

Febrile Illness

Nonspecific febrile illnesses are common with enteroviruses, especially in the 1st few months of life. GI symptoms are rare. If enteroviral infection is widespread in a community, a large number of infants < 4 weeks of age will likely present with "fever without focus."

Rashes

Hand-foot-and-mouth disease presents with fever and vesicles of the buccal mucosa, tongue, and, less commonly, the palate, lips, and gums. A red maculopapular rash may appear on the hands and feet and eventually may become vesicular. In infants, the diaper area is commonly involved with such a rash. Coxsackieviruses A16, A5, A10, and A6 (EV-71) are often involved.

Meningitis / Encephalitis

Fever, headache, and malaise are common in older children with viral (aseptic) meningitis/encephalitis. In all ages, fever to 104° F is common and may be gradual or abrupt in onset. Fever lasts 3–5 days. Focal findings are rare. The CSF is nonspecific, may have a predominance of PMNs early on, and can be confused with bacterial meningitis. Total protein is normal, and glucose is usually normal, although it may be diminished.

No long-term sequelae have been demonstrated in infants with enteroviral aseptic meningitis, but some types of enterovirus meningoencephalitis (especially EV-71) have now been associated with long-term neurologic sequelae.

Of concern are patients with agammaglobulinemia who cannot readily eradicate enterovirus infections from the CNS. These children have recurrent episodes and severe manifestations such as seizures, hemiparesis, hearing loss, and mental deterioration.

Paralytic Disease

Polioviruses are commonly associated with paralytic disease, but group B coxsackievirus and enteroviruses 70 and 71 have also been associated with paralytic disease and encephalitis. Classically, if paralysis is to occur, it is asymmetric with lower extremity and involves larger muscle groups. Atrophy of involved muscles becomes apparent, typically within 2 months. Variable degrees of recovery occur in most by 6–18 months.

Acute Hemorrhagic Conjunctivitis

Enterovirus Type 70 and coxsackievirus A24 cause subconjunctival hemorrhage. Swelling, redness, and tearing with pain are common. It resolves within 1 week without specific therapy.

Herpangina

Herpangina is most commonly associated with coxsackievirus group A infection. It presents with tiny vesicles or punched-out ulcers on the anterior pillars of the tonsils, uvula, and pharynx (in contrast to herpes simplex virus, which more commonly occurs in the front part of the mouth and extends out onto the lips). The lesions are 1–2 mm in diameter. They sometimes can enlarge and rupture with a shallow, yellow-gray ulcer. Herpangina presents with a high, abrupt fever, sore throat, and dysphagia.

Bornholm Disease (Pleurodynia, Epidemic Myalgia)

This acute illness presents with paroxysmal thoracic pain and is due to group B coxsackievirus. The pain is pleuritic in nature and is aggravated by deep breathing, coughing, or movement. It can last up to 14 days but usually is over in 4 days.

Myocarditis / Pericarditis

Myocarditis or pericarditis may occur in older children with group B1–B5 coxsackievirus or echovirus. It can be mild to fatal.

POLIO

Polioviruses are part of the *Enterovirus* genus and belong to the family *Picornaviridae*, a small RNA virus. 90% are self-limited, and a majority of those infected have asymptomatic or mild, nonspecific illness. CNS onset is characterized by an aseptic meningitis and/or an asymmetric, flaccid paralysis without reflexes. Paralysis begins proximally and progresses to involve distal muscle groups—known as a descending paralysis. Brain stem, spinal, mixed spinal bulbar, or bulbar involvement can result in respiratory muscle paralysis. It has essentially been eliminated in the western hemisphere and developed countries worldwide. The last case of wild-type polio in the U.S. occurred in 1979 among an outbreak of unimmunized people. Since 1986, the only reported cases of polio were associated with oral polio vaccine. In the U.S., institution of an all-IPV vaccine schedule in 2000 essentially ended vaccine-associated cases there.

Poliovirus is easily recovered from stool, throat swabs, or occasionally CSF for up to 3–6 weeks.

No specific therapy is available. If bulbar paralysis is present, respiratory support is required.

Late symptoms of acute paralytic poliomyelitis or post-polio syndrome become apparent anywhere between 1.5 and 40 years. It presents with acute muscle pain, weakness, or new paralysis.

ROTAVIRUS

Rotavirus is the most common viral cause of gastroenteritis worldwide. Rotaviruses are double-stranded RNA viruses with at least 7 antigenic groups A through G. Group A viruses are the major cause of rotavirus diarrhea around the world.

Before rotavirus vaccine was introduced in the U.S., rotavirus was the most common health-care–associated diarrhea in young children and an important cause of diarrhea in children attending day care.

Infection is characterized by the abrupt onset of fever and vomiting, followed in 24–48 hours by watery diarrhea. Infection occurs between November and April, and it is transmitted by fecal-oral spread, with an incubation period of 1–3 days. In moderate-to-severe cases, dehydration, electrolyte abnormalities, and acidosis can occur. Infection in immunocompromised children (congenital immunodeficiency, transplant recipients) can be severe and persistent.

2 rotavirus vaccines are currently available in the U.S. In 2006, a live, oral human-bovine pentavalent rotavirus vaccine (RotaTeq®) was licensed to be given to infants at 2, 4, and 6 months old. In 2008, a live, oral human-attenuated monovalent vaccine (Rotarix®) was licensed to be given in 2 doses, at 2 and 4 months of age. Some studies outside the U.S. have detected a low level of increased risk of intussusception following rotavirus vaccine shortly after the 1st dose. The level of risk is substantially lower than with the previous rotavirus vaccine, RotaShield®, which was taken off the market in 1999 due to its association with intussusception. The benefits of rotavirus vaccine, which include prevention of hospitalization for severe rotavirus disease in the U.S. and of death in other parts of the world, far outweigh the rare potential risks.

CALICIVIRUS (NOROVIRUS AND SAPOVIRUS)

Caliciviruses (CVs) are single-stranded RNA viruses. There are 5 genera in this family of viruses but only 2 (norovirus and sapovirus) cause disease in humans, who are the primary reservoirs.

Noroviruses—of which Norwalk is the only species—are the most common cause of outbreaks of gastroenteritis in the U.S. and tend to occur in closed populations such as nursing homes, child care centers, and cruise ships. Noroviruses are increasingly being recognized as a major cause of community-acquired and hospital-acquired viral gastroenteritis.

Transmission is by person-to-person spread via the fecal-oral route or through contaminated food or water. Common source outbreaks have occurred after eating ice, shellfish, salads, and bakery products contaminated by food handlers. Incubation period is 12–48 hours. It is the cause of about 50% of all infectious non-bacterial gastroenteritis outbreaks in the U.S.

Symptoms include abrupt onset of vomiting, watery diarrhea, abdominal cramps, and nausea that last 24–60 hours. Sometimes myalgia, malaise, and headache occur. Infection occurs year-round but is more common in colder months. Sapovirus infections cause acute diarrhea in children and are increasingly being recognized as a cause of outbreaks.

Diagnosis of norovirus can be made by quantitative, real-time PCR (RT-qPCR) assays for viral detection in stool and is available at all state and public health laboratories. Treatment is supportive, and contact precautions are recommended until 48 hours after symptoms resolve.

Note: Hepatitis viruses are covered in Gastroenterology & Nutrition, Book 4.

RABIES

Rabies is especially common in bats, but is also found in dogs, cats, wolves, ferrets, raccoons, skunks, and foxes. It is rare in squirrels, farm animals, and opossums. On the exam (and in real life), if a child wakes up and a bat is in the room, even without evidence of a bite, the child should be prophylaxed for presumed rabies (except in

Quick**Quiz**

- List the clinical case definition for a child with polio.

- How do you diagnose rabies?

- What time after exposure should rabies vaccine be given and in how many doses?

- Know the scenarios for rabies prophylaxis for bites due to: a) a wild animal; b) an immunized, non-rabid-appearing dog that had been provoked by a child, and the dog is available for observation; c) a case where a "street" dog bit a child in an unprovoked attack and then ran away and cannot be located. (The child says, "He acted funny.")

- Describe the clinical syndrome seen with mumps.

rabies-free Hawaii). Rabies is generally not found in rodents, rabbits, birds, and reptiles; and human rabies cases are rare. However, when it does happen, the fatality rate is ~ 100%. Rabies in humans presents as an acute encephalomyelitis, with symptoms of restlessness, excitation, and severe spasms of the larynx and pharynx—especially when the affected person sees food or water (hydrophobia).

Rabies is an RNA virus and a rhabdovirus. Bite wounds introduce the virus through infected saliva into abraded skin. Virus spreads via peripheral nerves to the brain, then via the sensory and autonomic nervous system to the eyes, salivary glands, skin, and viscera. The brain areas most commonly affected include the thalamus, hypothalamus, substantia nigra, pons, and medulla. Diagnose by finding pathognomonic Negri bodies (acidophilic inclusion bodies) in the cytoplasm of neurons.

80% of cases either have no known exposure to a rabid animal or their exposure to a suspect animal did not involve a bite or mucous membrane exposure.

Incubation period is shorter for bites to the head than to the extremities. The initial phase is apprehension, anxiety, and insomnia, with fever also common. In the initial "excitation" phase, or "furious" rabies, the patient has apprehension and terror. This results in hydrophobia and often seizures. The excitation phase is followed by the paralytic phase, with coma and death following soon thereafter.

Infection in animals can be diagnosed by demonstration of virus-specific fluorescent antigen in brain tissue. Any suspected rabid animal should be euthanized in a way that preserves the brain for appropriate laboratory testing. In humans, diagnosis is made by fluorescent microscopy of skin biopsy specimens from the nape of the neck, and is facilitated with assistance from the CDC. PCR is now available for blood, CSF, and saliva. Other testing can

include looking for rabies antibody in CSF or serum or for viral antigens and nucleic acids in infected tissues.

For exposures from pet dogs, cats, and ferrets without evidence of rabies, these animals should be observed by a veterinarian for 10 days; if they behave normally, immunization of the victim is unnecessary.

Consider wild animals listed in the first paragraph (skunks, bats, foxes, etc.) rabid, and initiate vaccine and RIG unless the animal is captured, euthanized, and tests negative for rabies. Livestock, rodent, and lagomorph (rabbits, hares) bites rarely require treatment. Preexposure prophylaxis is indicated for cave explorers and veterinarians but not for hunters or mail carriers.

After exposure to possible rabies via a bite or mucous membrane contamination—or contamination of a scratch or abrasion with saliva from an animal that is suspected of having rabies—initiate rabies immune globulin (RIG) and vaccine as soon as possible. Infiltrate the wound with as much RIG as you can and then administer the rest of the 20 IU/kg dose via the IM route (separate site from the vaccine!).

Rabies vaccine should be given on the 1st day of postexposure prophylaxis (day 0), and repeated doses are given on days 3, 7, and 14 after the 1st dose.

MUMPS

Mumps (RNA) occurs most commonly in winter and early spring (Image 5-40). Recent outbreaks in Iowa and the Midwest (2006) and New York (2009) increase the chance it will appear on exams. Although often asymptomatic, it can present with uni- or bilateral parotitis, aseptic meningitis, and/or encephalitis.

Mumps is most communicable 1–2 days before parotid swelling and continues until 5 days after parotid swelling begins. Patients are not infectious after 9 days of parotid swelling.

Because of the use of vaccine in younger children, the incidence of mumps has decreased markedly; the typical age of onset has increased to 10–14 years.

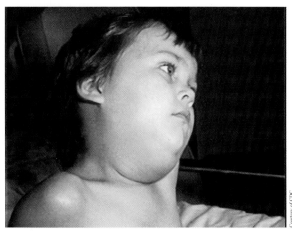

Image 5-40: Mumps

Vaccine "failure" occurs at a rate of 2–5%; use of the 2nd dose increases immunity considerably. Infection provides lifelong immunity.

The swelling usually involves both parotids but sometimes is unilateral, and may also involve the submandibular glands, with or without the parotids. The entire parotid swells, including the uncinate lobe, which extends to the back of the ear lobe. Anorexia and abdominal pain are common, indicating either pancreas or, in females, ovarian involvement.

In postpubertal males with mumps, 15–35% get an epididymoorchitis that is typically unilateral. Children as young as 3 years of age have been affected. Postinfection sterility is a rare occurrence. Mastitis occurs in 31% of adolescent females. Oophoritis occurs in ~ 7%.

CNS infection is very common. Headache, lethargy, and meningismus occur with CSF abnormalities. Most CSF counts are < 500 with mostly lymphocytes. The meningitis is usually self-limited without sequelae.

Deafness is a complication of mumps and, in 1 study, occurred in 4% of those affected. Most were unilateral and almost all recovered in a few weeks.

Mumps does not cause congenital malformation syndromes.

The mumps skin test is not effective for checking immunity.

To differentiate mumps from bacterial parotitis (most commonly due to *Staphylococcus aureus*), check a Gram stain of the parotid secretions. There are many WBCs and organisms in bacterial parotitis—but there are none in mumps.

Note: Another cause of enlarged parotid glands is frequent vomiting. Always consider bulimia in an adolescent with parotid gland enlargement.

PARVOVIRUS

Parvovirus is a small DNA virus. One parvovirus, B19, causes various disorders, ranging from erythema infectiosum to arthralgias/arthritis to aplastic anemia.

Erythema infectiosum (Fifth disease) is a mildly contagious, self-limited infection that causes a rash and arthritis. The facial component of the rash causes a "slapped cheek" appearance (Image 5-41). This rash is much more common in children; the arthritis is more common in adults. The rash on the extremities is "lattice-like" and becomes more prominent in the sun or with a warm bath (Image 5-42). Most children are not that ill but complain more of pruritus with the rash. The rash likely occurs in only ~ 50% of children with the infection.

The arthritis more commonly affects adults, especially women. Usually, it is a symmetric disease of the hands, knees, or wrists.

In patients with chronic hemolytic anemias or AIDS, it can cause aplastic anemia. In these persons, the bone marrow shows characteristic "giant pronormoblasts."

Pregnancy with parvovirus B19 is a special case to consider. Most mothers who are infected during pregnancy have infants without abnormalities. However, there is a risk of intrauterine hydrops and possibly fetal loss. To date, there is no reliable method to predict which fetuses will have poor outcomes.

Diagnosis is clinical. Test IgM antibodies to diagnose an acute infection. PCR is helpful in immunocompromised patients in both acute (sometimes they don't make antibody responses) and chronic/reactivation disease.

Treatment is symptomatic. For those who are immunocompromised, IVIG may be helpful.

In Fifth disease, once the rash appears, the child is no longer infectious and may return to day care. However, children with aplastic anemia due to parvovirus B19 are highly infectious. If hospital admission is required, place the child in negative-pressure room isolation with droplet precautions. Masks should be worn.

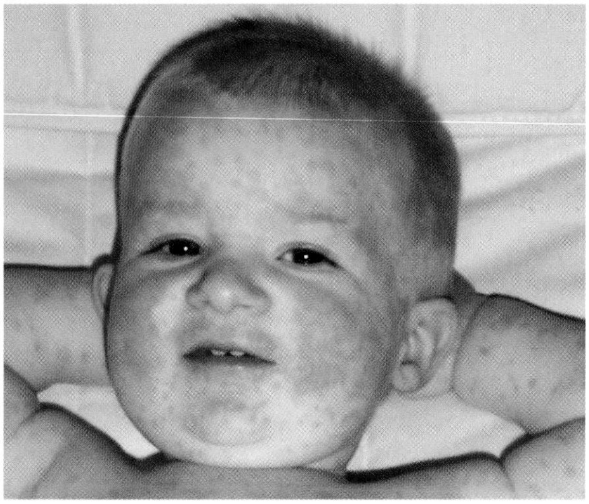

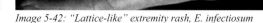

Image 5-41: "Slapped cheek" with E. infectiosum

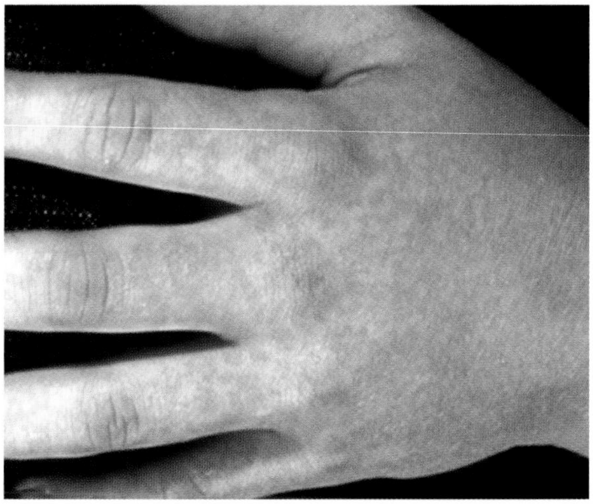

Image 5-42: "Lattice-like" extremity rash, E. infectiosum

Quick Quiz

- What complications of mumps can occur in adolescent males? In adolescent females?
- What sensory loss may occur with mumps?
- What infection does parvovirus B19 cause?
- Describe the rash of Fifth disease.
- What is the risk for a pregnant woman infected with parvovirus B19?
- When is a child with Fifth disease no longer infectious?
- In what geographic area of the U.S. has hantavirus most commonly been reported?

ARBOVIRUSES

Arboviruses are mainly transmitted by mosquitoes or ticks. Various arboviruses occur in the U.S., typically in the late spring and summer. Until recently, most cases occurred along the Gulf Coast in Louisiana and Florida. Now, with West Nile virus, the arboviruses are seen from coast to coast.

From 2002–2012, West Nile virus (WNV) was the most common arbovirus identified in the U.S. Colorado, Idaho, and California had the most cases during 2005–2009, and Texas had the most cases in 2012. Most cases are asymptomatic, but others may present as a febrile illness with flu-like symptoms. More severe neurologic disease presents as fever, headache, altered mental status, paresis, nerve palsies, or coma. The risk of CNS disease with WNV increases with age and is highest among adults > 60 years of age. A 4-fold rise in virus-specific serum antibodies or finding a positive IgM-CSF antibody titer is helpful for diagnosis. Treatment is supportive.

Other viruses besides West Nile, including LaCrosse, St. Louis, Eastern Equine (EEE), Western Equine (WEE), Venezuelan Equine, Powassan, and Colorado tick fever occur on occasion in the U.S. Almost all have similar symptoms with fever, headache, chills, and various severity of encephalitis or aseptic meningitis. However, many cases are asymptomatic; only ~ 1/100 infected may present with symptoms. Diagnose by finding virus-specific IgM antibody in the CSF or serum.

HANTAVIRUS

A hantavirus-associated disease, called hantavirus pulmonary syndrome (HPS), starts with severe myalgias, fever, headache, and cough and quickly progresses to ARDS (adult respiratory distress syndrome) and death. More than 50% die. The primary reservoir in the western and southwestern U.S. is the deer mouse. On the East Coast and in the Southeast, the cotton rat is the main reservoir.

The infection occurs when the excreta or saliva are inhaled. Transfer of the virus can also occur through broken skin. No person-to-person transfer is known to have occurred.

Symptoms:

- Early: Constitutional symptoms in all; ~ 50% have N/V, diarrhea, and abdominal pain.
- Late: 4–10 days later, coughing and shortness of breath as ARDS develops.

No rash is seen with hantavirus infection.

Suspect hantavirus on the examination in an adolescent who lives in the Desert Southwest presenting with severe hemorrhagic pneumonia, thrombocytopenia, and increased hematocrit.

DENGUE FEVER

Dengue fever, dengue hemorrhagic fever, and dengue shock syndrome are caused by 4 serotypes of the *Flavivirus*. It is a tropical disease that uses humans and the day-biting *Aedes* mosquitos (*Anopheles* carry malaria) in its life cycle. Dengue fever has had a resurgence in the past 10 years in Puerto Rico, Central and South America, and Mexico, with a few cases also in Florida and south Texas. No vaccine is available yet (but one is under development).

Symptoms are rapid onset of high fever, severe myalgias and arthralgias ("break-bone fever"), retro-orbital pain, and severe headaches with N/V, followed by a macular red rash, which covers most of the body. A 2nd rash that looks more like measles occurs later, along with a recurrence of fever ("saddleback fever"—up, down, up).

Suspect this in a traveler with these symptoms who has returned from tropical latitudes (including the Caribbean and Mexico).

Treatment is supportive.

SLOW VIRUSES

Overview

There are 2 classes of slow viruses:

1) Normal viruses such as papilloma (warts) and papovavirus (PML)
2) Defective viruses such as the defective measles virus, which causes subacute sclerosing panencephalitis

Papillomavirus

Human papillomavirus (HPV) causes warts. Genital warts are associated with an increased risk of cervical cancer. There are many variants. HPV types 1, 2, and 5 are common causes of plantar warts. HPV types 6, 11, 16, 18, and 31 are genital. HPV types 6 and 11 are the cause of the exophytic, grossly visible genital warts, but HPV types 16, 18, and 31 are associated with cervical cancer. (Remember: Higher numbers occur higher up on the body and are more cancer-prone!) The HPV types 16, 18, and 31 that cause cervical cancer are usually subclinical! So do not jump to "cervical cancer" when you see visible genital warts! All warts tend to recur. (More detail on the infection and vaccine can be found in Adolescent Health and Gynecology, Book 1.)

Polyomaviruses

BK virus (BKV) and JC virus (JCV) infections in immunocompetent children are usually asymptomatic.

BK virus has a tropism for the genitourinary epithelium and can cause asymptomatic hematuria or cystitis in healthy children. In immunocompromised patients (especially renal transplant and stem cell transplant recipients), it is more likely to cause hemorrhagic cystitis or interstitial nephritis.

JCV is the cause of progressive multi-focal leukoencephalopathy (PML) that occurs in severely immunocompromised patients (AIDS, patients on chemotherapy, or those receiving monoclonal antibody therapy for immune suppression).

SSPE

Subacute sclerosing panencephalitis (SSPE) is a rare form of encephalopathy thought to be due to a measles virus that changed but was not eradicated by the immune reaction to the primary infection. The average incubation period is 10.8 years. Occurrence is 1/300,000 cases of measles. Patients typically had measles at age < 2 years and present with dementia, myoclonus, and new-onset seizures ~ age 10. Most die within several months of onset.

Prion Disease

Prions are proteinaceous infectious particles that lack nucleic acid and constitute a previously unknown means of transmitting disease. Previously, these diseases were thought to be caused by a "slow virus."

Prion diseases include Kuru, Creutzfeldt-Jakob disease (CJD), new variant CJD (vCJD), Gerstmann- Sträussler-Scheinker (GSS) syndrome, and fatal familial insomnia. In animals: scrapie and mad cow disease (= bovine spongiform encephalopathy, = vCJD when transmitted to humans).

Human prion diseases can be sporadic (CJD), infectious (vCJD, Kuru, rare cases of CJD), or genetic (GSS syndrome, familial CJD, fatal familial insomnia).

Kuru was found in New Guinea, associated with cannibalism, and thought to be transmitted by ingestion of raw human brain tissue. It has an incubation period of up to 30 years. (Last case was 2008.)

Creutzfeldt-Jakob disease (CJD) is the most common prion disease. It is almost always sporadic, but ~ 5% are infectious (e.g., corneal transplants, cadaveric human

growth hormone) and very few are genetic. Its incubation period is ~ 18 months. Patients with CJD get myoclonus and severe dementia. Neurologic symptoms predominate. They generally die within 5 months! There is no effective therapy for either Kuru or CJD. The EEG is diagnostic.

A new variant of CJD (vCJD), transmitted from beef with bovine spongiform encephalopathy (mad cow disease), has been contracted by ~ 60 people in several European countries. No endemic U.S. human cases of vCJD have been reported. (Cases have occurred in the U.S. in immigrants, and cows imported from Canada have been infected.) These patients have early psychiatric symptoms and late-appearing neurologic symptoms (~ 6 months out with ataxia). Once neurologic symptoms appear, progression to death is rapid. Test: Look for a young adult from England with progressive psychiatric symptoms and ataxia.

HIV AND AIDS

OVERVIEW

Changes in the treatment and management of HIV infection are evolving rapidly. The following covers the basics—not the cutting edge.

VIRUS STRUCTURE

The HIV virus is composed of a dense, single-strand RNA core surrounded by a lipoprotein envelope. The RNA contains reverse transcriptase, which allows the RNA to be transcribed into DNA, which is then assimilated into the host's genome. The cell then becomes an HIV-producing machine.

The structure in the lipoprotein envelope that allows the HIV to attach to the CD4 cell is named gp120. As opposed to influenza, the envelope on HIV is very unstable. That's why it is much more difficult to make a vaccine against it.

HIV gp120 envelope glycoprotein binds to the CD4 receptors and co-receptors on the helper T cells, macrophages, and monocytes. The virus fuses with the cell, and the viral core material enters the cell. Immune dysfunction results from the ongoing destruction of CD4 lymphocytes, which are more fully described under Summary of Important Advances on page 5-62. The CD4 cells are the major regulator cells in the body. They can suppress the B lymphocytes and regulate the CD8/suppressor cells.

With the decrease in CD4+ counts, B cells become deregulated and are no longer suppressed, causing a polyclonal increase in total serum immunoglobulins—even though overall antibody function is decreased! For this reason, infectious diseases in AIDS patients include not only the cell-mediated infections (PCP, viruses, *Mycobacteria*, fungal), but also those seen with humoral deficiency (pneumococcus, meningococcus, *H. influenzae*, and *Giardia*).

Quick **Quiz**

- What HPV types are associated with an increased risk of cervical cancer?

- Which virus is associated with SSPE? Describe SSPE.

- Describe a typical patient with new variant CJD.

- A newborn of a mom with HIV needs to receive ZDV for how long to prevent infection?

- What are the early manifestations of undiagnosed HIV infection in infants?

The glial cells of the CNS may be directly infected by HIV, causing atrophy and dementia. The GI epithelium may also be directly infected, causing a wasting enteropathy with diarrhea. Marrow progenitor cell infection can cause anemia and thrombocytopenia.

PREVALENCE AND TRANSMISSION

Humans are the only known reservoir for HIV-1 (more common in the U.S.) and HIV-2. Modes of HIV transmission include:

- Sexual contact (vaginal, anal, or orogenital)
- Percutaneous blood exposure (contaminated needles/ sharp instruments)
- Mucous membrane exposure to contaminated blood or other body fluids
- Mother-to-child (vertical) transmission during pregnancy, around the time of labor and delivery or postnatally through breastfeeding, and
- Transfusion with contaminated blood products

Due to effective screening, blood, blood products, and clotting factor, virtually have been eliminated as a cause of HIV transmission in the U.S.

On the exams, think about HIV in IV drug users, gay and bisexual men, those with tuberculosis, and those seeking treatment for other STDs. Prevalence is < 1% in heterosexuals in the U.S., but in central Africa, heterosexual transmission is the primary route! HIV has also been transmitted in the course of treatment by an infected dentist.

Pediatric AIDS cases account for fewer than 1% of all reported cases of AIDS in the U.S. The number of HIV-infected children in the U.S. is currently estimated to be about 3,000. 90% of HIV-infected children and infants get their infection vertically; the CDC estimates that in the U.S., 215–370 infants are born annually with HIV. Most transmissions occur during labor and delivery. The risk of infection for an infant born to an HIV-positive mother who did not receive interventions to prevent transmission ranges from 12–40% (average 21–25% in the U.S.).

Prevention programs of mother-to-child transmission (including antiretroviral therapy [ART] during pregnancy, zidovudine [ZDV; previously AZT] during delivery, 6 weeks of ZDV therapy in newborns, and avoiding breastfeeding) can reduce the rate of transmission to < 1%. The dose of ZDV in newborns has recently been changed from 4 x day to 2 x day for 6 weeks and is adjusted according to gestational age. For infants born to HIV-positive women who have received no antepartum ART therapy, in addition to ZDV, nevirapine is given (3 doses in the 1st week of life). The risk of vertical transmission increases with each hour in the duration of ruptured membranes. C-section performed before onset of labor and before rupture of membranes has been shown to reduce mother-to-child transmission of HIV. Current U.S. guidelines recommend C-section before onset of labor and rupture of membranes for HIV-infected women with a viral load > 1,000 copies/mL (irrespective of use of ART during pregnancy) and for women with unknown viral loads at the time of delivery.

Note: In developed countries where infant formula is readily available, breastfeeding of the perinatally HIV-exposed infant is not recommended. For HIV-infected mothers in developing countries, 2010 WHO guidelines recommend breastfeeding as alternative sources of nutrition (i.e., only do if no infant formula is available).

Early manifestations of HIV infection in infants include:

- Chronic candidiasis
- Parotitis
- Persistent generalized lymphadenopathy
- Hepatosplenomegaly
- Fevers
- Failure to thrive
- Recurrent diarrhea
- Hepatitis
- CNS disease
- LIP (lymphoid interstitial pneumonia)
- Recurrent invasive bacterial infections
- Recurrent upper respiratory infections including otitis media or sinusitis
- Other opportunistic infections

About 20% of untreated HIV-infected infants present in the first 3–6 months of life with an AIDS-defining illness, such as *Pneumocystis jiroveci* (formerly *P. carinii*) pneumonia (PCP), serious bacterial infection, or serious fungal infection. CD4 count can even be normal at the time of PCP presentation in an infant.

Immune function is categorized in children based on age-specific CD4 counts:

Evidence of severe immune suppression:

- < 12 months of age: < 750 CD4 cells/μL (< 15%)
- 1–5 years of age: < 500 CD4 cells/μL (< 15%)
- 6 years of age: < 200 CD4 cells/μL (< 15%)

Although the rate of perinatally acquired HIV is decreasing, the rate of acquiring HIV during adolescence and young adulthood continues to increase. In adolescence, HIV disproportionately affects youth of minority race/ethnicity. Transmission of HIV among adolescents is usually through sexual exposure or illicit IV drug use. Young males acquire HIV through same-sex sexual contact, while infection among young women is generally heterosexual.

DIAGNOSIS

Older than 18 Months

Diagnosis of HIV infection in children ≥ 18 months is by the presence of antibody to the virus by means of the EIA test, which is 99% sensitive and 90% specific. Positive responders are confirmed by the Western blot. Antibody to HIV is typically detectable 2–3 months after inoculation, although there can be a window of up to 6 months! The earliest detectable sign of infection is a positive HIV DNA by PCR.

Note that the enzyme-linked immunosorbent assay (ELISA) and the enzyme immune assay (EIA) are 2 very similar tests that were developed independently and simultaneously and measure the same thing. The terms are often used interchangeably, but, with HIV testing, EIA is the more correct term.

Younger than 18 Months

For children < 18 months of age born to a mother who is HIV-infected, the presence of infection is more difficult to diagnose because of the presence of transplacentally acquired antibody to HIV. In these infants, diagnosis of HIV infection requires demonstrating viral nucleic acids (HIV DNA by PCR). Most centers perform 3 PCR tests over a period of 4 months, trying to determine if the child is truly infected. If all 3 tests are negative and the last one has occurred ≥ 4 months of age, the child is considered uninfected.

Note: Culturing the virus from the infant is rarely done today and no longer recommended.

There are several tests that measure HIV RNA by amplifying the RNA by oligonucleotide hybridization or enzymatic methods. These tests accurately determine viral load but are not generally used for diagnosis (especially in HIV-exposed infants receiving ART prophylaxis). They are discussed further below.

TREATMENT OF HIV INFECTION

Overview

According to the latest initial and recertification exam content specifications, knowledge of dosing HIV medications is no longer specifically listed. The specifications previously stated, "Plan antiretroviral therapy for a patient with HIV infection." So, unless you are actively treating patients with HIV, do not try to digest the whole HIV section being presented in this Core Curriculum. Rather, focus on only yellow highlighted areas. Pay particular attention to the drug side effects that are highlighted; those are likely fair game for the exams. Be sure to know how to screen for HIV, how it is spread (breast milk too!), and which vaccines to use in HIV-infected children!

Treatment of HIV infection: Adherence is a key determinant in the degree and duration of viral suppression! AIDS: Note that it is extremely important to actively involve the patient and/or the parent in the treatment decision-making process. Guide decisions regarding initiation or changes in antiretroviral therapy by monitoring plasma HIV RNA (viral load) and CD4 T-cell counts, in addition to the patient's clinical condition. First, we will review the major classes of anti-HIV drugs, then the treatment protocols.

Classes of HIV/AIDS antiretroviral drugs:

- Reverse transcriptase (RT) inhibitors interfere with reverse transcription. There are 2 types of RT inhibitors:
  - Nucleoside/Nucleotide RT inhibitors (NRTIs): "faulty" DNA building blocks that are incorporated into HIV DNA and act as terminators of proviral DNA synthesis
  - Non-nucleoside RT inhibitors (NNRTIs): bind to a hydrophobic pocket close to the RT active site, interfering with its ability to convert HIV RNA into HIV DNA
- Protease inhibitors (PIs): interfere with the protease enzyme that HIV uses
- Fusion/Entry inhibitors (FIs): interfere with the ability to fuse with the cellular membrane, thereby blocking entry into the host cell
- Integrase inhibitors (II): block integrase, the enzyme HIV uses to integrate genetic material of the virus into the host cell

OK—let's go into more detail!

Nucleoside Reverse Transcriptase Inhibitors (NRTIs)

NRTIs include ZDV, ddI, ddC, d4T, 3TC, FTC, and abacavir. These drugs inhibit the replication of HIV by interfering with the reverse transcriptase enzyme. These are all analogs of normally occurring nucleic acid bases.

Zidovudine (ZDV) = Azidothymidine (previously called AZT) = Retrovir®. This is the oldest of the antiretroviral drugs, but it still remains very useful. It is well tolerated at currently used doses but causes bone marrow suppression (e.g., anemia, granulocytopenia) and myopathy. A macrocytosis (elevated MCV) always occurs but has no clinical consequence. ZDV does not usually cause problems for the kidneys or lungs and does not cause pancreatitis.

As with all antiretroviral drugs, combination therapy is the standard of care to prevent resistance. Use ZDV

- How do you diagnose HIV in a child ≥ 18 months of age? < 18 months of age?
- What are the main side effects of zidovudine?
- What are the main side effects of didanosine?
- Which anti-HIV medication is teratogenic?

in combination with 3TC, ddI, or ddC, as well as protease inhibitors. Some studies have suggested antagonism between ZDV and d4T. The effectiveness of ZDV decreases over time due to development of resistance.

Give ZDV to pregnant HIV+ patients because ZDV decreases transmission of the HIV virus to the fetus by 25–35%. It is also given to newborns of HIV-infected mothers for 6 weeks after birth.

ddI (didanosine, Videx®) is useful in combination regimens—with ZDV and protease inhibitors. Viral resistance develops more slowly than with other reverse transcriptase inhibitors. A newer, enteric-coated tablet has replaced the regular preparation, eliminating the GI side effects of diarrhea and cramping, thus affording much better patient tolerance. The most severe side effects of ddI are pancreatitis, which can be life-threatening, and peripheral neuropathy. There is no bone marrow toxicity.

ddC (zalcitabine, Hivid®) can be used as part of a combination regimen (the combination with ZDV is best studied). It is very easy to take, and the only significant side effects are stomatitis, neuropathy, and—less commonly—pancreatitis. Since the availability of newer drugs, ddC is rarely used.

d4T (stavudine, Zerit®) has emerged as a very useful drug because it is very well tolerated over long periods of time, with little toxicity. Well-studied combinations include d4T/3TC, with or without protease inhibitors. Recent data have implicated d4T in lipodystrophy and mitochondrial toxicity syndromes. Also, do not use d4T in combination with ddI in pregnant women—fatal lactic acidosis! Side effects are pancreatitis and peripheral neuropathy.

3TC (lamivudine, Epivir®) is a very effective drug in combination therapy. Combinations with ZDV or d4T are often used. The drug is well tolerated. Side effects are rare.

FTC (emtricitabine, Emtriva®) is similar to 3TC but stays in the blood stream for a longer period of time.

Abacavir (Ziagen®) is very effective in combination therapy. Side effects: The most serious reaction is hypersensitivity and is associated with HLA-B57, which usually occurs within 4 weeks. The reaction consists of a generalized rash and/or a flu-like illness, with fever, chills, N/V, myalgias, cough, and shortness of breath. Take any patient off abacavir who develops this reaction, and

never prescribe it again for that patient; reactions will continue to worsen and could even be fatal.

Combos: Currently there are several combo drugs, including: Combivir® = ZDV + 3TC, Trizivir® = ZDV + 3TC + abacavir, and Truvada® = FTC + tenofovir.

Nucleotide Reverse Transcriptase Inhibitor

Tenofovir (Viread®) is a nucleotide RTI very similar to the above nucleoside analogs, except that tenofovir is chemically pre-activated, and therefore requires less biochemical processing than the nucleoside RTIs. Tenofovir has once-daily dosing and a good side-effect profile—mainly asthenia/headache/N/V/D/flatulence. It must be taken with an NRTI and at least 1 PI or NNRTI.

Non-Nucleoside Reverse Transcriptase Inhibitors (NNRTIs)

Nevirapine (Viramune®) is the 1st of this class of drugs. It is not useful as a single agent but is useful as part of a regimen with nucleoside reverse transcriptase inhibitors and/or protease inhibitors. Rash, which can be severe, is the primary toxicity.

Efavirenz (Sustiva®) is more potent than nevirapine. CNS toxicity is commonly seen. Efavirenz is teratogenic, so do not use—in any way—concurrent with pregnancy. Other side effects include rash and "weird dreams."

Protease Inhibitors (PIs)

The HIV protease inhibitors (saqui-, rito-, indi-, nelfi-, ampre-, fosampre-, lopi-, ataza-, darunavir) inhibit the HIV protease enzyme that is involved with processing the completed virus. They are frequently used in combination with each other (e.g., saquinavir + ritonavir) or with the just discussed NRTIs +/– NNRTI to prevent the emergence of resistance. Fat redistribution and lipid abnormalities (increased triglycerides and cholesterol), as well as new-onset diabetes, have been recognized as side effects with the use of PIs. However, in treating the lipid abnormalities, do not use simvastatin or lovastatin with any of the PIs! Avoid other interactions: rifampin, astemizole, cisapride, and St. John's Wort.

Saquinavir (Fortovase®) is highly effective, has minimum side effects, and is useful in combination protease inhibitor regimens.

Ritonavir (Norvir®) is a very potent drug, but patient tolerability is poor due to side effects. The main side effects are N/V, flushing, distorted taste, and paresthesias. There are many drug interactions because of interference with the p450 enzyme system. Low-dose ritonavir inhibits metabolism of—and, therefore, significantly boosts levels of—indinavir, saquinavir, amprenavir, and the NNRTI efavirenz. Ritonavir is now usually used in low doses to boost the levels of other PIs and efavirenz.

Indinavir (Crixivan®) has side effects that include an asymptomatic hyperbilirubinemia and a high incidence of nephrolithiasis. The drug should be taken on an empty stomach with adequate hydration—although boosting with ritonavir eliminates the food requirement.

Nelfinavir (Viracept®) is a PI with good potency and it is well tolerated. The most common side effect is diarrhea. If resistance to nelfinavir develops, treatment with indinavir or amprenavir may be effective.

Amprenavir (Agenerase®) is a PI with a resistance profile that is unique among protease inhibitors. 1% get serious skin reactions, including Stevens-Johnson syndrome. GI side effects are common.

Fosamprenavir (Lexiva®) is just the prodrug of amprenavir. It is not approved for children.

Lopinavir/ritonavir (Kaletra®) is a co-formulation of lopinavir and low-dose ritonavir. Lopinavir is available only in this co-formulation. It is very potent and well tolerated.

Atazanavir (Reyataz®) is a newer protease inhibitor on the market. It can be used in children > 6 years of age.

Darunavir (Prezista®) used in combination with ritonavir in children ≥ 3 years who are treatment-experienced and have resistance to the 1st line agents.

Integrase Inhibitors

Integrase strand transfer inhibitors (INSTIs; Ralte-, Dolutegravir) prevent the HIV integrase enzyme from inserting HIV's genetic information into the host cell's own DNA, halting this critical step in the life cycle of HIV. INSTIs must be used in combination with other antiretroviral drugs.

Raltegravir (Isentress®) is an oral agent. Raltegravir is now indicated for all lines of therapy, including naïve patients. Its twice-daily dosing is well tolerated with few drug interactions and no effect on lipids. It was approved in 2011 for pediatric use (ages 2–18 years).

Dolutegravir (Tivicay®) was approved in 2013 for treatment-naïve and treatment-experienced adolescents > 12 years and > 40 kg.

Key Words

Key words/phrases to remember for side effects:

- ZDV: bone marrow suppression, myopathy
- The "Ds" (ddI, ddC, and d4T): pancreatitis and peripheral neuropathy
- Abacavir (Ziagen®): potentially fatal hypersensitivity reaction
- Efavirenz (Sustiva®): teratogenic
- Indinavir (Crixivan®): kidney stones

Note: For the medications above, at least know the yellow highlighted areas! These are what they are most likely to ask on the exams!

State of Treatment

Summary of Important Advances

HIV RNA assays are available for accurately determining viral load. Prior to the availability of these assays, the HIV virus was thought to enter a prolonged latency period until the onset of symptoms. It turns out that there is continuous, high-level replication from the onset of infection to death.

Viral load is a good, long-term predictor of outcome. After primary infection, the rate of virus replication and turnover equilibrates to a certain set point for each individual—resulting in a pretty much constant plasma viremia of 100 to 10^6 HIV RNA copies/mL. This set point may endure for months or years, and it determines the rate of disease progression. Plasma viremia < 5,000 HIV RNA copies/mL is associated with near-normal CD4+ counts and minimal, if any, clinical progression of disease; whereas viral loads > 30,000 HIV RNA copies/mL indicate a greatly increased risk of disease progression. Barring treatment, a single HIV RNA count can establish a prognosis—similar to staging of certain malignancies.

The HIV protease inhibitors decrease viral load—sometimes tremendously—for prolonged periods when used in combination therapy.

Combination therapy is always used for HIV treatment—even for needlestick with an infected needle.

1st line therapy is:

- PI(s) and
- NRTI(s) and/or
- NNRTI(s).

Basis of Treatment Protocols

- Determining CD4 and viral load are key indicators for when to start therapy.
- Combination therapy is the standard of care; use monotherapy only in special circumstances.

Indications for Viral Load Testing

- Syndrome consistent with acute HIV
- Initial evaluation of newly diagnosed HIV
- Every 3–4 months for patients on and not on therapy
- 2–8 weeks after initiation of therapy
- Clinical event or substantial decline in CD4 Count

Indications for Using Drug-Resistance Assays

Resistance testing are a useful tool in selecting active drugs when changing antiretroviral regimens in cases of virologic failure or suboptimal reduction of viral load. Currently, 2 types of resistance testing are available—genotypic and phenotypic. These are expensive tests but are becoming more popular in determining optimal regimens. The genotypic test will detect specific genes in the individual patient's HIV virus known to confer

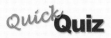

Quiz

- What renal abnormality is seen in patients taking indinavir?
- True or false? ZDV/d4T combined or ZDV therapy alone is acceptable for a child with symptomatic HIV.
- Which patients should be started on ART?

resistance toward a specific antiretroviral drug. The phenotypic test determines if the gene is operating and if resistance is being expressed. Currently, one is not recommended over the other, and some centers prefer to test for both. Drug-resistant assays are sort of like a crude antibiogram for the HIV virus—if resistance is determined, then you can switch from ineffective drugs. Drug-resistance assay use is very expensive, and it is not well standardized in pediatrics (or adults for that matter).

When to Start Antiretroviral Therapy (ART)

Definitely initiate ART in:

- Symptomatic (AIDS or significant symptoms): Start therapy no matter what the CD4 or viral load.
- All children < 12 months of age who are known to be HIV-infected (regardless of being asymptomatic or having a high CD4).
- HIV-infected children ≥ 1 year of age with minimal or no symptoms with the following CD4 values:
  - 1 to < 3 years of age: with CD4 cell count < 1,000 cells/mm^3 or CD4 percentage < 25%
  - 3 to < 5 years of age: with CD4 cell count < 750 cells/mm^3 or CD4 percentage < 25%
  - ≥ 5 years of age: with CD4 cell count ≤ 500 cells/mm^3

Consider ART in:
- HIV-infected children ≥ 1 year of age with minimal or no symptoms with the following CD4 values:
  - 1 to < 3 years of age: with CD4 cell count ≥ 1,000 cells/mm^3 or CD4 percentage ≥ 25%
  - 3 to < 5 years of age: with CD4 cell count ≥ 750 cells/mm^3 or CD4 percentage ≥ 25%
  - ≥ 5 years of age: with CD4 cell count > 500 cells/mm^3
  - Plasma HIV RNA levels > 100,000 copies/mL provide stronger evidence for initiation of treatment

[Also know:] A fingerstick from an infected needle requires immediate treatment with 3-drug antiretroviral therapy.

Make all decisions regarding the start of therapy on the basis of prognosis, as determined by CD4, viral load, and the willingness of the patient/parent to adhere to therapy.

Which Combination of Drugs to Use

"Strongly recommended" by the CDC:

- Use 1 of the following:
  - Efavirenz
  - Nevirapine
  - Lopinavir plus ritonavir

- With 1 of the following sets:
  - Abacavir plus lamivudine or emtricitabine
  - ddI plus emtricitabine
  - Tenofovir plus lamivudine or emtricitabine—only for those Tanner stage 4 or postpubertal
  - ZDV plus lamivudine or emtricitabine

Note: You are sweating this, right? How do you remember all of these? You don't!

Throw out any consideration that has:

- ZDV/d4T combined
- ddC anywhere in the choice
- Single-drug therapy

When to Change HIV Therapy

This is again controversial. However, 2 things to know:

1) Do not change drugs based on 1 viral load; always repeat a high viral load to be sure it is not lab error.
2) Intolerance to the medication should prompt evaluation for change of therapy.

Possible reasons to change therapy are based on treatment failure (various definitions and not standardized):

- Therapy has not suppressed viral RNA to undetectable levels (< 50 copies) within 4–6 months of starting therapy.
- An increase of ≥ 3-fold from the nadir of plasma HIV RNA.
- Previously undetectable levels now surpassing 5,000–10,000 copies.

The other problem: What drug to change to? Generally, just know you should probably change therapy based on resistance testing.

Postexposure Prophylaxis (PEP)

First, determine the exposure risk: Was the source material blood or bloody fluid? If so, determine if it was a percutaneous exposure (yes—PEP recommended), mucous membrane, or skin with compromised integrity (PEP probably recommended). It is easier (and frequently asked on tests) to remember to whom not to give PEP.

Do not give for intact-skin exposures and urine-source exposures. The latest CDC guidelines for health care workers date from September 2005. Generally: Use potent, combination therapy. Start treatment ASAP—within hours of exposure. The standard recommended regimen is ZDV, 3TC, +/– lopinavir/ritonavir for

4 weeks. Most would also offer PEP in cases of sexual assault or sharing needles by/with known HIV-infected individuals.

Know that new guidelines are pending and many experts now follow a different approach. In the U.S., you can get help choosing a regimen by calling the National Clinicians/ PEP hotline (PEPLine) at 888-448-4911.

Pregnancy

Both the AAP and CDC recommend that all pregnant women are tested for HIV, and many states mandate this. Most experts recommend that pregnant HIV+ patients receive antiretroviral therapy (ART) based on their immune status (CD4 count, HIV viral load). At this time, zidovudine (ZDV) is the only drug approved/recommended to prevent "vertical transmission." There are 3 interventions used in the U.S. for prevention of mother-to-child HIV transmission:

1) Antiretroviral prophylaxis (ARV)

2) Avoidance of breastfeeding

3) As indicated, C/S prior to ROM (if maternal viral load > 1,000 copies/mL)

Optimally, give the mother ZDV as one of her ART drugs as well as IV ZDV during labor and delivery. If the mother is well controlled on her current ART therapy, then she does not have to add ZDV but should receive IV ZDV during labor and delivery. The newborn should be treated with oral ZDV x 6 weeks.

Suppressing the viral load in the mother lowers the risk of transmission to the newborn. The bottom line for most pregnant women: Treat them with ART, include ZDV if possible, and do not use efavirenz (teratogenic) or a d4T/ddI combination (increased risk of lactic acidosis in pregnant women).

Immunization Recommendations

[Know!] All recommended childhood immunizations should be given to HIV-exposed infants. Children with confirmed HIV infection should be immunized as soon as is age appropriate with inactivated vaccines (e.g., DTap, Hib, PCV13, IPV, hepatitis B, hepatitis A). Live-virus vaccines (MMR, varicella) can be given to asymptomatic HIV-infected children and adolescents with appropriate CD4 T-cell percentages (i.e., greater than 15% in children 1–5 years of age). Rotavirus (a live-viral vaccine) can be given to HIV-exposed and HIV-infected infants regardless of their CD4 T-cell counts. Because of the increased risk of pneumococcal infection, HIV-infected children should all receive a dose of 23-valent polysaccharide vaccine (PPSV23) after 24 months of age (given at least 8 weeks after the last PCV13). Trivalent inactivated influenza vaccine (TIV) should be given annually to HIV-infected children (> 6 months of age) and their family contacts.

HIV-ASSOCIATED INFECTIONS AND CONDITIONS

Introduction

[Know these:] Signs of HIV disease include persistent or recurrent seborrheic dermatitis, tinea infections, psoriasis, molluscum contagiosum, folliculitis, and mucocutaneous infections (hairy leukoplakia, herpes, oral or vaginal candidiasis, and warts). EBV causes hairy leukoplakia. "Wasting" is a common presentation in children. Also, the older child with chronic ear infections should always be suspected on exam questions to have an immune deficiency, particularly HIV.

Kaposi lesions are a neoplasia of blood vessels and are due to human herpesvirus 8. Lesions are heaped up and well localized, often with some surrounding bruising. Kaposi lesions may occur in adolescents but are very rare.

Don't forget the acute retroviral syndrome: This is a flu- or mononucleosis-like syndrome that occurs 2–4 weeks after initial infection and lasts 1–2 weeks. Suspect the sexually active or IV drug-using adolescent! Patients present with fever, lymphadenopathy, pharyngitis, rash (usually erythematous maculopapular with lesions on face, trunk, or extremities, including palms and soles), mucocutaneous ulcerations involving the mouth, esophagus, or genitals—and myalgias/arthralgias. Consider it in a young person who has multiple sexual partners or an IV drug user who presents with signs/symptoms of mono or scarlet fever.

Immune Reconstitution Inflammatory Syndrome (IRIS)

The term "immune reconstitution inflammatory syndrome" (IRIS) describes a collection of inflammatory disorders associated with paradoxical worsening of preexisting infectious processes following the initiation of antiretroviral therapy (ART) in HIV-infected individuals. Common infections include: *Mycobacterium tuberculosis*, *Mycobacterium avium* complex, cytomegalovirus, *Pneumocystis*, herpes simplex, and hepatitis B. These preexisting infections may have been previously diagnosed and treated, or they may be subclinical and later unmasked by the child's regained capacity to mount an inflammatory response. If immune function improves rapidly following the commencement of ART, systemic or local inflammatory reactions may occur at the site or sites of the preexisting infection. This inflammatory reaction is usually self-limited, especially if the preexisting infection is effectively treated. However, long-term sequelae and fatal outcomes may rarely occur, particularly when neurologic structures are involved. Most patients with IRIS develop symptoms within 1 week to a few months after the initiation of ART. The decision to treat IRIS with corticosteroids is generally made with the assistance of a specialist.

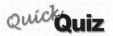

Quick Quiz

- A nurse is emptying a Foley catheter bag and some urine from an HIV patient spills on her ungloved hand. Should she take postexposure prophylaxis?

- What medication should an HIV-infected pregnant woman receive during labor and delivery?

- Describe the acute retroviral syndrome in an adolescent.

- What is the most common opportunistic infection in pediatric AIDS patients?

- What is the treatment for PCP?

- When should you start PCP prophylaxis?

PCP and HIV

Pneumocystis jiroveci infection produces subclinical infection in most "normal" children by the age of 4 years. Typically, only the immunocompromised are seriously affected by this organism.

Infantile form: The infection occurs in premature and debilitated infants ages 2–6 months. Onset is insidious with cough and mild tachypnea. Fever is absent. Over a period of 1–4 weeks, the infection progresses to a diffuse, bilateral, interstitial plasma cell pneumonitis with cyanosis and retractions. Without effective therapy, 50% of these infants die.

Immunocompromised older children and adolescents: *Pneumocystis jiroveci* pneumonia (PCP) is the most common opportunistic infection in patients with AIDS. It is the presenting illness in 50% of untreated patients. It is probably the most common lung infection overall in these patients, but, because prophylaxis is so effective, PCP incidence in these patients is decreasing to less than that of *S. pneumoniae* in some places.

Presentation of PCP: insidious onset of fever, shortness of breath, dry cough. ABG: pH > 7.40. A-a gradient is wide. Hypoxia is common. PCO_2 is low (from respiratory alkalosis). LDH is elevated (> 400), and liver enzymes are normal. The CXR usually shows a diffuse "batwing" infiltrate, although it may also be lobar or unilateral. Occasionally, the CXR is normal. Again, PCP generally has an insidious onset; if an AIDS patient presents with an acute onset of pulmonary symptoms, first get sputum for Gram stain and C+S, and start empirical treatment for community-acquired pneumonia. Patients who are most susceptible for PCP have fallen below their age-appropriate CD4 count threshold, so give all of these patients PCP prophylaxis!

[Know.] The threshold for starting PCP prophylaxis:

- All infants 1–12 months of age who are HIV-infected or are HIV-indeterminate
- HIV-infected children ages 1–5 years with a CD4 count < 500/mm³ (< 15%)
- HIV-infected children ≥ 6 years with CD4 count < 200/mm³ (< 15%)

The best method of diagnosis is by methenamine silver stain or PCR of samples taken by bronchoscopy or BAL, although induced sputum is effective in up to 50% in some hospitals.

Treat mild PCP with oral TMP/SMX—or atovaquone if the patient is unable to tolerate TMP/SMX.

Treat more severe PCP (PO_2 < 70 or A-a gradient > 35) with PO or IV TMP/SMX or IV pentamidine and high-dose corticosteroids (start on the 1st day). Inhaled pentamidine is not recommended for treatment of PCP. If there is no response after 1 week, or if severe side effects develop, switch. Alternative treatments are dapsone + trimethoprim, clindamycin + primaquine, or atovaquone alone for mild-to-moderate cases. PCP patients must receive 21 days of effective therapy. Remember: Include steroids for any patient with a PaO_2 < 70!

Side effects: Both TMP/SMX and pentamidine can cause neutropenia/leukopenia. TMP/SMX side effects include skin rash, nausea/vomiting, and, occasionally, fever. Pentamidine causes fever, nausea, vomiting, and diarrhea. Pentamidine also causes azotemia and renal failure. Recurrent courses of pentamidine destroy the islet cells of the pancreas, causing hypoglycemia that may not be reversible. (If a patient treated with pentamidine is seizing, check fingerstick glucometer!) Hyperglycemia may also occur with pentamidine. Patients on aerosolized pentamidine are at risk for apical pneumothorax. For some patients with AIDS, the reactions to either TMP/SMX or to pentamidine are intolerable, and the medication must be changed.

Indications for PCP prophylaxis:

- All perinatally HIV-exposed infants from 4–6 weeks of age until proven not to be infected
- All HIV-infected asymptomatic infants until 1 year of age
- HIV-infected (1–5 years of age) if CD4 count is < 500 cells/uL or CD4 is < 15%
- HIV-infected (6–12 years of age) if CD4 count is < 200 cell/uL or CD4 is < 15%
- History of prior PCP infection; give lifelong prophylaxis

Choice of prophylaxis: TMP/SMX is preferred (150 mg of TMP/m²/day with 750 mg SMX/m²/day PO divided bid, 3 x a week on consecutive days (e.g., MTW). Alternate regimens include once daily dosing or alternate day dosing.

Alternative regimens if TMP/SMX is not tolerated:

- Dapsone—2 mg/kg (not to exceed 100 mg) orally once daily. Screen for G6PD deficiency first!
- Aerosolized pentamidine (children > 5 years)—300 mg administered via Respirgard® II nebulizer monthly
- IV pentamidine—4 mg/kg every 2–4 weeks

Why TMP/SMX is the drug of choice for PCP prophylaxis:

- TMP/SMX is more effective than the alternatives.
- TMP/SMX is effective against extrapulmonary *Pneumocystis jiroveci*, whereas aerosolized pentamidine is not.
- TMP/SMX also prophylaxes against toxoplasmosis; the alternatives do not.

Mycobacterium and HIV

Tuberculosis is also common in AIDS patients, sometimes without infiltrates and hardly ever with cavitation. Patients usually respond very well to treatment. Do a TB skin test on all persons who are seropositive for HIV. Treat a positive PPD (> 5 mm) without sign of disease with INH for 9 months. Treatment of active TB in a patient with AIDS is the same as for regular patients. However, treat the TB (and MAC below) for a period of time before you start ART to help decrease the risk of IRIS!

M. avium complex (MAC, *M. avium-intracellulare*) is a common infection in patients with AIDS. It is typically disseminated, causing a wasting syndrome with fever, weight loss, and night sweats. There is no cure. Clarithromycin or azithromycin in combination with ethambutol, and sometimes other agents, including rifabutin, quinolones, clofazimine, or amikacin can be beneficial in terms of decreasing fever or improving bone marrow function.

Pulmonary: Other

Lymphocytic interstitial pneumonitis (LIP) is more common in perinatally acquired than in transfusion-acquired HIV. Before medications to prevent perinatal transmission of HIV infection became widely available in the United States, children with perinatally acquired HIV infection typically presented in the 2nd to 3rd year of life with an incidence of > 15%. The onset of HIV-related LIP generally is insidious. Cough and tachypnea are often noted. However, auscultation of the chest reveals few abnormalities. Digital clubbing may be observed in advanced cases. Extrapulmonary manifestations include generalized lymphadenopathy, hepatosplenomegaly, and salivary gland enlargement. Hypergammaglobulinemia is usually present. The clinical course is variable. Spontaneous clinical remission sometimes is observed. Exacerbation of clinical signs and symptoms may occur in association with intercurrent viral respiratory illnesses. In severe cases, progressive hypoxia and respiratory failure occur. Treat with steroids.

Streptococcus pneumoniae infection rates are much higher in HIV-infected individuals.

Cryptococcus involves the lung and can be disseminated, but it also commonly goes to the CNS. Cryptococcal meningitis is strongly associated with AIDS, Hodgkin disease, ALL, diabetes, and post-organ transplant. Treat with amphotericin B +/– flucytosine, then oral fluconazole. Fluconazole is a good choice for all but critical disease. Flucytosine (5-FC; 5-fluorocytosine) is sometimes not used along with amphotericin B in patients with AIDS because of the problem with bone marrow suppression.

Histoplasma can either affect the lung or disseminate in AIDS patients. (Only non-AIDS patients have the calcified lung lesions.) It can affect many organ systems, including the bone marrow. Think of this when an HIV-positive patient presents with interstitial pneumonia, palate ulcers, splenomegaly, and bone marrow suppression—especially if they live in an endemic area (Mississippi, Ohio, and St. Lawrence River valleys in U.S.). Treat with itraconazole or amphotericin B.

Coccidioides: Again, involves the lungs, but it also can disseminate. It is associated with arthralgias, arthritis, hilar adenopathy, erythema multiforme, and erythema nodosum (similar to sarcoidosis). Treatment suppresses but typically does not cure this disease; so chronic, suppressive treatment is needed (weekly fluconazole [1st choice] or amphotericin B).

[Know:] Both *Aspergillus* (especially associated with marijuana use) and *Mucor* can cause a necrotizing, cavitating pneumonia in AIDS patients.

Pseudomonas infections are seen more in granulocytopenic patients (leukemia, chemotherapy, and post-transplant) than in AIDS patients.

GI and HIV

Organisms to consider in AIDS patients with GI infections: *Candida*, especially with esophagitis. Not all *Candida* esophagitis is associated with thrush. If the patient does not respond to treatment for *Candida*, consider CMV esophagitis. Chronic diarrhea in AIDS patients is usually caused by *Cryptosporidium*, *Salmonella*, *Shigella*, *Cyclospora*, and *Isospora belli*. Other causes of diarrhea in HIV-infected patients include CMV, atypical mycobacteria (i.e., *Mycobacterium avium-intracellulare* [MAC], histoplasmosis). *Cryptosporidium* shows up as small, round, red organisms ("round bodies") against a green background on acid-fast staining of the specimen. *Cyclospora* and *Isospora belli* are also acid-fast (*I. belli* is large and oval); both are treated with TMP/SMX.

Neuro and HIV

Subacute, diffuse encephalitis (caused directly by HIV) is a common neurologic problem seen in AIDS. CNS disease is much more common in children and occurs quite early.

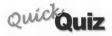
Quiz

- Which opportunistic infection causes meningitis in HIV patients?
- In a neonate < 60 days old, name the bacteria most commonly associated with bacteremia. With UTI? With diarrhea?

In as many as 25% of infants with HIV, CNS disease manifests as static encephalopathy, presenting as developmental delay in the 1st year of life. In ~ 1/3, progressive encephalopathy occurs, with loss of milestones and moderate-to-severe cognition defects. It appears that ART (antiretroviral therapy) prevents or slows progressive encephalopathy.

Toxoplasma gondii is the most common cause of "AIDS-associated enhancing focal-space-occupying lesions" (but the differential diagnosis also includes CNS lymphomas). CT scan shows CNS abscesses due to *Toxo* as ring-enhancing lesions. They are usually multiple but may be single. If these are seen in any AIDS patient, start empiric treatment for CNS toxoplasmosis with 1 of the following: long-term pyrimethamine + a sulfonamide, clindamycin, or trimetrexate. *Toxoplasma gondii* is rare in children.

Again: For suspected cryptococcal meningitis, get a cryptococcal antigen test (or India ink) of both the CSF and the blood! (The blood antigen is much more sensitive in patients with HIV.) Especially consider *Cryptococcus* in the patient with meningitis who has AIDS, Hodgkin disease, ALL, diabetes, or those who are post-organ transplant. Treat cryptococcal meningitis initially with amphotericin B, then oral fluconazole.

Syphilis, even if previously treated, may reactivate in AIDS patients and cause neurosyphilis!

Any eye problems are probably due to CMV retinitis.

Stopping Prophylaxis Guidelines (Adolescents and Older Only)

Stopping primary prophylaxis (no history of these infections):

- PCP: If CD4 > 200 for ≥ 3 months in response to ART, you can discontinue PCP prophylaxis.
- MAC: If CD4 > 100 for ≥ 3 months in response to ART, you can discontinue MAC prophylaxis.

Stopping secondary prophylaxis (+ history of these infections):

- PCP: If CD4 > 200 for ≥ 3 months in response to ART, you can discontinue PCP prophylaxis.
- MAC: controversial on whether and when you can stop MAC prophylaxis with a history of MAC.

COMMON ID SYNDROMES

FEVER WITHOUT A SOURCE (FWS) IN INFANTS AND CHILDREN

Infants < 60 Days of Age with FWS

Fever without a source (FWS) in this age group can indicate bacteremia in 2.5% and meningitis in 1%. Approximately 10% of these infants will have a serious bacterial infection, with UTI being most common. Group B *Streptococcus* and *E. coli* are the most common causes of bacteremia, meningitis, and osteomyelitis in this age group. *Listeria* may be an infrequent cause as well. UTIs are typically due to *E. coli*, and bacterial gastroenteritis is most commonly due to *Salmonella*.

Viruses also commonly cause infection in this age group and include HSV and enteroviruses.

For all infants with fever in this age group, do a complete history and physical, CBC, U/A, and blood/urine cultures. CSF evaluation is controversial in 30- to 60-day-old infants; some recommend it while others do not. UTIs are more common in uncircumcised vs. circumcised male infants, especially if < 3 months old. CXR is not indicated unless symptoms warrant it; some medical centers have guidelines such as WBC > 20K, ANC > 10K, or if there are respiratory symptoms.

If the infant appears "well," was previously healthy, and the laboratory values show a normal WBC, with absolute band count < 1,500, < 11 WBC/hpf on spun urine, and < 6 WBC/hpf on stool smear (if diarrhea is present), you can observe the infant (inpatient or outpatient) with or without antibiotics. If you give the antibiotics, you must first do a lumbar puncture.

If the infant appears ill, antibiotics and hospitalization with lumbar puncture are mandatory. Further workup depends on the symptoms/signs.

Infants 61–90 Days of Age with FWS

Management is the same as for the younger infant, but most are likely to be managed as an outpatient.

Children 3–36 Months of Age with FWS

Obtain blood cultures if you suspect occult bacteremia or if the patient is to receive empiric antibiotics. Some recommend getting blood cultures for temperatures > 39° C (102.2° F) without localizing signs of infection and with a WBC count > 15,000.

If *H. influenzae* or *N. meningitidis* is found with "occult" bacteremia, admit the child and perform full blood, urine, and CSF cultures. If *S. pneumoniae* is found and the child returns and is well, repeat the blood culture and continue observation. If the child is ill or worsening, repeat the blood cultures, do CSF, and give ceftriaxone.

Do lumbar puncture if you suspect meningitis. UTIs are present in 7% of boys ≤ 6 months of age and in 8% of girls < 1 year of age who present with fever and no localizing signs. Do urine cultures on all boys < 6 months and girls < 1 year. (More on UTIs in GU infections, see page 5-74) CXR is beneficial if the child has symptoms/signs. Obtain stool for those with bloody or mucoid diarrhea.

Admit any toxic-appearing child, begin antibiotics, and do blood, urine, and CSF cultures. A well-appearing child with fever < 39° C is unlikely to have occult bacteremia and does not require further laboratory testing.

COMMON ID SYNDROMES: ENDOCARDITIS

Introduction

Bacterial endocarditis—See Cardiology, Book 4, for prophylaxis indications and medications. Blood cultures are vital in diagnosing endocarditis of any type and should be drawn before empiric antibiotics are started. Blood cultures are commonly positive (95%!) due to continual bacteremia. If cultures are negative (and patient has not been partially treated with antibiotics), consider fungi, Q fever (*Coxiella burnetii*), *Legionella*, *Chlamydophila psittaci*, *Bartonella*, and the HACEK organisms (discussed below) as possible causes.

Surgery is required for endocarditis with fistula, abscess, pericarditis, embolic disease (brain abscess or stroke), or persistent fever—and for cases in which the resulting valve dysfunction causes ventricular failure. In the heart, the electrical conduction pathway passes just beside the aortic valve. A conduction disturbance in a patient with aortic valve endocarditis is another indication for surgery. Vegetations alone usually are not an indication for surgery (unless large in size).

Diagnosis

Modified Duke Criteria

Definite endocarditis is diagnosed when the patient has any of the following:

• Pathologic evidence of disease
• 2 major clinical criteria
• 1 major clinical criterion + 3 minor clinical criteria
• 5 minor clinical criteria

Pathologic evidence would be visible organisms from a vegetation or valve lesion or a positive culture from the same tissue.

Possible endocarditis is diagnosed with 1 major + 1 minor, or 3 minor.

Major Criteria

With a lot of qualifiers, the 2 major clinical criteria are:

1) Positive blood cultures
2) Abnormal echocardiogram

Qualifiers for blood cultures:

• To count as a major criterion, organisms grown in culture should be the "typical" ones we described previously (*S. aureus*, viridans strep, *S. bovis*, enterococci, HACEK) from 2 separate cultures at least 12 hours apart.

• Any other organism should be observed in at least 3 or a majority of ≥ 4 cultures, drawn from separate sites, with 1st and last culture drawn at least an hour apart.

• Any 1 blood culture that grows *C. burnetii* is significant. A positive serologic test for *C. burnetii* is also significant (anti-phase 1 IgG > 1:800).

Qualifiers for echocardiograms. Significant echo findings include any of the following:

• An oscillating intracardiac mass visible on a valve or on valve-supporting structures
• An oscillating mass in the path of regurgitant jets
• An oscillating mass on implanted intracardiac devices
• An abscess
• Prosthetic valve dehiscence
• New regurgitation of a valve

Minor Criteria

Minor clinical criteria:

• Predisposing condition (valve disease or injection drug use)
• Fever
• Vascular phenomena (arterial emboli, pulmonary infarcts, mycotic aneurysms, stroke, conjunctival hemorrhages, Janeway lesions)
• Immunologic phenomena (acute glomerulonephritis, Osler nodes, Roth spots, +RF)
• Positive blood culture that does not meet major criterion

Again: CHF with endocarditis is an indication for cardiac surgery. Mortality in endocarditis surgery correlates with the pre-op severity of ventricular failure. The most common cause of cardiac death due to endocarditis is congestive heart failure.

Acute Bacterial Endocarditis (ABE) vs. Subacute Bacterial Endocarditis (SBE)

There are 2 methods of classification of endocarditis in adults, but these are less commonly used in children. The classic method is based on acuity of presentation: acute (ABE) vs. subacute (SBE). The more recent method is based on pertinent etiologic factors: native valve, prosthetic valve, addict (i.e., IV drugs), and culture-negative. These may have acute or subacute presentations. Addict and culture-negative can also be thought of as subsets of native valve and prosthetic valve endocarditis.

In one series, 92% of children with endocarditis had an underlying heart defect (congenital or rheumatic).

Quick Quiz

- In children with fever without a source between the ages of 3 and 36 months, when should urine cultures be considered for girls? For boys?

- What laboratory test is the most important diagnostic test in endocarditis: a blood culture or echocardiogram?

- True or false? Most children with endocarditis have an underlying heart defect.

- What organism most commonly causes endocarditis in children?

- In patients with "normal valves," which organism is most likely to cause endocarditis?

- What are Janeway lesions? Roth spots? Osler nodes? How common are these in children with endocarditis?

Congenital defects made up > 80% of the total, with tetralogy of Fallot and ventricular septal defect (VSD) the most common. Other lesions included aortic stenosis, patent ductus arteriosus (PDA), and transposition of the great vessels.

Viridans streptococci are responsible for 40% of cases of infective endocarditis in children, with 20–30% due to *Staphylococcus aureus*. *S. aureus* is more likely to infect normal heart valves. Next most common, at nearly 5%, is coagulase-negative staphylococci, followed by gram-negative bacilli and enterococci. *S. pneumoniae* causes only ~ 3% of endocarditis in children. Pneumococcal endocarditis has a high mortality.

In adolescent and adult IV drug addicts, the major organism is, again, *S. aureus* (50%), with MRSA a major component, followed by enterococci (15%). The following 3 have a frequency of 7–8% in this group: streptococci, gram-negatives (usually *Pseudomonas* or *Serratia*), and *Candida*.

In prosthetic valve endocarditis occurring up to 1 year after surgery, by far the most common organism is *S. epidermidis*, (55–60%).

Acute bacterial endocarditis (ABE) is caused by virulent bacteria, often attacking normal valves. Without treatment, ABE has an acute course in which there is often rapid cardiac valve destruction and resultant ventricular decompensation. Children are most likely to present with fever, splenomegaly, and heart murmur. (But remember: Most of these children already had a murmur from their previous cardiac defect.)

Other findings that are common in adults are rare in children:

- The peripheral manifestation of ABE is **Janeway lesions**, which are small, nontender macules on the palms and soles (Image 5-43). With *Staphylococcus*,

peripheral ecchymoses sometime appear. Embolization (again, especially with *S. aureus*) of the heart vegetations leads to metastatic infection (especially to the CNS and kidney).

- Subacute bacterial endocarditis usually occurs in patients with underlying cardiac disease. Manifestations include low-grade fever, heart murmurs, conjunctival petechiae, splenomegaly (in 66%), splinter hemorrhages, Roth spots, and Osler nodes. But again, in children, only fever, splenomegaly, and heart murmurs are common.

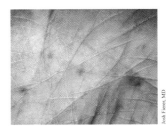

Image 5-43: Janeway lesions

- **Roth spots** are pale retinal lesions surrounded by hemorrhage. **Osler nodes** (= OUCHler nodes) are ~ 0.5-cm, tender nodules on the palms, fingertips, and soles. Roth spots and Osler nodes are late developments of SBE and are seen less frequently today because SBE is diagnosed and treated earlier. Remember: The Janeway lesions (nontender macules) are found in ABE, generally not SBE.

Streptococcus bovis, one of the group D streptococci, is easily killed by PCN alone. Enterococci require an aminoglycoside plus a beta-lactam antibiotic (2 cidal antibiotics).

There are some cases of fastidious, gram-negative organisms causing SBE. They are called the "HACEK" organisms (*Haemophilus*, *Actinobacillus*, *Cardiobacterium*, *Eikenella*, and *Kingella*) and usually are sensitive to beta-lactams. These are often the cause of "culture-negative" endocarditis, since they may require > 7 days to grow to detectable levels in culture media. Treat with PCN + gentamicin or ceftriaxone, or per culture results.

Also remember: Endocarditis in adults caused by either *S. bovis* or *Clostridium septicus* is often associated with colon cancer, so a thorough GI workup in these patients would be warranted—especially in adults.

Prosthetic Valve

Prosthetic valve endocarditis (PVE) can be acute or subacute in presentation. Early PVE (< 2 months postsurgery) is typically due to seeding during the surgery. An acute presentation means emergent surgery is generally necessary. Even with surgery, it still has a 40% mortality.

Late type PVE (> 2 months postsurgery) has a subacute presentation. The infection often invades the annulus and requires surgery. *S. epidermidis* is the culprit in 55–60% of the cases of PVE in the 1st year after surgery. If the infecting organism is viridans streptococci, the prosthetic valve infection may be cured with antibiotics alone.

Treatment of Bacterial Endocarditis

Treatment of native valve endocarditis:

- PCN-sensitive *Streptococcus*: 2 weeks of PCN G or ampicillin + gentamicin or 4 weeks of PCN/ampicillin, cefazolin, or ceftriaxone. Note: For this, vancomycin is less effective than beta-lactam antibiotics and should be used only for severe PCN allergy. Reliably compliant patients may be discharged from the hospital on a once-daily IM dose of ceftriaxone.
- PCN-insensitive *Streptococcus* (including *Enterococcus faecalis*): The treatment is 4 weeks of PCN G or ampicillin + gentamicin x 4 weeks if *Enterococcus* (2 weeks otherwise)—or vancomycin if PCN-allergic.
- Treat *S. aureus* (MSSA) endocarditis with oxacillin or cefazolin x 6 weeks (optional addition of gentamicin); again: If the *S. aureus* is methicillin-resistant, use vancomycin +/– gentamicin.

Treatment of prosthetic valve endocarditis:

- Methicillin-resistant *Staphylococcus* (especially *S. epidermidis*) requires vancomycin, rifampin, and gentamicin—all 3—for 14 days, followed by vancomycin + rifampin for 4 weeks. The gentamicin prevents the emergence of resistance to rifampin. Remember: Gentamicin is nephro- and ototoxic.
- *S. aureus*: Nafcillin/oxacillin or cefazolin + gentamicin for 5 days (however, adding an aminoglycoside became controversial in 2010 because of data showing that inclusion of an aminoglycoside did not change outcome and increased nephrotoxicity), followed by the beta-lactam for a total of 6 weeks.

COMMON ID SYNDROMES: CNS

Bacterial Meningitis

Overview

Acute bacterial meningitis—if suspected, do the following CSF tests: Gram stain, C+S, cell count with differential, protein, and glucose. Culture results are the gold standard. Bacterial antigen tests should be reserved for pretreated cases with a negative Gram stain and culture x 48 hours. PCR can also be used if cultures are negative.

The etiology of meningitis is age-dependent (Table 5-6):

- In neonates (< 1 month of age), think group B *Streptococcus* (*S. agalactiae*), gram-negatives, and *Listeria*.
- *S. pneumoniae* is the most common cause of meningitis in children ≥ 3 months to < 10 years of age.
- *Neisseria meningitidis* is the most common cause in children 10–19 years of age.
- *Listeria monocytogenes* is the 3rd most common cause of meningitis overall; it is more prevalent in infants, organ transplant recipients, immunodeficiency patients, and patients who are > 60 years old.

In the U.S., meningococcal serogroups C, B, and Y account for approximately 35, 32, and 26 percent of isolates. The main culprit in infants is group B (B for bad). There are effective vaccines against A, C, Y, and W-135, but not type B.

Prior to 1990, *H. influenzae* was, by far, the most common cause of bacterial meningitis in children. The Hib vaccine has had a wonderfully dramatic effect on *H. influenzae* in the U.S. Its prevalence has decreased from ~ 40% to ~ 2%!

A similarly dramatic effect was seen from 1998 (pre-PCV7) to 2007, when the incidence of vaccine-type invasive pneumococcal disease (IPD) infections decreased by 99%, and the incidence of all IPD decreased by 76% in children < 5 years of age! (IPD is basically confirmed when *S. pneumoniae* is found in blood or CSF, but not sputum. So, IPD can be caused by meningitis, endocarditis, pneumonia, etc.)

Treatment of Bacterial Meningitis

In partially treated, gram-positive meningitis, the bacteria stain poorly, and they may even look gram-negative! A bloody tap (contaminated) has increased protein and decreased glucose.

Effective treatment requires an antibiotic that both crosses into the CSF and has bactericidal activity.

Antibiotics that do not cross into the CSF well at any time are:

- Erythromycin
- Tetracycline
- Clindamycin
- Cefoxitin
- 1st generation cephalosporins

These are common distractors on exam questions asking about meningitis treatment—pick something else!

Start empiric treatment of meningitis while Gram stain and/or culture results are pending. If the LP cannot be done immediately, start antibiotics even before the LP! [Know:]

- Meningitis in children > 3 months of age is empirically treated with ceftriaxone or cefotaxime (3rd generation cephalosporin) and vancomycin because of resistant *S. pneumoniae*.
- For empiric treatment of the neonates (< 3 months of age), add ampicillin (for *Listeria*) to the above treatment. Many recommend all 3 drugs as empiric therapy for this age group, especially if the neonate is in day care or has older siblings.
- More specifically, in neonates (< 1 month), use cefotaxime as the 3rd generation cephalosporin because ceftriaxone may exacerbate hyperbilirubinemia.

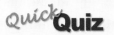

Quiz

- What are the treatments for native valve endocarditis?
- Which organisms are the most common cause of meningitis in a 1-month-old? 6-year-old? 17-year-old?
- What is the empiric treatment for meningitis in infants > 3 months of age? < 3 months?
- What is the antibiotic therapy for pneumococcal meningitis?
- When are glucocorticoids approved for use in meningitis?

If you have a suspicion of 1 of the following, the empiric therapy may change:

- For presumed pneumococcal meningitis (especially if Gram stain is suspicious), be sure to add vancomycin to the 3rd generation cephalosporin; rifampin if vancomycin-allergic.
- Treat confirmed meningococcal meningitis with high-dose PCN (3rd generation cephalosporin if PCN-allergic), and ensure contacts receive prophylaxis.
- The 3rd generation cephalosporins cover gram-negative meningitis.

Prophylaxis with rifampin is also indicated for invasive *Haemophilus influenzae* disease. You do not need to give chemoprophylaxis to contacts of someone with pneumococcal meningitis because prophylaxis won't get rid of the carrier state.

Dexamethasone is approved for use in *H. influenzae* meningitis to reduce neurologic complications (including hearing loss) and must be started prior to or concurrent with the 1st dose of antibiotics. Data in pediatrics for *S. pneumoniae* are lacking, and the 2012 Red Book is noncommittal on its use.

In adolescent patients with AIDS, ALL, or Hodgkin disease, think *Cryptococcus* and do a cryptococcal antigen and/or India ink. Consider amebic meningitis (e.g., *Naegleria fowleri*) 1st when the meningitis patient has been swimming in brackish (cow ponds) water.

Aseptic Meningitis

Aseptic meningitis is manifested by headache, meningismus, and CSF lymphocytosis—many, many causes. On the CSF, do the same tests as for acute meningitis and add testing for HSV PCR, enteroviral PCR (in summer/early fall), *Coccidioides* (in endemic areas), VDRL, acid-fast smear and culture, and either the India ink or cryptococcal antigen test. Test results that make aseptic meningitis unlikely are CSF glucose < 40, CSF protein > 150, and CSF WBC count > 1,200.

Viruses are the most common etiologies of aseptic meningitis (indeed, the most common cause of all meningitis)—including enteroviruses and mosquito-borne arboviruses in the summer/early fall, mumps in the spring, and HSV. Suspect *Coccidioides* and *Histoplasma* in endemic areas (arid Southwest and Mississippi/Ohio River valleys, respectively). Chronic neutrophilic meningitis is unusual—think of *Nocardia*, *Actinomyces*, or fungus as possible causes. Treat *Cryptococcus*—common in AIDS, Hodgkin disease, and ALL (i.e., cell-mediated)—with IV amphotericin B + oral flucytosine (5-FC; 5-fluorocytosine), followed by oral fluconazole.

Classic presentation and findings for acute viral meningitis:

- Fever
- Headache
- Nuchal rigidity
- Nonfocal exam
- Normal CT
- LP showing increased lymphocytes

Table 5-6: Bacterial Etiologies of Meningitis in the U.S.						
0–2 mos	**%**	**3 mos–15 yrs**	**%**	**Adult**	**%**	**Notes on > 60 yrs**
Gram-negative (*E. coli & Klebsiella*)	20–30	*S. pneumoniae* esp 3 mos to < 10 years	30–50	*S. pneumoniae*	30–50	*S. pneumoniae* *N. meningitidis*
Strep (group B) (*S. agalactiae*)	40–50	*N. meningitidis* esp 10–19 years	10–35	*N. meningitidis*	10–35	See more often: *Listeria* *E. coli*
Listeria	2–10	*H. influenzae*	0–7	Listeria	2–11	*H. influenzae*
Staphylococci	2–5	Streptococci	2–4	Gram-negative	1–10	*Pseudomonas*
S. pneumoniae	0–5	Gram-negative	1–2	Streptococci	5	
H. influenzae	0–3	Staphylococci	1–2	Staphylococci	5	
N. meningitidis	0–1	*Listeria*	1–2	*H. influenzae*	1–3	

Remember, for the newborn and adults > 60 years, empiric treatment is usually ceftriaxone or other 3rd generation cephalosporins and ampicillin. (Cephalosporins have no effect against *Listeria*!)

TB Meningitis

Tuberculous meningitis is sometimes manifested by cranial nerve palsies, especially the 6th cranial nerve. CSF typically shows only mild-to-moderate WBC elevation, very high protein, and low glucose. Look especially for basilar enhancement on CT scan of the head. Other causes of aseptic basilar meningitis include spirochetal (secondary syphilis and Lyme disease).

Lyme Meningitis

Lyme meningitis can cause peripheral and cranial nerve palsies (especially of the 7th cranial nerve), so think of Lyme disease when a patient presents with Bell's palsy, and/or foot drop, and a suggestive history. Treat meningitis with ceftriaxone 2 g qd x 21 days. Bell's palsy can be treated with oral agents alone. Alternative is high-dose PCN G.

Encephalitis

Acute encephalitis—the cause of most of these cases is unknown! The most commonly identified cause of encephalitis in the U.S. is arboviruses (West Nile, LaCrosse, etc.). HSV is responsible for the highest number of deaths due to encephalitis. Suspect HSV especially if there are focal seizures localized to the temporal lobes. The CSF may be bloody due to hemorrhagic necrosis of the temporal lobes, but blood in the CSF is not pathognomonic for herpes! If you suspect HSV, you should empirically start the patient on IV acyclovir.

Spinal Epidural Abscess

Spinal epidural abscesses may be caused by either hematogenous spread or local extension (e.g., from osteomyelitis). *S. aureus* is the most common cause. Patients present with fever, spinal pain, and nerve compression problems. Do an MRI. CT is not as good as MRI because CT is susceptible to bony artifacts. Drainage is usually required.

Neurosyphilis

CSF-VDRL test is the test of choice for neurosyphilis; it is 100% specific but only 50% sensitive. A positive test confirms neurosyphilis, but a negative test cannot be used to rule it out. CSF FTA-ABS is very sensitive—unfortunately, it is so sensitive that a positive result often reflects contamination of CSF with peripheral blood, so it is not used. Often, treatment must be based on suspicion.

Brain Abscess

Diagnosis: CT/MRI with contrast is the procedure of choice (> 95% sensitivity). If the abscess is accessible, you would most likely aspirate it and give antibiotics. You may need to surgically excise the lesion. Lumbar puncture is absolutely contraindicated if signs of increased intracranial pressure are present—such as focal neurologic signs. There is an increased risk of herniation.

Cysticercosis (caused by ingesting the pork tapeworm, *Taenia solium*) is the most common cause of brain lesions in developing countries, and imported cases are often seen in the U.S. Symptoms, especially seizures, are seen when the cysticerci (larval forms of *T. solium*) die, causing an inflammatory reaction. On an exam, if you are presented with a teenager from Mexico with new onset seizures and a ring-enhancing lesion on CT scan, think neurocysticercosis! *Toxoplasma* is the most likely etiologic agent if the patient is immunodeficient—especially if there are multiple lesions. Infection is usually due to a reactivation of dormant cysts.

Location of the abscess is often related to the source. Frontal lobe—think paranasal sinus: pneumococcus, *H. influenzae*, and anaerobes. Temporal or cerebellum—think middle ear: pneumococcus, *H. influenzae*, *S. aureus*, gram-negative. Both frontal and parietal abscesses can be due to hematogenous spread from such things as lung infections and endocarditis.

Treatment of brain abscesses is always initially empiric:

- In general, vancomycin, cefotaxime, and metronidazole.
- If an oral source is suspected: high-dose penicillin G plus metronidazole.
- If an ear or sinus source is suspected: either ceftriaxone or cefotaxime plus metronidazole.
- If there was a neurosurgical procedure, penetrating head trauma, or acute endocarditis, think MRSA and add vancomycin to cephalosporin and metronidazole above. (*Pseudomonas* also occurs after neurosurgery.)

Nocardia pulmonary disease can spread and cause focal lesions in the brain. It is also a rare cause of neutrophilic aseptic meningitis.

COMMON ID SYNDROMES: GI

Overview

Diarrhea is a symptom of a variety of diseases. These diseases usually last only a few days but can cause dehydration and electrolyte imbalance. In infants, diarrhea is a doubling of the number of stools per day. In older children, it is ≥ 3 watery/loose stools per day.

Causes of infectious diarrhea:

1) Viral (80%): rotavirus, norovirus
2) Bacterial (10–20%): *E. coli*, *Campylobacter*, *Salmonella*, *Shigella*
3) Parasitic (< 10%): *Giardia* (many more if patient has been traveling!)

Common clinical scenarios:

- Fever with nonbloody diarrhea—think viral gastroenteritis

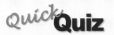

- Afebrile with nonbloody diarrhea—may still be viral but also may be antibiotic associated, or due to over-feeding (during first 6–12 months of life)
- Febrile with bloody or mucous diarrhea—generally have bacterial enteritis with some exceptions:
  - Pseudomembranous colitis (previous antibiotics, systemic toxicity, abdominal distention) + bloody stools
  - Amebiasis—immigrants or travelers to endemic areas (India, Africa, Mexico, Central and South America)
  - Inflammatory bowel disease—history of recurrent abdominal pain, weight loss
- Afebrile with bloody diarrhea—think intussusceptions, HUS, pseudomembranous colitis

Viral Causes of Acute Diarrhea

Rotavirus is frequently found in children. It is the most important cause of severe diarrhea in infants and is easily found in their stools. It is nonbloody in character. It most commonly occurs between November and April and is transmitted by fecal-oral spread, with an incubation period of 1–3 days.

Adenovirus types 40 and 41 make up the 2nd most common cause of gastroenteritis in children. Adenovirus is similar to rotavirus in that it mainly affects children < 2 years of age, but adenovirus infection is year-round. Incubation is 3–10 days, which is longer than most other GI viruses.

Human caliciviruses (norovirus and sapovirus) cause abrupt onset vomiting and watery diarrhea, lasting 24–60 hours. Noroviruses infections are associated with clams and oysters, causing "winter vomiting disease," but they can also be waterborne. Identify noroviruses with an ELISA test. Infections are typically epidemic, and recent cruise ship outbreaks underscore this. Noroviruses cause ~ 50% of infectious viral gastroenteritis outbreaks in the U.S. It is spread fecal-orally and in contaminated food and water; it has a 1–2-day incubation period.

Bacterial Causes of Acute Diarrhea

E. coli is the most common cause of bacterial diarrhea (commonly without blood or WBCs) affecting both the resident children and travelers in developing countries. There is an enterohemorrhagic, Shiga toxin–associated *E. coli* (serotype O157:H7) that causes localized out-breaks of hemorrhagic colitis, TTP, and HUS (hemolytic uremic syndrome)—usually after eating undercooked beef or unpasteurized milk. Do not treat diarrhea caused by *E. coli* O157:H7 with antibiotics because you may increase the risk of HUS and antibiotics do not shorten the duration of illness.

Traveler's diarrhea is most often caused by enterotoxi-genic *E. coli*. Treat with azithromycin or daily quinolone or TMP/SMX.

Vibrios—think seafood and shellfish. *V. cholerae* 01 (causes cholera) is occasionally associated with Gulf Coast crabs. The non-01 *V. cholerae*, *V. parahaemolyti-cus*, and other *Vibrios* are even more frequent causes of shellfish-associated diarrhea. These are usually self-limited. *Vibrio vulnificus* causes skin infections and sepsis, especially in the immunocompromised or those with chronic liver disease.

Antibiotic-associated colitis is caused by **Clostridium difficile**. (Antibiotic-associated diarrhea is just a side effect of the medicine with change in normal flora.) Symptoms can occur up to 3 weeks after the antibiotics are stopped. See page 5-10 for more on *C. difficile*.

Cryptosporidia is known to cause prolonged diarrhea in AIDS patients and a self-limited diarrhea in travelers. It is found with acid-fast stains of the stool (small, round, red organisms on a green background). Animals (including humans) are the reservoirs.

Salmonella and **Shigella** were previously discussed under Gram-Negative Bacteria, page 5-12.

When to Do Stool Studies

Do stool cultures in febrile children with bloody or mucous stools, immunocompromised patients, those with prolonged symptoms, in epidemic outbreaks, and in those with foreign travel. Routine cultures of stool are not recommended for nonbloody diarrhea of brief duration in otherwise healthy children.

When ordering stool culture, especially in patients with blood or mucus in their stool, add:

- Fecal WBCs if you suspect invasive bacterial enteritis (severe diarrhea, fever)

- O+P if the patient has a history of foreign travel
- *C. difficile* PCR if the patient has recently been on antibiotics and develops diarrhea
- Other pathogens such as *Cryptosporidia* and *Microsporidia* if the patient is immunocompromised

Additional studies:

- If only mild-to-moderate dehydration, additional labs are likely unnecessary.
- If more severely ill or dehydrated, then obtain labs to assess electrolytes and renal function.
- If the child is toxic appearing and has bloody diarrhea with abdominal pain, imaging studies (ultrasound/CT) may be indicated.

Treatment

Treatment protocol overview:

- Antibiotics should not be used for children with acute bloody diarrhea unless a specific pathogen has been identified.
- Antibiotics may prolong *Salmonella* infection and are relatively contraindicated in *E. coli* O157:H7 infections.

Do not give antimotility agents for any diarrhea when there are fecal WBCs. *Campylobacter* is resistant to TMP/SMX, so give azithromycin/erythromycin or quinolones instead. Prolonged, intermittent diarrhea with malaise and flatus suggests giardiasis or *Cyclospora*.

Treatment for antibiotic-associated colitis: Stop the antibiotics and give 10–14 days of metronidazole or oral vancomycin. 1st line treatment is metronidazole because it is just as effective as oral vancomycin yet much less expensive. Relapse rate on either drug is ~ 30%. This is usually due to the spores becoming active; just repeat the same treatment!

Treatment for Traveler's Diarrhea Only

Mild: loperamide and single-dose quinolone. In children < 18 years of age, azithromycin may be used for 3 days. Rifaximin, a luminal nonabsorbable agent, is useful in children > 12 years of age. Bismuth-containing agents (Pepto-Bismol®) are generally avoided in children because of their co-mixture with salicylates.

Severe: same—except quinolone or azithromycin is more commonly used.

COMMON ID SYNDROMES: GU INFECTIONS AND STDs

Note about STDs

There are many causes of STDs. Know the treatment of all STDs! Many of them have similar manifestations consisting of genital ulcerations with regional adenopathy (gonorrhea does not have these). STDs are covered in Adolescent Health and Gynecology, Book 1.

Urinary Tract Infection (UTI)

Urinary tract infection (UTI) is one of the most common infections in pediatrics. The 2 broad clinical categories of UTI are pyelonephritis (upper UTI) and cystitis (lower UTI). The incidence of UTI varies based on age, sex, and gender. In the U.S. each year, it is estimated that UTIs affect 2.4–2.8% of children. Occurrence of 1st time, symptomatic UTI is highest in boys and girls during the 1st year of life and then decreases markedly after that. Boys with UTI are also more likely to have anatomic urinary tract abnormalities (e.g., posterior urethral valves or vesicoureteral reflux). The risk of UTI is also higher in uncircumcised boys (2.15%) vs. in circumcised boys (0.22%). Other risk factors for UTI in both sexes include: genetic predisposition, alteration of GU flora by antibiotics, diabetes, anatomic abnormalities, bowel and bladder dysfunction (e.g., neurogenic bladder), indwelling urinary catheters, and constipation.

Signs and symptoms of UTI may vary with the child's age. Neonates and infants up to 2 months of age with pyelonephritis do not have symptoms localized to the urinary tract, and often UTI is diagnosed as part of a sepsis evaluation. Neonates with UTI may have fever, jaundice, failure to thrive, poor feeding, vomiting, and irritability. Older children (2 months–2 years) may additionally have strong-smelling urine or abdominal pain. Preschoolers (2–6 years of age) may have more common UTI symptoms such as dysuria, urgency, frequency. Still, older children and adolescents display flank/back pain, enuresis, and incontinence. On exam, patients will have costovertebral angle tenderness, abdominal or suprapubic tenderness, palpable bladder or dribbling, or poor urinary stream.

Bacterial infections are the most common etiology of UTI:

- *E. coli* causes the majority of infections (75–90%)
- *Klebsiella* species
- *Proteus* species
- *Enterococcus* species
- *Staphylococcus saprophyticus* (female adolescents and sexually active females)
- Group B *Streptococcus* (neonates and pregnant women)
- *Pseudomonas aeruginosa*

Fungi (especially *Candida*) may also cause UTIs, especially after instrumentation (indwelling urinary catheters) of the urinary tract. Adenovirus can also cause hemorrhagic cystitis.

Diagnosis and Management of UTI in Young Children (2–24 Months)

In 2011, the AAP revised their clinical practice guidelines regarding diagnosis and management of febrile UTIs in infants and children 2–24 months of age. The prevalence of UTI in this age group is high (~ 5%).

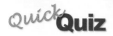

Quick Quiz

- What is a risk factor for UTIs in boys?
- Which bacterial cause of UTI is associated with kidney stones?
- What is the "fish tank bacillus"? Characterize the infection it causes.

Uncircumcised male infants with fever are 4-8x more likely to have a UTI than those who are circumcised.

Diagnosis is made on the presence of both pyuria and at least 50,000 colonies/mL of a single urologic pathogen in an appropriately collected urine specimen (e.g., suprapubic aspiration [SPA] or catheterized urine). The old definition of UTI required at least 100,000 colonies/mL of a single uropathogen, but this was based on studies in adult women with UTI. A bagged urine is frequently contaminated (high false-positive rate) and is useless unless it is negative.

Empiric antibiotic choices should cover the most common causes of UTI in this age group (e.g., *E. coli*, *Klebsiella*, other gram-negatives) and can usually be given orally. If patients are "toxic" appearing or unable to take oral medications, they should be treated with IV antibiotics. Once culture and sensitivity results are known, antibiotics can be tailored appropriately.

Antibiotics should be administered x 7–14 days. Febrile infants with UTI should undergo renal and bladder ultrasound (RBUS) to look for hydronephrosis or other anatomic abnormalities. A voiding cystourethrogram (VCUG) is indicated if the RBUS reveals hydronephrosis, renal scarring, or findings suggestive of high-grade vesicoureteral reflux (VCUR) or obstructive uropathy. VCUG should be performed if there is a recurrence of a febrile UTI.

Treatment of UTIs in Older Children and Adolescents

Routine UTI: TMP/SMX x 3 days in adolescents/adults and longer in those younger (7–14 days). (TMP/SMX is more effective than amoxicillin.)

Uncomplicated pyelonephritis: The treatment is oral TMP/SMX or 3rd generation cephalosporin x 14 days.

Complicated pyelonephritis (including pregnant patients): 3rd generation cephalosporin, IV ampicillin + gentamicin, TMP/SMX, or fluoroquinolones (not in pregnant). Use gentamicin or 3rd generation cephalosporin alone if the Gram stain shows no gram-positive cocci. Recommend follow-up urine analysis after the antibiotic treatment ends. Fluoroquinolones are alternate therapy for complicated, or recurrent, cystitis or pyelonephritis.

Note: The CDC recommends ciprofloxacin for 2nd line therapy of UTI and pyelonephritis in children 1–17 years of age. Consider if *Pseudomonas* is an issue. For community-acquired UTIs with extended-spectrum beta-lactamase (ESBL)-producing *E. coli*, a carbapenem is the drug of choice.

UTI organisms to know:

- *Proteus* infections are associated with stones (so do a KUB to check for stones) and hyperammonemia.
- *Streptococcus agalactiae* (Group B *Streptococcus*) infections are seen in pregnancy and infants < 3 months.
- *Staphylococcus saprophyticus*: Although coagulase-negative staphylococci are usually considered skin contaminants, UTI due to *S. saprophyticus* in adolescent females is considered a pathogen and should be treated. Treat with TMP/SMX, nitrofurantoin, or cephalothin. Note that 2nd and 3rd generation cephalosporins are not effective against *S. saprophyticus*.

Treatment of Pregnant Women

[Know:] Treat asymptomatic bacteriuria in pregnant women (1/3 go on to pyelonephritis), neutropenic patients, diabetics, and transplant patients. Also, always admit pregnant patients with pyelonephritis and treat as a complicated pyelonephritis (see above).

[Also know:] Pregnancy-safe antibiotics to use for pyelonephritis are ampicillin, aminoglycosides, cephalosporins, and TMP/SMX; but you should not give TMP/SMX in late pregnancy or to early nursing mothers because it might cause kernicterus in the child. Also, do not use tetracycline/doxycycline or quinolones.

COMMON ID SYNDROMES: SOFT TISSUE INFECTIONS

Vibrio is found especially in shellfish. *V. vulnificus* causes large hemorrhagic bullae, followed by necrosis and lymph-adenopathy +/– septicemia. Patients who are immunocompromised or have chronic liver disease are especially susceptible.

Mycobacterium marinum is also called "fish tank bacillus." It causes nonhealing skin ulceration in people who work around fish tanks. Infection may present as a single granuloma, but the organism often invades the lymphatics and can cause a series of lesions over a lymph vessel similar to the lesions seen in sporotrichosis. Lesions tend to localize in the distal extremities because the organism does not grow well at body temperature. Diagnosis: Look for acid-fast bacilli in the lesion biopsy. Treat with ethambutol + rifampin or clarithromycin + rifampin.

Erysipelothrix rhusiopathiae is another cause of skin infection in fishermen and meat handlers. Treat with PCN G, ampicillin, or fluoroquinolones.

COMMON ID SYNDROMES: BONE INFECTIONS

Osteomyelitis

Osteomyelitis is an infection of bone that is usually bacterial in origin. Microorganisms can be introduced into bone in 3 ways:

1) Hematogenous
2) Direct inoculation (trauma or surgery)
3) Local invasion from a contiguous infection (decubitus ulcer or periodontal disease)

Acute hematogenous osteomyelitis occurs most commonly in children < 6 years of age and is more common in boys. Frequently, there is a history of minor trauma or intercurrent URI. Hematogenous osteomyelitis most commonly affects the long bones, with the lower femoral and upper tibial metaphyses being the most commonly affected, followed by the proximal femoral metaphysis and distal metaphyses of the radius and humerus.

Initial symptoms can be nonspecific and are associated with bacteremia, such as malaise and fever. Once infection becomes established in the bone, warmth, swelling, and point tenderness of the involved site are the classic physical findings. Typical laboratory findings include an elevated white blood cell count (WBC), and elevation of acute phase reactants such as erythrocyte sedimentation rate (ESR), C-reactive protein (CRP), or procalcitonin.

The diagnosis of osteomyelitis can be confirmed with imaging. Start with plain radiographs of the suspected site of infection; however, these may be negative early in the course of osteomyelitis. Usually it takes 10–14 days to see plain x-ray changes (periosteal reaction/elevation), but they are helpful to exclude fracture or bone tumors. Bone scans may be helpful in patients without localizing findings. They are readily available in most hospitals and do not require sedation in young children. However, MRI is the modality of choice because it is the most sensitive and specific. It can show bone marrow edema (early in the course of osteomyelitis) and can be helpful in identifying subperiosteal or intraosseous abscesses, which bone scans cannot. Most young children require sedation in order to achieve an optimal study.

It is important to attempt isolation of a pathogen from bone, periosteal collection, joint fluid, or by blood culture prior to starting empiric antibiotic therapy. However, do not delay antibiotics in children who have signs of systemic illness or "toxicity." A bacteriologic diagnosis can be confirmed in 50–80% of cases, but sometimes a causative pathogen cannot be identified, especially if the patient was pretreated with antibiotics prior to obtaining cultures.

Acute infection is typically caused by *S. aureus* and group A *Streptococcus*. *H. influenzae* used to be very common but now has disappeared. *S. pneumoniae* and *Kingella* are also pathogens—typically seen in younger children.

In neonates, *S. aureus*, group B *Streptococcus*, and gram-negatives are most common.

In IV drug abuser, think *Pseudomonas*, especially if the infection involves the vertebrae or pelvis.

If a puncture wound through a tennis shoe, again think *Pseudomonas*.

In patients with sickle cell disease, think *Salmonella*.

In children with chronic granulomatous disease, small bone osteomyelitis can be caused by *Serratia*, *S. aureus*, and *Candida*.

In vertebral osteomyelitis, think about *S. aureus*, TB, or even *Bartonella*!

Treat uncomplicated acute hematogenous osteomyelitis with IV antibiotics directed at the pathogen for 5–14 days, followed by oral antibiotics to complete 4–8 weeks. If there is evidence of a subperiosteal or bone abscess, surgical drainage is indicated. Length of therapy is based on clinical response, the pathogen found, and any complications.

Septic Arthritis

Septic arthritis is most common in children < 3 years of age. It typically involves a single large joint (knee or hip most commonly) and more commonly affects boys.

Children present with pain and refusal to move or bear weight on the joint. The involved joint is often swollen, red, and warm to the touch. Neonates may have a swollen, red extremity that they won't move (pseudoparalysis). In young children, it is often hard on physical exam to localize where the involved joint is, so you should x-ray the joint above and below where you think the problem is. Fever is common. *S. aureus* is the leading cause.

In neonates, group B *Streptococcus* (usually late-onset) and gram-negatives are implicated as well.

In children < 5 years of age, *S. aureus*, *S. pyogenes*, and *S. pneumoniae* are the most common; in those > 5 years of age, *S. pneumoniae* diminishes as a common cause.

Don't forget: *N. gonorrhoeae* in the sexually active adolescent, especially if she is menstruating! *Salmonella*, again, is common in patients with sickle cell disease.

Do joint aspiration quickly to discern the diagnosis and send the fluid for Gram stain, culture, and cell count. WBC count > 50,000 is common with mostly PMNs. Also obtain blood cultures. MRI or ultrasound of the joint may be helpful in discerning the presence of fluid.

Treatment involves drainage of the infected joint and starting antibiotics directly against the most likely organism. Open drainage is sometimes recommended (especially with deep-seated joints like the hip). Continue antibiotics for 3–6 weeks.

- How long does it take before you can see plain x-ray changes in osteomyelitis?
- What imaging test is most sensitive and specific for the workup of osteomyelitis?
- What is the most common cause of osteomyelitis in children? In neonates? In patients with sickle cell disease?
- What is the most common cause of septic arthritis?
- What is a common cause of septic arthritis in a sexually active teenager who is menstruating?
- What vector is responsible for most nosocomial ICU infections?
- What organisms commonly cause IV catheter-related infections?

COMMON ID SYNDROMES: NOSOCOMIAL INFECTIONS

Order of frequency: UTI > post-op wound infection > pneumonia.

Nosocomial pneumonia is often bacterial and has the highest mortality rate of all the nosocomial infections. It is usually caused by gram-negative organisms; next most frequently, by *Staphylococcus aureus.* If there is an outbreak of bacterial pneumonia (or almost any illness) in the ICU, the most likely vector of transmission is the hands of the ICU workers.

IV catheter-related infections: There are 3 types, and all 3 can cause bacteremia/fungemia:

1) Asymptomatic
2) Localized
3) Septic thrombophlebitis (rarest)

Secondary endocarditis is more likely to occur in patients with catheters that extend into the heart. IV lines become infected after ~ 3 days! Metal needles are less likely than plastic angiocatheters to become infected. IV catheter infections are commonly due to *S. epidermidis* and *S. aureus.* Some other causes are *Candida, Corynebacterium jeikeium* (especially in bone marrow transplant units), and gram-negative rods.

Treatment: Remove catheter and give antibiotic therapy for 2 weeks. Septic thrombophlebitis often requires removal of the affected vein. If there is gram-positive septicemia, start with vancomycin in case it is methicillin-resistant. Exception: If there is a gram-positive bacteremia in a patient with a Hickman or Broviac catheter, you can try to treat with antibiotics for 2–4 weeks without removing the catheter. Again, start with vancomycin until culture results are back.

ANTIBIOTIC THERAPY

OVERVIEW

Review of Protein Synthesis

Most antibiotics work either by interrupting protein synthesis or cell wall synthesis (Figure 5-1). First, let's review protein synthesis.

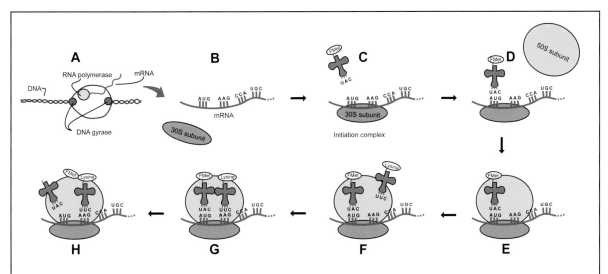

A represents transcription. DNA gyrase is targeted by **quinolones** and **metronidazole**. **Rifampin** binds to RNA polymerase.
B to C shows attachment of the 30S subunit to the mRNA. **Tetracyclines** bind reversibly and **aminoglycosides** bind irreversibly to the 30S subunit.
C to D shows attachment of the 50S subunit to form the 70S ribosome. **Oxazolidinones** and **macrolides** bind to the 50S subunit.

Figure 5-1: Antibiotic Effects on Protein Synthesis

Protein Synthesis—Transcription

The DNA particle must be unwound from its supercoiled arrangement before it can be "read" by RNA polymerase. This involves cutting the strand, holding onto the cut ends to prevent them being damaged, allowing the double helix to uncoil and the DNA to be copied, then precisely gluing the cut ends back together again. The key enzyme that carries out this process in bacteria is DNA gyrase.

RNA polymerase moves along a section of DNA (a gene), uncoiled by the DNA gyrase and, following the coded messages on the deoxyribonucleotides, forms a string of complementary-paired ribonucleotides, i.e., a piece of RNA—more specifically pre-mRNA. With the removal of an intron, the pre-mRNA becomes mRNA (messenger RNA). This is called transcription because the DNA code is transcribed into a complementary RNA code.

Protein Synthesis—Translation

Ribosomes are the translation units that convert the coded message in the mRNA to a specific sequence of amino acids. A 30S ribosomal subunit attaches to the mRNA at the "ribosome binding site," then moves along it until the start codon (AUG) is reached. Here a tRNA (with anticodon UAC) carrying an altered methionine (f-Met) binds with this subunit and mRNA to form the "initiation complex." A 50S ribosomal subunit then comes along and binds to this complex to form the 70S ribosome.

Amino acid-specific transfer RNAs (tRNAs) attach to the 20 amino acids used in making protein. The bottom loop of these "inverted cloverleaf-shaped" tRNAs have 3 unpaired bases called anticodons.

As the 70S ribosome moves along the mRNA, tRNAs attach one at a time, bringing these amino acids with them. The amino acids are bound together, forming a gradually lengthening protein chain.

When the ribosome reaches the end of the coded message, translation stops. The ribosomal subunits then separate and detach from the mRNA, and the completed protein is released.

Antibiotics That Block Protein Synthesis

There! Now we can see what is affected by the antibiotics that interfere with protein synthesis.

Rifampin binds to RNA polymerase and blocks initiation of the transcription of DNA to mRNA.

Quinolone antibiotics specifically target the DNA gyrase of bacteria. This allows the DNA gyrase to cut the double helix but then prevents the cut ends from being rejoined.

Metronidazole, a very important antianaerobic and antiprotozoal agent, probably has a similar primary mode of action to the quinolones, although it also affects cell membrane function.

Aminoglycosides bind irreversibly (bactericidal) to the 30S subunit and prevent the 50S subunit from attaching.

Tetracyclines bind reversibly to the 30S subunit, distorting it so that the anticodons of the tRNAs cannot align properly with the codons on the mRNA.

Oxazolidinones are a new class of antibiotic, of which linezolid (Zyvox®) is the 1st available. The drug binds to the 50S ribosomal subunit, thereby preventing attachment to the initiation complex.

Macrolides bind reversibly to the 50S subunit. They prevent peptide bond formation between the amino acids and hence keep the 70S ribosome from translocating down the mRNA.

Antibiotics Affecting Cell Wall Synthesis

Peptidoglycan is an exclusively bacterial polymer and is a component of bacterial cell walls. There are a variety of antibiotics that act at one or more stages of peptidoglycan synthesis.

Beta-lactams (see next) are a class of antibiotics that focus on attacking the cell wall. These antibiotics contain a structure similar to that found in amino acids, which when administered can then cross-link and destabilize the bacterium cell wall. Because there is no analogous structure in human cells, these antibiotics can be given at much higher doses without fear of toxicity.

Note

To replicate DNA, folic acid is required. Bacteria are required to make their own folic acid from para-aminobenzoic acid (PABA). Trimethoprim and the sulfonamides block this process.

[Know:] Antibacterial agents must be 'cidal for effective treatment of endocarditis, meningitis, and for treatment of infected neutropenic patients. Bactericidal antibiotics are the beta-lactams (PCNs, imipenem, and cephalosporins), fluoroquinolones, vancomycin, aminoglycosides, rifampin, and metronidazole. Bacteriostatic agents are erythromycin, tetracycline, and clindamycin. Chloramphenicol is unusual in that it is normally bacteriostatic, but it is 'cidal against *H. influenzae*, pneumococci, and meningococci!

BETA-LACTAM ANTIBIOTICS

Overview

The 1st of the beta-lactam antibiotics was penicillin (PCN). They now include the semisynthetic PCNs (methicillin, oxacillin, and cloxacillin), carbapenems, and cephalosporins. Because the bacteria rupture when the integrity of the cell wall is decreased, these drugs are also bactericidal.

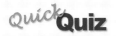

Quick Quiz

- Name an antibiotic that targets the DNA gyrase of bacteria.
- Which antibiotics bind to the 50S ribosomal subunit?
- Which antibiotics interfere with folic acid production/recycling in the bacteria?
- What are the bacteriostatic agents?
- What organism is common in cat bites?
- What are the criteria for implementing antibiotics for a bite?
- What is the drug of choice for bite wounds?
- Name common infections for which penicillin is still the drug of choice?
- True or false? IV cefazolin is a good choice for VP shunt infections.

Penicillins

Penicillin, as noted above, has the beta-lactam ring. It is very active against meningococci, most streptococci (groups A and B, viridans group, and *S. pneumoniae*), *Pasteurella* (dog and especially cat bites), and many *Neisseria* species. It is also active against many anaerobes (such as *Clostridium*), but not *B. fragilis*. [Know:] Even though PCN is indicated for meningococcal infections, ceftriaxone, rifampin, or quinolones are better for eradication of the carrier state. Rifampin concentrates in the upper respiratory mucosa.

Resistance develops via production of beta-lactamases (*Haemophilus influenzae*) and alteration in penicillin-binding proteins (*Streptococcus pneumoniae*).

More on cat/dog bites—when to give antibiotics:

- Moderate or severe bite wounds
- Crush injury
- Puncture wounds (nearly all cat bites)
- Facial bites
- Hand and foot bites
- Genital area bites
- Immunocompromised child

Besides *Pasteurella*, *Staphylococcus aureus* is a likely organism, so most recommend amoxicillin-clavulanate as the drug of choice for bite wounds; if PCN-allergic, use cephalosporin or TMP/SMX + clindamycin. For human bites, the main organisms are streptococci, *S. aureus*, *Eikenella corrodens*, and anaerobes. Always treat human bites with antibiotics.

PCN is still the drug of choice for many infections. [Know:]

- Periodontal infections
- Erysipeloid (*Erysipelothrix rhusiopathiae*)
- Group A and group B streptococci
- Rat-bite fever
- Syphilis
- Yaws
- Leptospirosis
- Actinomycosis
- Meningococcal meningitis and meningococcemia

Ampicillin has a spectrum similar to that of PCN, but its spectrum extends to include certain gram-negative rods—especially some *E. coli*, *H. influenzae*, *Salmonella*, *Shigella*, and *Proteus mirabilis*. However, it does not cover *Klebsiella*, and many of the *H. influenzae*, *E. coli*, and *P. mirabilis* are now resistant to it.

Ampicillin is the drug of choice for:

- *Listeria monocytogenes* meningitis
- Salmonellosis—if sensitive (increasing resistance though!)
- UTIs due to susceptible organisms
- Enterococcal infections

Penicillinase-resistant semisynthetic PCNs like nafcillin and oxacillin are needed against *S. aureus* because 85% have beta-lactamase. (Note: Penicillinase is just a specific type of beta-lactamase.) Unfortunately, there has been a rapidly expanding resistance to these in staphylococci; i.e., "methicillin-resistant". Nafcillin is similar to methicillin, but it is not as likely to cause interstitial nephritis (so methicillin is rarely used). Nafcillin and oxacillin are drugs of choice only for staphylococcal infections.

Antipseudomonal PCNs (AP-PCN: ticarcillin-clavulanate, piperacillin-tazobactam) are better against the gram-negative organisms (including *Pseudomonas*) and anaerobes (including *B. fragilis*).

Antipseudomonal PCNs: They are the only PCN drugs effective against infections caused by:

- *P. aeruginosa*
- *Acinetobacter*

Cephalosporins

Note

Cephalosporins also contain the beta-lactam ring but are penicillinase-resistant. In general, cephalosporins have no activity against enterococci, *Listeria*, and methicillin-resistant staphylococci.

1st Generation

1st generation cephalosporins (cefazolin, cephalothin, cephapirin) are active against most *Staphylococcus aureus* (including the lactamase-producing strains, excluding the methicillin-resistant strains) and most streptococci. Really, there is no anaerobic activity or reliable CNS penetrations, so do not use for meningitis or ventriculoperitoneal (VP) shunt infections. 1st generation are also effective against many of the community-acquired *E. coli*, *Klebsiella*, and *Proteus*. (The gram-negative coverage is superior to ampicillin.) Cephalothin increases the nephrotoxicity of concurrently administered aminoglycosides. Commonly given for:

- Skin and soft tissue infections
- Some surgical prophylaxis

2nd Generation

All 2nd generation cephalosporins are more active against the gram-negative organisms (e.g., good against *H. influenzae*) and less active against gram-positive bacteria.

Parenteral: All of the 2nd generation cephalosporins—cefoxitin, cefotetan, cefamandole, etc. (except cefuroxime [Zinacef®]) have variable activity against gut anaerobes. None of the 2nd generation cephalosporins consistently cross into the CSF; so, they are not used to treat meningitis.

2nd generation cephalosporins have good activity against *H. influenzae*, *Neisseria* (although gonococcal resistance is increasing), and gram-positive organisms. They are among drugs of choice for:

- PID (Although gonococcal resistance is increasing, the CDC now recommends 3rd generation ceftriaxone + azithromycin or doxycycline as gonococcal treatment of choice.)
- Abdominal surgery

Know that 3rd generation cephalosporins have largely replaced 2nd generation. Exception: abdominal/pelvic infections, because of the better anaerobic coverage of the 2nd generation cephalosporins.

3rd Generation

3rd generation cephalosporins (3GCs) are especially resistant to beta-lactamase and are especially effective against *N. gonorrhoeae* and *H. influenzae*. They also are effective against most of the *Enterobacteriaceae* (*E. coli*, *Klebsiella*, *Proteus*, *Enterobacter*, and *Serratia*).

3GCs are not active against *S. aureus*. Of all of the cephalosporins, only some of the 3GCs are active against *Pseudomonas*—especially ceftazidime (Fortaz®). But ceftazidime is not reliably effective against *S. pneumoniae*.

Note, however, that in the latest febrile neutropenia guidelines, ceftazidime is no longer recommended as a 1st line agent for empiric therapy because of inferior outcomes with this agent! Recommended gram-negative coverage for patients with fever and neutropenia include piperacillin-tazobactam (Zosyn®), cefepime, or a carbapenem.

Ceftriaxone (Rocephin®) has the longest half-life and is effective against most *S. pneumoniae*, but it is not effective against *Pseudomonas*.

There are four 3rd generation cephalosporins that can cross an inflamed blood-brain barrier and thus are indicated as the primary therapy for meningitis caused by *Enterobacteriaceae*. These are:

1) Ceftriaxone
2) Cefotaxime (Claforan®)
3) Ceftizoxime (Cefizox®)
4) Ceftazidime

Remember: Ceftriaxone is no longer used as a single agent for empiric treatment of meningitis. For neonatal, elderly, and pregnant patients, add ampicillin to cover *Listeria* and enterococci. For patients with presumed resistant *S. pneumoniae* meningitis, add vancomycin until proven otherwise.

Advanced Generation

Advanced generation cephalosporins. Cefepime (Maxipime®) is a broad-spectrum antibiotic with enhanced stability to cephalosporinases. It has the gram-negative activity of 3rd generation cephalosporins and the gram-positive activity of 1st generation cephalosporins. Plus, it has limited anaerobic coverage. Ceftaroline (Teflaro®) was approved in 2011 for community-acquired pneumonia and skin and soft tissue infections in patients ≥ 18. It is the 1st cephalosporin with activity against MRSA.

Carbapenems

Carbapenems have the broadest spectrum of antibacterial activity of the beta-lactams antibiotics. Carbapenems are very resistant to beta-lactamases and are the drugs of choice for extended-spectrum beta lactamase (ESBL) producing organisms—which are resistant to penicillins and cephalosporins.

Imipenem is a very broad-spectrum carbapenem antibiotic. It is very active against *B. fragilis*. It kills most *Enterobacteriaceae*, *Pseudomonas*, and gram-positive organisms and is inhibitory for *Listeria* and *Enterococcus faecalis*. The few organisms resistant to it include *Enterococcus faecium*, *Corynebacterium jeikeium* (JK), *Stenotrophomonas maltophilia*, and methicillin-resistant staphylococci. Now, ~ 20% of *P. aeruginosa* are also resistant. [Know:] Imipenem can lower the seizure threshold, so it should be used only as a last resort in seizure patients or in patients with renal insufficiency.

Imipenem is always formulated with equal amounts of cilastatin (combo = Primaxin®). Cilastatin causes metabolism of imipenem to be blocked in the renal tubule, thereby increasing its half-life to 1 hour! Cilastatin has no effect on beta-lactamases.

Meropenem is a similar carbapenem with a longer half-life, so there's no need for an enzyme inhibitor. It is also less likely than imipenem to cause seizures. Meropenem is also the drug of choice for *Burkholderia cepacia* infections (seen in patients with CF and chronic granulomatous disease).

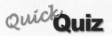

Quiz

- What antibiotics are good for PID?
- Which is better for *S. pneumoniae*—ceftriaxone or ceftazidime?
- Which is better for *Pseudomonas*—ceftriaxone or ceftazidime?
- What group of patients should receive imipenem only as a last resort?
- Why is cilastatin combined with imipenem?
- What is the "red man syndrome"?
- Which antibiotics have "the postantibiotic effect"?

Ertapenem is approved for intraabdominal infections, skin infections, community-acquired pneumonia, complicated UTI/pyelonephritis, and acute pelvic infections. It is not active against *Pseudomonas*. Its seizure risk is 0.5%.

Doripenem was approved in 2012 for treatment of complicated intraabdominal or complicated urinary tract infections. Doripenem also does not require cilastatin. It has very strong activity against *Pseudomonas*.

Aztreonam

Aztreonam is a monobactam, which is good only against aerobic and facultative, gram-negative bacteria. Its spectrum is similar to aminoglycosides (gram-negative aerobes). It is effective against most *Enterobacteriaceae* and *Pseudomonas*, but it is not active against gram-positive cocci or anaerobes.

Beta-lactamase Inhibitors

Beta-lactamase inhibitors include:

- Sulbactam
- Clavulanic acid
- Tazobactam

These inhibitors bind irreversibly to the beta-lactamase made by some bacteria. They increase the activity of drugs against beta-lactamase producing bacteria such as *B. fragilis*, *Klebsiella*, and *S. aureus* (variably).

Formulations using the beta-lactamase inhibitors:

- Clavulanic acid mixed with amoxicillin (Augmentin®, Clavulin®)
- Clavulanic acid mixed with ticarcillin (Timentin®)
- Sulbactam mixed with ampicillin (Unasyn®)
- Tazobactam mixed with piperacillin (Zosyn®, Tazocin®)

OTHER ANTIBIOTICS

Vancomycin

Vancomycin is, in general, bactericidal, although less so than beta-lactams. Vancomycin is effective against most gram-positive organisms, including methicillin-resistant staphylococci, *Clostridia*, and *Corynebacteria*. There are some vancomycin-resistant strains of enterococci and recent reports of vancomycin-resistant *S. aureus*. (Yikes!) *Staphylococcus haemolyticus* and a few *Staphylococcus epidermidis* are resistant (causing serious trouble in some endocarditis patients).

Vancomycin sometimes causes the "red man syndrome," which consists of tachycardia, flushing, occasional angioedema, and generalized pruritus. You can prevent this either by slowing down the infusion time or by pretreatment with antihistamines (but not H_2 blockers). Nephrotoxicity is also a common side effect, especially when an aminoglycoside is used concurrently.

Aminoglycosides

Aminoglycosides are effective against many gram-negative organisms. They require the aerobic mechanism of the cell to be effective, so they are no good against anaerobes. Aminoglycosides have a persistent, antigram-negative effect after removal of the drug—known as the postantibiotic effect! So, it is possible to dose aminoglycosides q 24 hours with equivalent or better results than the same total daily dosage given more often. Because they irreversibly inhibit ribosomal protein synthesis, they are bactericidal.

Aminoglycosides are effective against *Yersinia pestis* plague and *Francisella tularensis* (streptomycin or gentamicin), *M. tuberculosis* (streptomycin or amikacin), and *M. avium-intracellulare* (amikacin). Gentamicin is often used in combination with a beta-lactam antibiotic for the treatment of subacute bacterial endocarditis. Gentamicin can be given along with rifampin to prevent the rapid development of resistance to rifampin (as in prosthetic valve endocarditis). It is also given to febrile neutropenic patients, along with either a 3rd generation cephalosporin or antipseudomonal penicillin.

Major side effects of aminoglycoside treatment are ear toxicity and kidney toxicity—these are more likely if either amphotericin B or cephalothin is also used!

Fluoroquinolones

Fluoroquinolones (ciprofloxacin, norfloxacin, ofloxacin, levofloxacin, sparfloxacin, moxifloxacin, gemifloxacin) are a set of very-wide-spectrum antibiotics that inhibit bacterial DNA synthesis. They are very good against gram-negative, aerobic organisms—including rods. They are not FDA-approved for children < 18 years of age, except in special cases (e.g., CF, topical therapy for external otitis, anthrax exposure). However, in 2004, ciprofloxacin was approved for children < 18 years of age as 2nd line therapy for complicated UTI and pyelonephritis. To date there have been no published reports of cartilage damage in children as in adults.

An important fluoroquinolone adverse effect is Achilles tendon rupture when used concurrently with steroids and in patients who have received renal, heart, or lung transplants.

Indications for fluoroquinolones in adults:

• Ciprofloxacin, ofloxacin, and the newer agents can be used for systemic infections.
• Fluoroquinolones are also good against all the usual causes of bacterial gastroenteritis (*Salmonella, Shigella, Campylobacter*, and *Yersinia enterocolitica*).

Fluoroquinolones are not effective in the following instances:

• They are not good against anaerobes (*B. fragilis*, etc.).
• Ciprofloxacin and ofloxacin have only intermediate activity against gram-positive organisms, including *S. pneumoniae*. Hence, they are not a good choice for empiric treatment of pneumonia. (On the other hand, levofloxacin, moxifloxacin, and gatifloxacin are alternative choices for community-acquired pneumonia. The newer fluoroquinolones are also effective treatment for atypical pneumonias.)
• They are not used for MRSA because of the widespread, rapid development of resistance to them.
• Again, do not give to children. (The FDA says give to no one < 18 years of age, except for anthrax and UTI. The CDC has approved quinolone use in adolescents for STDs, but they are no longer approved for treatment of gonorrhea!)
• Never use in pregnant patients.

[Know:] Some fluoroquinolones increase the levels of theophylline and cyclosporine by decreasing metabolism and increasing the effect of warfarin by an uncertain mechanism. They do not increase the elimination of any drug.

Macrolides

Erythromycin is a drug to consider for community-acquired pneumonia because it is effective against *S. pneumoniae* (although there is increasing resistance), *Mycoplasma pneumoniae*, and *Legionella pneumophila*. It is also effective against *Chlamydophila pneumoniae*, *Campylobacter* (diarrhea), diphtheria, and pertussis. It is not so good against *H. influenzae* and is not effective against Q fever (*Coxiella burnetii*), which is treated with tetracycline or chloramphenicol. Like the quinolones, erythromycin increases the effect of theophylline, cyclosporine, and warfarin. Erythromycin also has been shown to increase risk of pyloric stenosis.

Azithromycin has the same indications as erythromycin—and it has better *H. influenzae* coverage. It has a very long half-life (hence, a once-per-day dosage) and is available in an IV form.

Tetracyclines

Tetracyclines (including doxycycline) are the drugs of choice for RMSF, *Ehrlichia*, and *Anaplasma* infections. They are also used to treat cholera and anthrax, as well as for malarial prophylaxis. Remember that prolonged use results in teeth staining in children < 8 years of age, but single therapeutic courses can be justified in children for the above indications.

Trimethoprim/Sulfamethoxazole

Trimethoprim/sulfamethoxazole is effective in therapy of most outpatient UTIs and is the drug of choice for *Pneumocystis*. It can cause bone marrow suppression and hypersensitivity reactions, including Stevens-Johnson syndrome. Do not use in children < 2 months of age.

Clindamycin

Clindamycin is the drug of choice for anaerobic lung infections. It is useful for MSSA and MRSA as well as streptococcal infection; thus, it is quite beneficial in treatment of bone infections in children. However, *S. aureus* clindamycin-resistance rates are rising, which may limit its use in the future.

Rifampin

Rifampin is bactericidal. It is never given alone to treat an acute infection because organisms rapidly develop resistance to it. Rifampin is used for prophylaxis, as in meningococcal infection or invasive *Haemophilus influenzae* infection. Rifampin causes secretions and urine to turn orange. Rifampin also interacts with other drugs and can make birth control pills ineffective.

Oxazolidinones

Oxazolidinones are an entirely new class of antibiotic, of which linezolid (Zyvox®) is the 1st available. They have a unique mechanism of action for the blocking of protein synthesis. The drug binds to the 50S ribosomal subunit, thereby preventing attachment of the 30S + mRNA subunit; so, the 70S ribosome initiation complex is not made and no protein is produced.

Linezolid is active against gram-positive organisms, including MRSA (methicillin-resistant *S. aureus*) and multidrug resistant pneumococcus. It is also effective against VRE (vancomycin-resistant enterococci) and anaerobes. Linezolid is available in oral (with 100% bioavailability) and IV preparations. The oral form makes it a desirable alternative to vancomycin for MRSA. However, concerns of developing resistance and the cost make this drug an unlikely 1st line agent. Toxicities include bone marrow suppression and neuropathy (including optic neuritis).

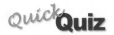

• For what indications have fluoroquinolones been approved for children?

• What electrolyte abnormalities are associated with amphotericin B use?

• Which systemic imidazoles are usually given for serious fungal infections?

Streptogramins

Quinupristin/dalfopristin (Synercid®) is the 1st of this new class of antibiotics. It was the 1st antibiotic approved for the treatment of serious infections with vancomycin-resistant *Enterococcus faecium*. The main side effects with this antibiotic are severe myalgias and arthralgias.

Cyclic Lipopeptides

Daptomycin (Cubicin®) is approved for skin/soft tissue infections and bacteremia or right-sided endocarditis due to MSSA or MRSA in adults. Do not use for pneumonia.

ANTIVIRAL AGENTS

Acyclovir is a nucleoside analog that selectively inhibits the replication of HSV (Types 1 and 2) and VZV. After intracellular uptake, it is converted to acyclovir monophosphate by virally encoded thymidine kinase; this step does not occur to any significant degree in uninfected cells and thereby lends specificity to the drug's activity. The monophosphate derivative is subsequently converted to acyclovir triphosphate by cellular enzymes. Acute renal failure can occur by the precipitation of the IV form in the renal tubules; this is prevented by adequate hydration. Valacyclovir and famciclovir have similar indications.

Ganciclovir (previously DHPG) is used for the treatment of CMV infections in AIDS patients, especially for chorioretinitis and colitis. Leukopenia is a side effect. Because it has only a suppressive effect against CMV, it usually needs to be given until the CD4 lymphocytes are > 200. Valganciclovir is also used to treat CMV (oral).

Foscarnet is used in patients with acyclovir-resistant herpes infection or as an alternative to ganciclovir for CMV. However, it is associated with nephrotoxicity and electrolyte abnormalities.

Ribavirin is indicated for the treatment of RSV (not used much anymore) and is used as part of combination therapy for hepatitis C.

Amantadine and rimantadine may or may not be effective against influenza A, depending on the strain, and definitely are not effective for influenza B!

Oseltamivir (Tamiflu®—oral) and zanamivir (Relenza®—powder for inhalation) are neuraminidase inhibitors and are useful for treatment of many influenza A and B strains (but resistance can develop).

ANTIFUNGAL AGENTS

Overview

There are 4 major classes of antifungal medicines: polyenes, imidazoles, triazoles, and the echinocandins.

Polyenes

Systemic polyene: Amphotericin B is the standard treatment for most systemic mycoses. Systemic amphotericin B can be given only by IV, and it has many side effects: fever, renal failure, phlebitis, acidosis, and low K^+ and Mg. Again! Amphotericin B is associated with electrolyte abnormalities—especially hypokalemia, hypomagnesemia, and renal tubular acidosis. Some recommend giving a test dose first. Hypotension with the 1st dose may occur (decrease in peripheral vascular tone).

Lipid-associated amphotericin B preparations are less nephrotoxic but much more expensive. Depending on the center, some have switched to lipid-associated formulations, while others prefer to use them only when toxicity has become a problem with regular amphotericin.

Topical polyene macrolides: Nystatin and amphotericin topical formulations are good only against cutaneous candidiasis (not ringworm). Both are also available in liquid form for oral and esophageal candidiasis.

Imidazoles

Systemic Imidazole

Ketoconazole for systemic use is given orally—increased gastric pH (low acid) decreases absorption. Absorption is not affected by food. Ketoconazole does not penetrate CSF well. It is occasionally used for palliative treatment of Cushing syndrome caused by ectopic production of ACTH (i.e., cancer) because it blocks the 11-hydroxylase enzyme in the adrenal gland, thereby decreasing the amount of cortisol produced.

Ketoconazole increases levels of indinavir and digoxin—and potentiates benzodiazepines. Side effects of ketoconazole include nausea and hepatitis. It also causes a decrease in androgen production, so patients may have decreased libido and males may develop gynecomastia.

Ketoconazole is cheaper than fluconazole and itraconazole but has largely been replaced by these 2 drugs for serious fungal infections. It has many interactions with common drugs—sometimes dangerous.

Topical Imidazoles

Clotrimazole and miconazole are available in both cutaneous and vaginal preparations. Other cutaneous imidazoles are ketoconazole, econazole, sulconazole, and oxiconazole. Other vaginal formulations are butoconazole and tioconazole. Spectrum and efficacy are the same. All are effective in the treatment of cutaneous candidiasis, tinea versicolor, and ringworm.

Triazoles

Systemic Triazoles

Itraconazole (Sporanox®) is a triazole analog of ketoconazole and is generally more effective and safer. The liquid formulation has much better bioavailability. Food enhances absorption. Indications are the same as ketoconazole (histoplasmosis, blastomycosis, coccidioidomycosis, esophageal candidiasis, and chronic mucocutaneous candidiasis), but also include aspergillosis, cryptococcosis, sporotrichosis, and onychomycosis.

[Know.] Fluconazole (Diflucan®): The main side effect is N/V. A single 150 mg oral dose is effective in vulvovaginal candidiasis. Fluconazole is also effective treatment for oral and esophageal candidiasis and candidemia. It has excellent penetration into the CSF, and it is often used for maintenance therapy in AIDS patients with cryptococcal meningitis—after an initial 2-week course of IV amphotericin B. Fluconazole is the treatment of choice for chronic coccidioidomycosis.

Voriconazole (Vfend®): The FDA approved the clinical use of voriconazole in May 2002 for primary treatment of acute, invasive aspergillosis and salvage therapy for rare, but serious, fungal infections caused by the pathogens *Scedosporium apiospermum* and *Fusarium.*

Posaconazole (Noxafil®) is approved for those ≥ 13 years of age for oropharyngeal candidiasis and prophylaxis in immunocompromised for *Aspergillus* and *Candida*.

Topical Triazoles

Vaginal formulation: terconazole (Terazol®).

Echinocandins

Caspofungin acetate (Cancidas®) is the 1st of a new class of drugs called echinocandins—a glucan synthesis inhibitor. In patients 3 months and older, it is used to treat esophageal or invasive candidiasis. It is also approved as empiric antifungal therapy in febrile, neutropenic patients.

In adults, it is used to treat aspergillosis.

Caspofungin acetate has poor CSF and renal parenchyma penetration.

Micafungin (Mycamine®) is approved by the FDA to treat esophageal candidiasis and prophylaxis of invasive *Candida* infections in patients undergoing hematopoietic stem cell transplantation. Anidulafungin (Eraxis™) is approved for treatment of candidemia and esophageal candidiasis.

Other Antifungals

Other Systemic Antifungals

Flucytosine (5-fluorocytosine; 5-FC) is highly soluble and penetrates well into the CSF. Upon entering a fungal cell, it is metabolized to the antimetabolite 5-fluorouracil. If used alone, drug resistance develops quickly. For this reason, and because it may have a synergistic antifungal effect with amphotericin B, it is combined with amphotericin B to treat cryptococcosis and serious forms of candidiasis. It can cause serious GI, hepatic, renal, and bone marrow toxicities—the latter usually presents as neutropenia and thrombocytopenia. Drug levels should be monitored. Slight decreases in renal function can increase 5-FC to toxic levels.

Other Topical Antifungals

Undecylenic acid and **tolnaftate** are effective only against ringworm. The following cutaneous preparations have the same efficacy and clinical spectrum as the imidazoles: naftifine, terbinafine, haloprogin, and ciclopirox olamine.

ANTIPARASITIC DRUGS

Praziquantel (Biltricide®) is the only drug effective against all species of *Schistosoma*, and so it is the drug of choice for schistosomiasis. It is also good against flukes and tapeworms (i.e., used to treat neurocysticercosis caused by the pork tapeworm, *T. solium*).

Albendazole is now used for cysticercosis and schistosomiasis.

Niclosamide is also used for the treatment of tapeworm, but it affects only those in the intestine.

Pentamidine, which is used for treatment (IV form) and prophylaxis (inhaled form) of *Pneumocystis jiroveci* (which is most likely a fungus), has many side effects, including azotemia (25%), leukopenia, pancreatitis, and hypo- or hyperglycemia. It causes no significant skin reactions.

Nitazoxanide (Alinia®) is approved in children ≥ 1 year for diarrhea due to *Cryptosporidium* or *Giardia*.

Antimalaria drugs: See malaria on page 5-34.

VACCINES

For vaccines, see Growth and Development/Preventive Pediatrics, Book 1.

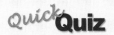

Quick**Quiz**

- What is the drug of choice for schistosomiasis?
- Which antibiotics should you never give to a pregnant woman?

ANTIBIOTICS AND THE PREGNANT OR BREASTFEEDING WOMAN

Many antibiotics cross the placenta or into breast milk. Only tetracycline has definite contraindications in the breastfeeding mother. And tetracycline and quinolones are definitely not given to pregnant women. Also, many avoid the use of aminoglycosides and chloramphenicol in pregnant or nursing mothers because of the concern of side effects with these drugs in the infant. Sulfa drugs are generally avoided near term. Do not give mothers of breastfeeding infants who have G6PD nitrofurantoin or primaquine to minimize the risk of hemolysis in the infant.

PREVENTION OF INFECTIOUS DISEASES

OVERVIEW

Know measures to control the spread of infections, including appropriate use of the different types of precautions and which illnesses require and do not require exclusion from child care centers.

Child Care Centers

Infants and children cared for in child care settings have an increased rate of communicable infectious diseases as well as an increased risk of acquiring antibiotic-resistant organisms. Child care programs should require that all enrollees and staff members receive age-appropriate immunizations and routine health care. Most mild or minor illnesses do not require exclusion from child care.

General recommendations for exclusion of children from child care include:

- Illness preventing participation in activities
- Illness requiring need for care greater than staff can provide
- Severe illness with fever, behavioral changes, lethargy, persistent crying, difficulty breathing, progressive rash
- Persistent abdominal pain (≥ 2 hours) or intermittent pain with fever, dehydration, or systemic signs
- Vomiting in preceding 24 hours
- Diarrhea if stool not contained in diaper, stool frequency > 2 or more stools above normal for that child, or stools containing blood or mucus
- Oral lesions (if unable to contain drool)
- Skin lesions (especially if on exposed skin and unable to cover)
- Fever (Many day cares exclude children with temperatures > 100.4° F.)

Disease-specific exclusions of children from child care:

- Hepatitis A virus: exclusion until 1 week after onset of jaundice
- Impetigo: exclusion until 24 hours after antibiotic started; cover lesions with watertight dressing
- Measles: exclusion until 4 days after onset of rash
- Mumps: exclusion until 5 days after onset of parotid swelling
- Pediculosis capitis (head lice): treatment at end of program day and readmission on completion of 1st treatment
- Pertussis: exclusion until 5 days of appropriate antibiotics completed
- Rubella: exclusion until 6 days after onset of rash for postnatal infection
- *Salmonella* typhi: exclusion until diarrhea resolves and 3 negative stool cultures are obtained
- Non-typhi *Salmonella*: exclusion until diarrhea resolves; negative stool cultures not required for readmission
- Scabies: exclusion until after treatment is given
- Shiga toxin-producing *Escherichia coli* (STEC) including *E. coli* O157:H7, or *Shigella* infection: exclusion until diarrhea resolves and 2 negative stool cultures
- *Staphylococcus aureus* infections: exclusion only if skin lesions are draining and cannot be covered by a watertight dressing
- Streptococcal pharyngitis: exclusion until 24 hours after antibiotics have been started
- Tuberculosis (active): exclusion until deemed not infectious by physician or health department; no exclusion for latent TB
- Varicella-zoster virus: exclusion until all lesions have dried and crusted (usually 6 days after rash onset in the immunocompetent but may be longer in the immunocompromised)

Hospital and Office Infection Control

For the exams and actual patient care, you should know the appropriate use of the following infection control measures.

Standard (Universal) Precautions

Used for all patients to prevent transmission of all infectious agents through contact with any body fluid, nonintact skin, or mucous membranes. Includes the following practices:

- Hand hygiene (before and after all patient contact).
- Gloves (clean, nonsterile) should be worn when touching blood, body fluids, secretions, excretions, and items contaminated with these fluids.

- Masks, eye protection, and face shields should be worn to protect mucous membranes during procedures and patient care activities.
- Nonsterile gowns that are fluid-resistant to protect skin and prevent soiling of clothing during procedures and patient care activities.
- Patient care equipment that has been used should be handled in a manner that prevents skin or mucous membrane exposure or contamination of clothing.
- All used textiles (linens) are considered to be contaminated and should be handled, transported, and processed appropriately.
- Follow safe injection practices when handling needles, scalpels, or other sharp instruments to avoid bloodborne pathogen exposure.
- Mouthpieces, resuscitation bags, and other ventilation devices should be available for all patients. No mouth-to-mouth resuscitation.

Transmission-Based Precautions

Transmission-based precautions are designed for patients with documented or suspected colonization or infection with pathogens for which additional precautions beyond standard precautions are necessary.

Airborne Transmission

Airborne transmission occurs by dissemination of airborne droplet nuclei (≤ 5 μm), which contain microorganisms that remain suspended in the air (e.g., *Mycobacterium tuberculosis*, rubeola [measles], and varicella-zoster virus). Patients should be in a room with special ventilation (negative pressure) and health care personnel (HCP) should wear N95 respirators.

Droplet Transmission

Droplet transmission occurs when droplets containing microorganisms generated from an infected person during coughing, sneezing, talking, or during a procedure (suctioning or bronchoscopy) are propelled a short distance (≤ 3 feet) and deposited onto mucous membranes. HCP should wear masks and gowns if coming within 3 feet of the patient. Examples of infections requiring droplet precautions include adenovirus conjunctivitis/pneumonia, diphtheria (pharyngeal), influenza, *Mycoplasma*, invasive *Neisseria meningitidis* or *Haemophilus influenzae* type b, and pertussis.

Contact Transmission

Contact transmission can be direct (person-to-person) or indirect (contact of susceptible host to inanimate object or fomite). HCP should wear gowns and gloves. Some infections where contact precautions are advised include *C. difficile*, MRSA, herpes simplex virus, herpes zoster, RSV, rotavirus.

Infections Transmitted Via Breast Milk

Mothers who are positive for human T-cell lymphotrophic virus type I or II or untreated brucellosis should not breast-feed nor give expressed breast milk to their infants.

Mothers who have untreated tuberculosis (infectious) or have HSV lesions on their breast should not breast-feed but can provide expressed milk for their infants. Breastfeeding can resume when a mother with TB has been treated x 2 weeks or is documented to be no longer infectious.

Mothers with onset of varicella 5 days before through 2 days after delivery should be separated from their infants but can provide them with expressed breast milk.

In developed countries, where infant formula is readily available, HIV-infected women should not breastfeed. In developing countries, where mortality is increased in nonbreastfed infants from a combination of malnutrition and infectious diseases, breastfeeding may outweigh the risks of acquiring HIV and is recommended by the WHO.

CMV can be shed intermittently in human milk. Very-low-birth-weight infants are at the greatest risk of developing symptomatic disease. Decisions about breastfeeding premature infants by mothers known to be CMV-seropositive should take into consideration the benefits of breast milk and risk of CMV transmission.

In infants born to HBsAg positive women, immunoprophylaxis with HBV vaccine and HBIG should effectively eliminate the risk of HBV transmission from breastfeeding. Maternal hepatitis C virus (HCV) infection is not a contraindication to breastfeeding because this mode of transmission has not been documented.

EVALUATION OF INTERNATIONAL ADOPTEES

OVERVIEW

Know how to perform an appropriate infectious disease screening and immunization schedule for an internationally adopted child.

In recent years, more than 90% of international adoptees are from Asia (China, South Korea, Vietnam, India, Kazakhstan, and the Philippines); Latin America and the Caribbean (Guatemala, Columbia, and Haiti); Eastern Europe (Russia and Ukraine); and Africa (Ethiopia, Nigeria, Liberia, and Ghana). Many of these children have unknown medical histories prior to adoption and have had limited health care; evaluation can be a challenge.

Before arriving in the U.S., all internationally adopted children are required to have a medical evaluation performed by a physician designated by the U.S. Department of State in their country of origin. This exam is limited to screening for certain communicable diseases and examination for serious defects or mental defects. Immigrants

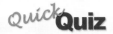

Quiz

- For which infections should mothers not breastfeed?
- How are tuberculin skin tests evaluated differently in an international adoptee who was vaccinated with BCG as an infant?

are also required to provide "proof of vaccination" with vaccines recommended by the Advisory Committee on Immunization Practices (ACIP) prior to entry into the U.S. Parents of internationally adopted children < 10 years of age or from countries not part of the Hague Convention can sign a waiver of exemption from vaccination prior to entering the U.S.; however, they have to sign another waiver indicating they will have the child vaccinated in the U.S. according to ACIP guidelines.

Infectious diseases are common in international adoptees, and it is recommended that they be screened for the following (preferably within 2 weeks) after arrival to the U.S:

- HBsAg
- Hepatitis C serology
- RPR
- HIV
- CBC
- Stool for ova and parasites (especially for *Giardia* and *Cryptosporidium*)
- TB skin test
- *Trypanosoma cruzi* serology (in children from countries with endemic infection)
- Serology for lymphatic filariasis (children > 2 years of age from endemic countries)
- In children with eosinophilia and negative stool ova and parasite exams:
  - *Strongyloides* serology
  - *Schistosoma* serology (for sub-Saharan Africa, Southeast Asia, certain Latin American adoptees)

Immunizations

In general, only written documentation of vaccines given to an adoptee with the date of administration, number of doses, intervals between doses, and age of the child at the time of immunization are acceptable evidence of adequacy of immunization. Bacille Calmette-Guérin (BCG), DTP or DTaP, poliovirus, measles, and hepatitis B vaccines are given routinely in many parts of the world. Other vaccines such as *Haemophilus influenzae* type b (HIB), *Streptococcus pneumoniae* (Prevnar® or Pneumovax®23), mumps, rubella, varicella, and hepatitis A are given less often and may not be part of routine immunization in some countries. Although there are some vaccines with less potency used in some countries, most vaccines worldwide are of adequate quality and are reliable.

When evaluating these children, give the parents the option of either:

- testing for antibody response to the vaccines that were documented and then doing "catch–up" immunizations for what they are lacking, or
- if the child is still an infant, starting the immunization schedule all over again according to U.S. standards.

Remember, many of these children are vaccinated with BCG as infants, and if they ever have to be evaluated for TB exposure, you should ignore this fact and interpret their TST test as if they never had BCG!

FOR FURTHER READING

BACTERIA: GRAM-POSITIVE

American Academy of Pediatrics. Staphylococcal Infections. In: Pickering LK, Baker CJ, Kimberlin DW, Long SS, eds. *Red Book®: 2012 Report of the Committee on Infectious Diseases*, 29th edition. Elk Grove Village, IL: 2012: 653–668.

Berk DR, Bayliss SJ. MRSA, staphylococcal scalded skin syndrome, and other cutaneous bacterial emergencies. *Pediatr Ann*. 2010 Oct;39(10):627–633.

Jackson MA, Newland JG. Staphylococcal infections in the era of MRSA. *Pediatr Rev*. 2011 Dec;32(12):522–532.

Liu C, et al. Clinical practice guidelines by the Infectious Diseases Society of America for the treatment of methicillin-resistant *Staphylococcus aureus* infections in adults and children: executive summary. *Clin Infect Dis*. 2011 Feb 1;52(3):285–292.

Liu C, et al. Clinical practice guidelines by the Infectious Diseases Society of America for the treatment of methicillin-resistant *Staphylococcus aureus* infections in adults and children. *Clin Infect Dis*. 2011 Feb 1;52(3):e18–e55.

American Academy of Pediatrics. Staphylococcal Food Poisoning. In: Pickering LK, Baker CJ, Kimberlin DW, Long SS, eds. *Red Book®: 2012 Report of the Committee on Infectious Diseases*, 29th edition. Elk Grove Village, IL: 2012: 652.

Rogers KL, et al. Coagulase-negative staphylococcal infections. *Infect Dis Clin North Am*. 2009 Mar;23(1):73–98.

Nuorti JP, et al. Prevention of pneumococcal disease among infants and children—use of 13-valent pneumococcal conjugate vaccine and 23-valent pneumococcal polysaccharide vaccine—recommendations of the Advisory Committee on Immunization Practices (ACIP). *MMWR Recomm Rep*. 2010 Dec 10;59 (RR-11):1–18.

Baker CJ, et al. Policy statement—recommendations for the prevention of perinatal group B streptococcal (GBS) disease. *Pediatrics*. 2011 Sep;128(3):611–616.

Doern CD, Burnham CA. It's not easy being green: the viridans group streptococci, with a focus on pediatric clinical manifestations. *J Clin Microbiol*. 2010 Nov;48(11):3829–3835.

Weinberg AN. Group C and group G streptococcal infection. *UpToDate*. 2010.

Bottone EJ. *Bacillus cereus*, a volatile human pathogen. *Clin Microbiol Rev*. 2010 Apr;23(2):382–398.

Cohen SH, et al. Clinical practice guidelines for *Clostridium difficile* infection in adults: 2010 update by the Society for Healthcare Epidemiology of America (SHEA) and the Infectious Diseases Society of America (IDSA). *Infect Control Hosp Epidemiol*. 2010 May;31(5):431–455.

Dubberke ER, et al. Strategies to prevent *Clostridium difficile* infections in acute care hospitals. *Infect Control Hosp Epidemiol*. 2008 Oct;29 Suppl 1:S81–S92.

BACTERIA: GRAM-NEGATIVE

American Academy of Pediatrics. Meningococcal conjugate vaccines policy update: booster dose recommendations. *Pediatrics*. 2011 Dec;128(6):1213–1218.

Centers for Disease Control and Prevention. Disseminated Gonococcal Infection (DGI). From: Sexually Transmitted Diseases Treatment Guidelines, 2010.

Centers for Disease Control and Prevention (CDC). Gonococcal infections. From: Sexually Transmitted Diseases Treatment Guidelines, 2010.

Centers for Disease Control and Prevention (CDC). Updated recommendations for use of meningococcal conjugate vaccines—Advisory Committee on Immunization Practices (ACIP), 2010. *MMWR Morb Mortal Wkly Rep*. 2011 Jan 28;60(3):72–76.

Centers for Disease Control and Prevention (CDC). Recommendation of the Advisory Committee on Immunization Practices (ACIP) for use of quadrivalent meningococcal conjugate vaccine (MenACWY-D) among children aged 9 through 23 months at increased risk for invasive meningococcal disease. *MMWR Morb Mortal Wkly Rep*. 2011 Oct 14;60(40): 1391–1392.

Centers for Disease Control and Prevention (CDC). Updates to: Sexually Transmitted Diseases Treatment Guidelines, 2010: Oral Cephalosporins No Longer a Recommended Treatment for Gonococcal Infections, 2012.

U.S. Preventive Services Task Force (USPSTF). Ocular prophylaxis for gonococcal ophthalmia neonatorum: U.S. Preventive Services Task Force reaffirmation recommendation statement. Rockville (MD): Agency for Healthcare Research and Quality (AHRQ); 2011 Jul:6.

American Academy of Pediatrics. Pertussis (whooping cough). In: Pickering LK, Baker CJ, Kimberlin DW, Long SS, eds. *Red Book®: 2012 Report of the Committee on Infectious Diseases*, 29th edition. Elk Grove Village, IL: 2012: 553–566.

American Academy of Pediatrics. *Kingella kingae*: an emerging pathogen in young children. *Pediatrics*. 2011 Mar;127(3):557–565.

Doran TI. The role of *Citrobacter* in clinical disease of children: review. *Clin Infect Dis*. 1999 Feb;28(2):384–394.

BACTERIA: ANAEROBES

Riordan T. Human infection with *Fusobacterium necrophorum* (necrobacillosis), with a focus on Lemierre's syndrome. *Clin Microbiol Rev*. 2007 Oct;20(4):622–659.

Wexler HM. Bacteroides: the good, the bad, and the nitty-gritty. *Clin Microbiol Rev*. 2007 Oct;20(4):593–621.

BACTERIA: ACID FAST

American Academy of Pediatrics. Tuberculosis. In: Pickering LK, Baker CJ, Kimberlin DW, Long SS, eds. *Red Book®: 2012 Report of the Committee on Infectious Diseases*, 29th edition. Elk Grove Village, IL: 2012: 736–759.

Blumberg HM, et al. American Thoracic Society/Centers for Disease Control and Prevention/Infectious Diseases Society of America: treatment of tuberculosis. *Am J Respir Crit Care Med*. 2003 Feb 15;167(4):603–62.

Taylor Z, et al. Controlling tuberculosis in the United States. Recommendations from the American Thoracic Society, CDC, and the Infectious Diseases Society of America. *MMWR Recomm Rep*. 2005 Nov 4;54(RR-12):1–81. Erratum in: *MMWR Morb Mortal Wkly Rep*. 2005 Nov 18;54(45):1161.

BACTERIA: OTHER

Baron S (ed). *Chlamydia. Medical Microbiology*, 4th Ed, Chapter 39. University of Texas Medical Branch at Galveston, 1996.

Centers for Disease Control and Prevention (CDC). Chlamydial infections. From: Sexually Transmitted Diseases Treatment Guidelines, 2010.

U.S. Preventive Services Task Force. Screening for chlamydial infection. *Ann Intern Med*. 2007 Jul;147(2):128–134.

SPIROCHETES

Centers for Disease Control and Prevention (CDC). Syphilis. From: Sexually Transmitted Diseases Treatment Guidelines, 2010.

FUNGI

Montenegro BL, Arnold JC. North American dimorphic fungal infections in children. *Pediatr Rev*. 2010 Jun;31(6):e40–e48.

Marcon MJ, Powell DA. Human infections due to *Malassezia* spp. *Clin Microbiol Rev*. 1992 Apr;5(2):101–119.

PARASITES

Pearson RD. Approach to parasitic infections. *Merck Manual for Health Care Professionals*. 2012.

Baron S (ed). *Chlamydia. Medical Microbiology*, 4th Ed, Chapter 77. University of Texas Medical Branch at Galveston, 1996.

Centers for Disease Control and Prevention (CDC). Trichomoniasis. From: Sexually Transmitted Diseases Treatment Guidelines, 2010.

Baron S (ed). *Chlamydia. Medical Microbiology*, 4th Ed, Chapter 86. University of Texas Medical Branch at Galveston, 1996.

VIRUSES

Centers for Disease Control and Prevention (CDC). Genital HSV infections. From: Sexually Transmitted Diseases Treatment Guidelines, 2010.

American Academy of Pediatrics Executive Summary. Kimberlin DW, Baley J, et al. Guidance on management of asymptomatic neonates born to women with active genital herpes lesions. *Pediatrics*. 2013 Feb;131(2):e635–e646.

Kimberlin DW, et al. Oral acyclovir suppression and neurodevelopment after neonatal herpes. *N Engl J Med.* 2011 Oct;365:1284–1292. October 6, 2011.

American Academy of Pediatrics. Cytomegalovirus Infection. In: Pickering LK, Baker CJ, Kimberlin DW, Long SS, eds. *Red Book®: 2012 Report of the Committee on Infectious Diseases,* 29th edition. Elk Grove Village, IL: 2012: 300–305.

Kimberlin DW, et al. Pharmacokinetic and pharmacodynamic assessment of oral valganciclovir in the treatment of symptomatic congenital cytomegalovirus disease. *J Infect Dis.* 2008;197(6): 836–845.

Caselli E, Di Luca D. Molecular biology and clinical associations of roseoloviruses human herpesvirus 6 and human herpesvirus 7. New *Microbiol.* 2007 Jul;30(3):173–187.

Casper C. New approaches to the treatment of human herpesvirus 8-associated disease. *Rev Med Virol.* 2008 Sep–Oct;18(5):321–329.

Baron S (ed). *Chlamydia. Medical Microbiology,* 4th Ed, Chapter 62. University of Texas Medical Branch at Galveston, 1996.

Treanor JJ. Clinical presentation and diagnosis of rotavirus infection. *UpToDate.* 2013.

American Academy of Pediatrics. Rabies. In: Pickering LK, Baker CJ, Kimberlin DW, Long SS, eds. *Red Book®: 2012 Report of the Committee on Infectious Diseases,* 29th edition. Elk Grove Village, IL: 2012: 600–607.

Centers for Disease Control and Prevention (CDC). Human papillomavirus (HPV) infection. From: Sexually Transmitted Diseases Treatment Guidelines, 2010.

Garg RK. Subacute sclerosing panencephalitis. *Postgrad Med J.* 2002 Feb;78(916):63–70.

HIV AND AIDS

Chaudhry AA, et al. Update in HIV medicine for the generalist. *J Gen Intern Med.* 2011 May;26(5):538–542.

National Institutes of Health. Clinical Guidelines Portal. Federally approved HIV/AIDS medical practice guidelines. *Aidsinfo.*

Prendergast AJ, et al. Treatment of young children with HIV infection: using evidence to inform policymakers. *PLoS Med.* 2012;9(7):e1001273.

Thompson MA, et al. Antiretroviral treatment of adult HIV infection: 2010 recommendations of the International AIDS Society-USA Panel. *JAMA®.* 2010 Jul 21;304(3):321–333.

Watkins DI. Update on progress in HIV vaccine development. *Top Antivir Med.* 2012 Jun–Jul;20(2):30–1.

Mofenson LM, et al. Guidelines for the Prevention and Treatment of Opportunistic Infections among HIV-exposed and HIV-infected children: recommendations from CDC, the National Institutes of Health, the HIV Medicine Association of the Infectious Diseases Society of America, the Pediatric Infectious Diseases Society, and the American Academy of Pediatrics. *MMWR Recomm Rep.* 2009 Sep 4;58(RR-11):1–166.

Lawn SD, Meintjes G. Pathogenesis and prevention of immune reconstitution disease during antiretroviral therapy. *Expert Rev Anti Infect Ther.* 2011 Apr;9(4):415–430.

COMMON ID SYNDROMES

Fleisher,GR. Evaluation of diarrhea in children. 2013 *UptoDate.*

Guerrant RL, et al. Practice guidelines for the management of infectious diarrhea. *Clin Infect Dis.* 2001 Feb 1;32(3):331–351.

Juckett G, Trivedi R. Evaluation of chronic diarrhea. *Am Fam Physician.* 2011 Nov 15;84(10):1119–1126.

Pawlowski SW, et al. Diagnosis and treatment of acute or persistent diarrhea. *Gastroenterology.* 2009 May;136(6): 1874–1886.

World Gastroenterology Organisation (WGO). WGO practice guideline: acute diarrhea. Munich, Germany: World Gastroenterology Organisation (WGO); 2008 Mar. 28.

American Academy of Pediatrics, Subcommittee on Urinary Tract Infection, Steering Committee on Quality Improvement and Management. Urinary Tract Infection: Clinical Practice Guideline for the Diagnosis and Management of the Initial UTI in Febrile Infants and Children 2 to 24 Months. *Pediatrics.* 2011;128(3):595-610.

Hooton TM, et al. Diagnosis, prevention, and treatment of catheter-associated urinary tract infection in adults: 2009 international clinical practice guidelines from the Infectious Diseases Society of America. *Clin Infect Dis.* 2010 Mar 1;50(5):625–663.

Yokoe D, et al. A compendium of strategies to prevent healthcare-associated infections in acute care hospitals. The Society for Healthcare Epidemiology of America. 2008 Oct; 29:S1–S92.

Mermel LA, et al. Clinical practice guidelines for the diagnosis and management of intravascular catheter–related infections: 2009 Update by the Infectious Diseases Society of American. *Clin Infect Dis.* 2009 July;49:1–45.

O'Grady NP, et al. Guidelines for the prevention of intravascular catheter–related infections. *Clin Infec Dis.* May 2011;52(9): e162–e193.

ANTIBIOTIC THERAPY

Leekha S, et al. General principles of antimicrobial therapy. *Mayo Clin Proc.* 2011 Feb;86(2):156–167.

Levison ME. Aminoglycosides. *Merck Manual for Health Care Professionals.* 2012.

Pearson RD. Merck Manual for Health Care Professionals (Online). Bacteria and Anti-bacterial Drugs 2009.

Calderwood SB. Beta-lactam antibiotics: mechanisms of action and resistance and adverse effects. *UpToDate.* 2013.

Schilling A, et al. Vancomycin: a 50-something-year-old antibiotic we still don't understand. *Cleve Clin J Med.* 2011 Jul;78(7):465–471.

Drew RH. Aminoglycosides. *UpToDate.* 2012.

American Academy of Pediatrics. The use of systemic and topical fluoroquinolones. *Pediatrics.* 2011 Oct;128(4): e1034–e1045.

Hooper DC. Fluoroquinolones. *UpToDate.* 2013.

Zuckerman JM. Macrolides and ketolides: azithromycin, clarithromycin, telithromycin. *Infect Dis Clin N Am.* 2004;18:621–649.

Razonable RR. Antiviral drugs for viruses other than human immunodeficiency virus. *Mayo Clin Proc.* 2011 Oct;86(10):1009–1026.

Sugar AM. Antifungal drugs. *Merck Manual for Health Care Professionals.* 2012.

Kappagoda S, et al. Antiparasitic therapy. *Mayo Clin Proc.* 2011 Jun;86(6):561–583.

ANTIBIOTICS AND THE PREGNANT OR BREASTFEEDING WOMAN

Moses S. Antibiotics in Pregnancy. *Family Practice Notebook.* 2011.

Moses S. Medications in Lactation. *Family Practice Notebook.* 2011.

American Academy of Pediatrics. Policy Statement: Breastfeeding and the Use of Human Milk. Section on Breast-feeding. *Pediatrics* Vol. 129, No. 3, March 2012.

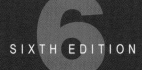

MedStudy®

PEDIATRICS REVIEW

CORE
CURRICULUM

6

SIXTH EDITION

ALLERGY & IMMUNOLOGY

Section Editor:

Peter Huynh, MD
Clinical Physician of Allergy and Immunology
Kaiser Permanente
Panorama City, CA

Medical Editor:

Mark Yoffe, MD
Internal Medicine Specialist
York Hospital
York, PA

Reviewers:

Edward Hu, MD
Assistant Professor of Clinical Medicine
Medical Director, Center for Asthma,
    Allergy, & Clinical Immunology
Keck Medical Center of
    University of Southern California
Los Angeles, CA

Breck Romine Nichols, MD, MPH
Residency Program Director,
    Combined Internal Medicine & Pediatrics
University of Southern California
Keck School of Medicine
Los Angeles, CA

Table of Contents
Allergy & Immunology

THE IMMUNE SYSTEM

OVERVIEW

Because pediatrics—more than any other medical specialty—focuses on primary or congenital immune deficiencies, it makes sense to spend a little time briefly reviewing the immune system.

THE INNATE IMMUNE SYSTEM

Components of the innate immune system include complement, macrophages, and natural killer (NK) cells. The innate immune system is the 2nd line of defense against pathogens, after the skin. It is rapid acting, nonspecific, and has no memory.

THE ADAPTIVE IMMUNE SYSTEM

The adaptive immune system consists of T cells, B cells, and immunoglobulins (Igs). It is the 3rd line of defense and is activated by the innate immune system. Unlike the innate system, it is much slower to get started but is very specific and has memory.

The adaptive immune system can be further broken down into 2 main components:

- **Humoral**: B cells, plasma cells, and immunoglobulins
- **Cell-mediated**: T cells

INNATE vs. ADAPTIVE IMMUNITY

The innate immune system is the foundation on which the more sophisticated adaptive immune system sits. The innate system not only protects the body while the adaptive immune system gears up, but it also helps direct the response. The innate immune system, in general, needs messages to prevent it from killing while the adaptive immune system needs messages (usually from the innate immune system) to allow it to kill.

The key difference between the 2 systems can be found in their receptors:

- **Innate** immune system receptors are generic, ready-made receptors such as the Toll-like receptors. These receptors allow a quick but nonspecific response— one that is rapid but may not be able to recognize all pathogens. Think of these as the "first responders" to a new attack.
- **Adaptive** immune system receptors are custom-made receptors (T cell receptors [TCRs] and Igs) that are refined to be as specific as possible for the pathogen. They provide the immune system with the ability to recognize a seemingly infinite variety of pathogens. Once these custom-made receptors have served their purpose, the body keeps a few of them around in case it needs them again in the future, enabling a quicker reaction next time based on memory.
- So the innate immune system provides a quick generic response while the adaptive provides a slower but more powerful and specific response to the foreign pathogen. Thanks to immunologic memory, if the pathogen is encountered again in the future, the adaptive system can mount a quicker and more robust response.

INNATE AND ADAPTIVE OVERLAP

It is important to understand that there is significant overlap between the innate and adaptive immune systems. For example, the macrophages and NK cells function as part of the innate system initially, but then they become further activated by T cells and can then act as part of the adaptive immune system. Similarly, the classical pathway of the complement system uses antibody (Ig) to initiate its activity. This antibody involvement in the complement system is also an example of how the adaptive immune system provides immunological memory.

INNATE-LIKE CELLS

Another example of overlap is a group of innate-like cells that, although part of the adaptive immune system, are more rapid acting and less specific.

Examples of innate-like immune cells are:

- γ:δ T cells
- Natural killer T (NKT) cells
- B-1 cells (an innate-like version of B cells)

CELLS OF THE IMMUNE SYSTEM

There are 2 major categories of cells in the immune system:

1) **Lymphoid cells**
   - Lymphocytes
     - B cells
       - B-1 cells (innate-like)
       - B-2 cells (aka conventional B cells)
       - Marginal B cells (innate-like)
     - T cells
       - α:β T cells
       - CD4 T cells
       - CD8 T cells
       - Natural killer T (NKT) cells (innate-like)
       - γ:δ T cells (innate-like)
   - Natural killer (NK) cells (different from the similarly named T cells!)
2) **Myeloid cells**
   - Granulocytes
   - Neutrophils
   - Eosinophils
   - Basophils

- Professional antigen-presenting cells
  - Monocytes/Macrophages
  - Dendritic cells
- Other
  - Mast cells
  - Erythrocytes
  - Platelets

HLA ANTIGENS

The histocompatibility molecules are the antigens required by the body to determine self vs. nonself material. The genes for the antigens are on chromosome 6, and this complex of genes is called the major histocompatibility complex (MHC). The human MHC is called HLA (human lymphocyte antigens). There are 3 classes of HLA antigens (I, II, and III). T cells are able to recognize antigens if, and only if, either class I or class II HLA antigens present them. This is the key concept of MHC restriction!

Class I HLA antigens (HLA-A, HLA-B, and HLA-C) are on all cells (including the antigen-presenting cells mentioned below)—except for mature RBCs, where they are never found. Class I antigens present nonself material to the CD8+ T cells—as with transplant rejection, neoplasms, and viruses.

Class II HLA antigens are on professional antigen-presenting cells: monocytes/macrophages, dendritic cells (e.g., Langerhans cells), and B cells. These HLA antigens mediate the interactions among macrophages, T cells, and B cells. The CD4+ T cells recognize material presented only by the class II antigens.

Class III HLA antigens consist of several complement component structures, cytokines, and heat shock proteins (not discussed much in reviews).

LYMPHOID CELLS

LYMPHOCYTES

T Cells

2 major functions of T cells:

1) They destroy intracellular and other bacteria (especially gram-negative), viruses, fungi, parasites, and mycobacteria.
2) They regulate antibody production by B cells.

All T cells have receptors (T-cell receptor = TCR), which are antigen-specific binding sites composed of 2 subunits (the majority being alpha and beta, and a minority being the innate-like gamma and delta). The TCR is similar to an immunoglobulin, and it is always found with a CD3 complex.

Again: All T cells recognize an antigen only if it is presented properly; that is, along with the HLA antigen of the presenting cell. CD8+ T cells recognize an antigen only if it is presented with a class I HLA antigen, whereas CD4+ T cells recognize an antigen only if it is presented with a class II HLA antigen. (A nice way to remember this: CD8 x MHC-I = 8, CD4 x MHC-II = 8).

On the T cell, the TCR, in association with the CD3 protein, recognizes the [(HLA antigen)—(foreign antigen) complex] on the presenting cell.

All T cells are CD2+, and most are CD3+. T cells also usually have either a CD4 or CD8 protein on their surface.

Review: CD stands for "clusters of differentiation." CD markers are like "nametags" and allow us to "differentiate" one immune cell from another. For example, T cells are CD2+ and CD3+. Mature B cells are CD19+ and CD20+. Natural killer cells are CD16+ and CD56+.

CD4+ T Cells

CD4+ T cell subsets

CD4+ T cells are the primary defense against exogenous antigens. The CD4+ T cells are roughly divided into 2 subsets: **TH1** (which induce CD8+ T cells and lead to cell-mediated immunity, transcription factor T-bet) and **TH2** (which induce B cells to produce antibody and humoral immunity, transcription factor GATA-3). They can be activated only by antigens presented along with class II HLA antigens.

Again: These class II antigens are on the professional antigen-presenting cells (monocytes/macrophages, dendritic cells, and B cells). For example, a macrophage ingests a foreign particle or microorganism, then extrudes an antigen (onto the macrophage surface) from the particle, which, along with the class II HLA antigen, is presented to the CD4+ T cell. These T cells, after being activated, induce B cells to convert to plasma cells and produce specific antibodies against that antigen.

HIV targets all CD4+ cells, including CD4+ T cells and other cells that express CD4, such as macrophages, monocytes, and microglial cells. By targeting and attacking CD4+ cells, HIV weakens the immune system, allowing opportunistic infections to occur.

Natural Killer T Cells: A Subtype of CD4+ T Cells

Natural killer T cells are not just MHC-restricted; they are actually restricted to an MHC-like molecule called CD1, which recognizes primarily lipids and glycolipids.

They are so named because they share several features with natural killer cells, such as granzyme production and CD16 and CD56 expression.

Name alert: There are also innate lymphoid cells with a very similar name—natural killer (NK) cells.

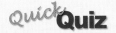

Quick Quiz

- What is the function of class I HLA antigens?
- Which cell types have class II HLA antigens?
- What is the difference between NK and NKT cells.

CD8+ T Cells

The CD8+ cells are cytotoxic T cells. They are important in the defense against viruses and neoplastic cells. They are activated by neoplastic antigens and other antigens presented in association with class I HLA antigens (so most cell types can present antigen to CD8+ T cells!).

T Regulatory / Suppressor Cells

These can be a confusing group of cells because they are still an area of active research and are made up of several different types of T cells (usually CD4 but also CD8 and others). These cells suppress, or more accurately, regulate the immune response by secreting cytokines like IL-10, TGF-β, and IFN-α. The expression of the transcription factor FOXP3 controls the development and function of T regulatory cells.

Review: Interleukins (IL) and cytokines are the "language" of immune cells. Different interleukins and cytokines are expressed by immune cells to communicate to other immune cells. For example, as discussed above, T regulatory cells express IL-10 and TGF-β to tell the immune system to "down-regulate" and "suppress."

B Cells

Some B cells, upon stimulation, become plasma cells (antibody-producing cells). B cells are "surface membrane immunoglobulin-positive (SmIg+)": B cells have IgG and IgD on their surface, which distinguishes them from T cells, B-cell precursors, and plasma cells.

B cells can be stimulated to convert to plasma cells by either antigen alone or activated CD4+ T cells. The specific antibody produced coats the microorganism. This coating either identifies it as edible to the macrophages (opsonization) or initiates the terminal part of the complement cascade, which builds a mechanism to drill a hole in the cell wall of the microorganism.

Again, remember that even though all B cells are SmIg+, the B-cell precursors and plasma cells may be SmIg–.

B cells, like monocytes/macrophages, have the class II major histocompatibility (HLA) antigens on their surfaces, so they also can present foreign antigens to the CD4+ (helper) T cells. The activated T cells then induce other B cells to convert to plasma cells and produce antibodies. B cells are the most specific antigen-presenting cells. Mature B cells are CD19+ and CD20+.

NATURAL KILLER (NK) CELLS

There are also non-B, non-T lymphoid cells that are not lymphocytes called natural killer cells (NK cells).

NK cells play a major role in the innate immune system response to tumors and viruses. They express CD16 and CD56 but not TCRs (T-cell receptors) nor their associated CD3 molecules (an important difference between NK and NKT cells). They are called natural killers because they are always in kill mode and must be presented in a particular fashion not to kill.

NK cells are an important component of the immune system because some viruses reduce MHC-I expression, effectively making them invisible and protecting them from recognition and destruction by cytotoxic T cells. With natural killer cells, it is precisely this absence or reduction of MHC-I that causes the natural killer cells to kill the infected cell (usually by inducing apoptosis).

In comparison, NKT cells, like all other T cells, require the antigen to be presented in association with an HLA antigen before they can become activated to kill. Thus they, like other T cells and unlike NK cells, would also miss the infected cells that were not expressing MHC-I.

MYELOID CELLS

Granulocytes—white blood cells with identifiable granules in their cytoplasm:

- **Neutrophils** = polys = PMNs = segs (mature) and bands (immature). They phagocytize microorganisms, especially if coated with antibodies (like an "M&M" coating of immunoglobulin, or more properly called "opsonization"). If PMNs are absent, patients are susceptible to overwhelming pyogenic infections.
- **Eosinophils**: involved in the pathology of allergic reactions but also in the immunologic defense against parasites.
- **Basophils**: may be involved with the late-phase response of IgE-mediated Type I hypersensitivity.

Professional antigen-presenting cells—cells expressing MHC-I and MHC-II. This is an exclusive group of cells consisting of B cells and the 2 described below:

1) **Monocytes/Macrophages**: eat opsonized microorganisms; process and present antigens to T cells.

2) **Dendritic cells** are scavengers; when they ingest a pathogen, they change confirmation, travel to a lymph node, and activate lymphocytes.

Other:

1) **Mast cells** are discussed later under Type I: Immediate Hypersensitivity Reaction on page 6-14.

2) **Erythrocytes** are covered in Hematology, Book 5.

3) **Megakaryocytes/Platelets** are discussed in Hematology, Book 5.

ANTIBODIES

All antibodies (immunoglobulins) have the same basic structure (Figure 6-1). Each monomer is composed of 2 heavy and 2 light chains that are held together by disulfide bonds. There are 5 immunoglobulin isotypes: **G**, **A**, **M**, **E**, and **D**. These isotypes are determined by differences in the structure of the constant regions of the heavy chains. All antibodies have 1 of 2 types of light chains, kappa or lambda.

Remember the following:

* **IgG** (chronic infection) is the main antibody in serum, and it is the major antibody in the immune response. It readily passes the placenta, providing protection against infection in the newborn. It has 4 subclasses (IgG1, IgG2, IgG3, and IgG4).
* **IgM** (acute infections) is the 1st antibody produced in response to an infection. It is a monomer on the cell surface but is secreted as a pentamer (5 immunoglobulins), in which each monomer is connected by a J chain. Because IgM is a pentamer, it is the best antibody for complement activation. IgM is useful to confirm recent illness and can help distinguish acute versus chronic infection.
* **IgA** is the antibody in secretions, and is usually a dimer (2 immunoglobulins) with the J chain and a secretory component, which is actually just a piece of the epithelial or liver-cell receptor attached to locally produced IgA. It is the main antibody secreted in breast milk. It has 2 subclasses (IgA1 and IgA2).
* **IgE** (atopy and parasites) is the antibody with the lowest concentration in normal serum but has a major role in allergic conditions, including atopy, asthma, allergic rhinitis, and food allergies.
* **IgD** (unknown) is found in trace amounts on adult B cells; its function has yet to be defined.

The variability in the specificities of the antibodies is due to the rearranging of several regions of the antibody genes: the variable (V), diversity (D), joining (J), and constant (C) regions.

Immunoglobulins (antibodies) bind specific antigens in the Fab region, and then activate either cells or complement (discussed next) by means of the Fc region to destroy the antigen-bearing material.

COMPLEMENT

THE 3 COMPLEMENT PATHWAYS

First, a brief review of the complement system (Figure 6-2): The complement system is a core component of both the innate and adaptive immune responses. It is now known to have 3 main pathways: classical, lectin, and alternative. Although they all start with different mechanisms, they each end up the same—they opsonize target cells with C3b and then form the "membrane attack complex (MAC)."

CLASSICAL PATHWAY

The immunoglobulins (usually IgG and IgM) activate the classical pathway: C1 complex (with q, r, and s subunits) initiates this response when a C1q subunit attaches to antibody in an antigen-antibody complex. C1q binds to the Fc portion of at least 2 IgGs (or 1 IgM pentamer) or it binds to the surface of the pathogen itself. Binding changes the conformation of the C1q. This activated C1 will cleave many C2 and C4, subcomponents of which (C2a and C4b) combine and form C4b2a ("C3 convertase"), which in turn activates many C3.

Again: 1 IgM pentamer can initiate the classical pathway, but it normally takes at least 2 IgGs.

LECTIN (OR MANNOSE-BINDING) PATHWAY

Lectins (mannose-binding lectin [MBL]; also called mannose- or mannan-binding proteins) bind mannose on the surface of pathogens. Then associated proteases cleave C2 and C4, and further steps are similar to the classical pathway. These MBLs are produced by an acute-phase response and are fairly nonspecific.

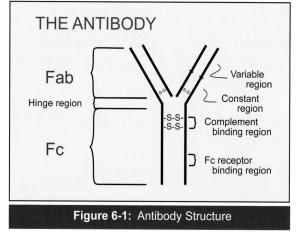

Figure 6-1: Antibody Structure

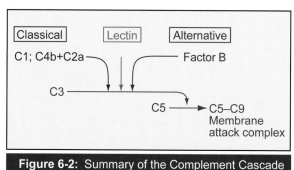

Figure 6-2: Summary of the Complement Cascade

Quick Quiz

- Describe the function of immunoglobulins G, A, M, and E.
- What is the 1st antibody produced in an infection?
- What is the main antibody in secretions and breast milk?
- Which antibody plays a major role in allergies?
- Be familiar with the categories of immunodeficiencies and the common type of infections associated with each group.

ALTERNATIVE PATHWAY

In the alternative pathway, C3 is spontaneously cleaved by bacterial cell wall hydroxyl groups. The cleaved C3 combines with a factor "B." This complex then activates more C3 and factor B, causing a cascade, which is normally kept under control by the inhibitory regulatory proteins "H" and "I." Both gram-positive and gram-negative cell walls directly activate the alternative pathway by spontaneous cleavage of C3.

COMMON TERMINAL PATHWAY— MEMBRANE ATTACK COMPLEX

C3, when combined with either C4b2a or factor B, will activate C5, which causes the formation of a C5-6-7-8-9 membrane attack complex (MAC). The MAC can poke holes in bacterial cell wall membranes.

IMMUNODEFICIENCIES

OVERVIEW

There are more than 150 described immunodeficiencies with many more waiting to be discovered. These as yet undescribed immunodeficiencies probably account for the large number of likely inappropriately labeled "immunocompetent" patients with odd and opportunistic infections that can be found in the literature.

Immunodeficiencies should be suspected when the patient has had recurrent and/or severe infections.

It is helpful to break these immunodeficiencies down into categories based on the overall structure of the immune system.

- **Adaptive**
  - Combined B- and T-cell deficiencies
  - T-cell deficiencies
  - B-cell deficiencies
- **Innate**
  - Phagocyte disorders
  - Toll-like receptor defects
  - Complement deficiencies

The following categories of immunodeficiencies are useful for guiding the workup because certain infections are classic for each category:

- **T-cell deficiency**: opportunistic infections
  - Bacteria (mostly intracellular): *Salmonella*, syphilis
  - Mycobacteria: tuberculosis, *Mycobacterium avium*-complex
  - Viruses: cytomegalovirus (CMV), herpes simplex virus (HSV), varicella-zoster virus (VZV), Epstein-Barr virus (EBV), hepatitis, human papillomavirus (HPV), molluscum contagiosum
  - Fungi: *Candida*, *Aspergillus*, coccidioidomycosis, *Cryptococcus*, histoplasmosis
  - Protozoa: *Pneumocystis*, toxoplasmosis, cryptosporidiosis, isosporiasis, microsporidiosis
- **B-cell deficiency**: recurrent sinopulmonary infections
  - Bacteria: *Streptococcus pneumoniae*, *Haemophilus influenzae*, *Staphylococcus aureus*, *Pseudomonas*
  - Virus: enterovirus
  - Protozoa: *Giardia*
- **Phagocytic disorder**: skin and organ abscesses
  - Bacteria: *Staphylococcus aureus*
- **Complement deficiency**: overwhelming sepsis
  - Bacteria: *Neisseria meningitidis*
- **Toll-like receptor defects**:
  - Bacteria: pyogenic bacteria, *Mycobacteria*
  - Virus: herpes virus

To work up these deficiencies, the 1st step is always the history and physical. The next step is to get a quantitative and qualitative test in each category (Table 6-1).

Children with immunodeficiency are also prone to developing cancers such as leukemias and lymphomas. Lymphomas are common in the brain and the GI tract. Today, malignancy is a more common cause of death than infection in some of the milder forms of immunodeficiency. The risk for cancer is increased by exposure to ionizing radiation, so minimize x-rays in these patients.

Patients with immunodeficiency are also at risk for autoimmune disorders.

The immune system is a complicated system that serves 3 major functions: prevention of infections, tumors, and autoimmune disease. When there is an abnormality in the immune system, it becomes less effective in all 3 functions. So patients with immunodeficiencies are not only more prone to infections but also to cancer and autoimmune disease.

COMBINED B- and T-CELL IMMUNODEFICIENCIES

Example Diseases

It is difficult to dissect out T-cell and combined B- and T-cell deficiencies because, in order for B cells to function, they need functioning T cells. So the more severe the T-cell deficiency, the more it also affects the B cells.

	Table 6-1: Test for Immunodeficiencies		
Category	**Quantitative**	**Qualitative**	**Tertiary Tests**
T cell	Flow cytometry	Delayed-type hypersensitivity (*Candida*, mumps)	Specific enzyme measurement, mitogens
B cell	Quantitative immunoglobulins	Response to vaccines	Neoantigen studies, mitogens
Phagocyte	CBC with diff	Neutrophil oxidation (NBT or DHR)	Surface glycoproteins
Complement	C3, C4	CH50	Individual complement (C5, C6, ...)

Some examples of combined B- and T-cell deficiencies are:

• SCID
• Wiskott-Aldrich syndrome
• Ataxia-telangiectasia
• Bloom syndrome
• Nijmegen breakage syndrome

Severe Combined Immunodeficiency

Overview

SCID, like many disorders, is actually a collection of different immune defects that all present similarly:

• **Cytokine receptor defect**
  ◦ Interleukin-2 receptor gamma (IL-2Rγ) defect (X-linked)
  ◦ Interleukin-7 receptor alpha chain (IL-7Rα) defect
• **T- and/or B-cell receptor defect**
  ◦ Recombinase activating gene (*RAG*) deficiency
  ◦ T-cell/CD3 receptor defect
• **T-cell receptor signaling defect**
  ◦ Janus kinase 3 (Jak3) deficiency
  ◦ Zeta-chain-associated protein kinase 70 (ZAP-70) deficiency
• **Metabolic defect**
  ◦ Adenosine deaminase (ADA) deficiency
  ◦ Purine nucleotide phosphorylase (PNP) deficiency
• **Other**
  ◦ Reticular dysgenesis
  ◦ Omenn syndrome
  ◦ Bare lymphocyte syndrome

Most common forms of SCID:

• 50% IL-2 receptor gamma (IL-2Rγ) defect (X-linked)
• 25–30% Recombinase activating gene (*RAG*) deficiency
• 15–20% Adenosine deaminase (ADA) deficiency
• < 10% all other forms of SCID combined

Most babies with SCID present in the 1st few months of life, but, depending on the severity of their immune dysfunction and their exposure, some may present later. These infants characteristically present with over-whelming sepsis, eczematous-like skin lesions, chronic lung infections, diarrhea, and failure to thrive. Absence of thymus shadow on CXR is commonly described on test questions. Infants with SCID are almost universally lymphopenic for age, but this often goes unrecognized because infant lymphocyte counts are much higher than in older children. So be sure to check age-appropriate normal values.

Children with SCID are at risk of infections with almost every conceivable microorganism, including bacteria, fungi, viruses, and protozoa.

Early in the disease process, look for candidiasis of the mouth, esophagus, and skin. Rotavirus can be persistent, and RSV may cause giant-cell pneumonia in these patients. *Pneumocystis jiroveci* pneumonia (formerly known as *P. carinii* pneumonia, or PCP) and CMV pneumonia are common.

Do not give these children live-attenuated virus vaccines! Such vaccines can be fatal. If children with SCID need transfusions, give them irradiated blood because nonirradiated blood contains T lymphocytes, which could lead to fatal graft-versus-host disease (GVHD).

Another useful way to subdivide SCID is during the workup. Typically, flow cytometry shows the level/presence of the different types of lymphocytes—T cells, B cells, and NK cells.

The configuration helps define the type of abnormality present:

T–, B–, NK– (no T cells, no B cells, no NK cells)
  ADA, reticular dysgenesis

T–, B–, NK+ (no T cells, no B cells, present NK cells)
  RAG, Omenn syndrome

T–, B+, NK– (no T cells, present B cells, no NK cells)
  X-linked SCID (IL-2Rγ), Jak3, PNP

T–, B+, NK+ (no T cells, present B cells, present NK cells)
  TCR/CD3, IL-7Rα, CHH

T+, B+, NK+ (present T cells, B cells, and NK cells)
  ZAP-70, bare lymphocyte syndrome

X-Linked SCID

X-linked SCID is the most common form of SCID and accounts for nearly 50% of SCID cases. Since it is

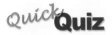

Quiz

- What finding is nearly universal in infants with SCID with regard to the lymphocyte count?
- What unusual organism is a common cause of pneumonia in children with SCID?
- Should children with SCID get live-attenuated virus vaccines?
- What type of blood transfusions should children with SCID receive?
- Which inheritance pattern occurs most commonly in patients with SCID?
- Patients with SCID due to purine nucleoside phosphorylase deficiency have what associated autoimmune diseases?

X-linked, only males are affected. It results in the total failure of T-cell and natural killer cell development (T–, NK–) and the complete absence of infant-produced T cells from the circulation and lymph tissues. Maternal T cells can be engrafted and may appear in large numbers, but they do not function correctly. B cells produced by the child are present (B+), but they also do not function normally.

Boys with X-linked SCID have mutations in the cytokine receptor subunit known as gamma (γ) chain—or gamma-c (γc). This chain is a component of several cytokine receptors, including those for IL-2, IL-4, and IL-7 (interleukins). Normal function of this protein is necessary for T-cell development.

The diagnosis is presumed in boys with absent T-cell function and confirmed by molecular analysis of the gene for γc. You can determine the carrier status in females by the same techniques.

Bone marrow transplantation restores normal T-cell development and function, but B-cell function is usually not restored. Thus, these patients still require intravenous immunoglobulins (IVIG) for antibody replacement.

Autosomal Recessive Forms of SCID

Autosomal recessive (AR) SCID may result from mutations in several genes important in lymphoid maturation. Genes that may be implicated in SCID include those for the Jak3 kinase, which is physically associated with the γc chain and mediates its signaling function, and the IL-7Rα chain, a critical signaling molecule in the development of the T-cell lineage. Defects in the purine salvage pathway also lead to profound immunodeficiency (see next topic). Other causes of AR SCID include lesions in the genes ZAP-70, RAG1, RAG2, and others.

SCID Due to Purine Salvage Pathway Disorders

Two purine salvage pathway disorders manifest as SCID:

- Adenosine deaminase (ADA) deficiency
- Purine nucleoside phosphorylase (PNP) deficiency (rare)

ADA deficiency accounts for 15–20% of the cases of SCID; PNP deficiency is immunologically less severe and much less common.

ADA deficiency affects T cells, B cells, and NK cells (T–, B–, NK–). ADA is located on chromosome 20, and most deficiency cases are due to point mutations or deletions; ADA deficiency is transmitted as an autosomal recessive disorder. ADA normally catalyzes the deamination of adenosine and deoxyadenosine to inosine and deoxyinosine. If ADA is deficient, the deoxyadenosine and its metabolite, deoxyadenosine trisphosphate (dATP), accumulate in the lymphocytes, a process that is toxic to the cell. A spectrum of disease has been identified with milder forms diagnosed even in adults, but most patients with ADA deficiency present within months of birth with recurrent infections, profound lymphopenia, and hypogammaglobulinemia. The most common infections are *Pneumocystis* pneumonia; oral, esophageal, and intestinal candidiasis; severe *Candida* diaper rash; CMV, EBV, and varicella virus; and severe enterovirus infections. Lymph nodes are not palpable and tonsils are small. Skeletal abnormalities are common, particularly cupping and flaring of the costochondral junctions and pelvic dysplasia. Low ADA in RBCs and high deoxyadenosine and dATP in blood and urine are diagnostic. Infants die early without bone marrow transplant or enzyme replacement therapy with polyethylene glycol-modified bovine ADA.

PNP deficiency is often associated with delayed diagnosis since the immune deficit may not be as profound as with most ADA SCID cases. These patients also have neurologic disorders and autoimmune diseases such as autoimmune hemolytic anemia and thrombocytopenia. Bone marrow transplant has been successful in a few patients.

RAG Deficiency
(T–, B–, NK+ SCID; Swiss-Type SCID)

RAG deficiency is an autosomal recessive disorder associated with fatal infections due to severe lymphopenia. It is the most severe form and accounts for 25–30% of all cases of SCID. RAG deficiency results from the mutation or deletion in the recombination activating genes 1 and 2 (RAG1, RAG2). It is a selective failure of lymphoid cell lines, due to the inability to rearrange the genes for immunoglobulin or the T-cell antigen receptor. T and B cells are absent, but natural killer (NK) cells are normal (T–, B–, NK+), as are nonlymphoid hematopoietic cell lines. Bone marrow transplant is both the treatment and the cure.

ALLERGY & IMMUNOLOGY

Reticular Dysgenesis
(T–, B–, NK– SCID)

Reticular dysgenesis is a very rare form of SCID. It occurs when the lymphoid and myeloid lines do not develop, but the erythroid and megakaryocytic cell lines develop normally. These infants do not have lymphocytes or granulocytes. A bone marrow transplant is curative; those without it die in infancy.

Omenn Syndrome

Omenn syndrome is a variant of RAG deficiency. These children present with severe erythroderma, diarrhea, hepatosplenomegaly, and failure to thrive (FTT). Affected infants have hypogammaglobulinemia, elevated IgE, and marked eosinophilia. B cells are depleted or absent, and T cells are produced only in the TH2 phenotype, which results in a large number of eosinophils and IgE. These patients have a partial inactivation of either the *RAG1* or *RAG2* genes.

SCID with MHC Class II Deficiency

SCID with MHC class II deficiency, also known as "bare lymphocyte syndrome," is an autosomal recessive disorder primarily in children of Mediterranean descent; it is rare in North America. It results from the failure to express MHC class II molecules, which include HLA-DP, HLA-DQ, and HLA-DR. Those affected present with chronic diarrhea and have recurrent, severe viral infections. Even with bone marrow transplantation, the prognosis is guarded because the thymic epithelium lacks HLA class II molecules and does not function properly in thymocyte selection.

Wiskott-Aldrich Syndrome

Wiskott-Aldrich syndrome is an X-linked disease with a classic triad of 1) thrombocytopenia, 2) eczema, and 3) susceptibility to encapsulated bacteria and opportunistic infections. Remember **EXIT** (**e**czema, **x**-linked, **i**mmunodeficiency, and **t**hrombocytopenia). There are different phenotypes of this disorder, depending on the severity of the eczema and immunodeficiency. The genetic cause maps to Xp11.22. The affected gene codes for *WASP*, the Wiskott-Aldrich syndrome protein gene.

Boys may present in early infancy with abnormal bleeding. Classic clinical scenario: boy with prolonged bleeding from circumcision site. Bloody diarrhea is also common. Look for mucosal bleeding or petechia. Eosinophilia and increased IgE are common when the eczema is prominent. Staphylococcal skin infections are frequent with the eczema. Immunodeficiency also may manifest as recurrent sinopulmonary infections, chronic otitis media, or severe viral skin infections such as varicella.

The thrombocytopenia may be profound. Small platelets are diagnostic for this disorder. Splenectomy returns the platelet count to normal but should be reserved for severe thrombocytopenia. The immune dysfunction is both cellular and humoral. T-cell proliferation to mitogens and specific antigens is decreased and worsens with time. Anergy is common. Under the electron microscope, you will see the paucity of microvilli on the T lymphocyte. On the humoral side, IgM is decreased, and IgA and IgE are elevated. IgG may be normal, but antibody response to immunization is poor and requires IVIG replacement.

Treatment of Wiskott-Aldrich syndrome: bone marrow transplant from an HLA-matched donor. Splenectomy is effective in improving the platelet count if bone marrow transplant cannot be done. The problem with splenectomy, though, is that it worsens the humoral deficit problem and increases the risk of infection with encapsulated organisms. You must prescribe antibiotic prophylaxis (amoxicillin or trimethoprim/sulfamethoxazole) to prevent these types of infections.

Ataxia-Telangiectasia

Ataxia-telangiectasia (A-T) is an AR disorder with 2 main characteristics (can you guess from its name?):

• Cerebellar ataxia
• Oculocutaneous telangiectasia

Immunodeficiency, a high incidence of cancer, and increased sensitivity to ionizing radiation are also associated with A-T. The gene responsible is known as *ATM* (A-T mutated); it maps to chromosome 11q22-23. The ATM protein is responsible for monitoring and repairing DNA. If it is not functioning, this leads to the accumulation of DNA strand breaks, resulting in programmed cell death (apoptosis). The incidence of A-T is 1/20,000 to 1/100,000, but nearly 2% of Caucasians in the U.S. carry one defective *ATM* gene. "Carrier" status increases risk for malignancy but does not cause clinical manifestations of A-T.

Clinically, the A-T syndrome generally presents with ataxia 1st, usually occurring by age 5 years. Telangiectasias start in the bulbar conjunctivae and also appear in the skin by age 5. You probably also will see telangiectasias around the ears, neck, and antecubital fossae. Other endocrine abnormalities, especially DM, are common.

Sinopulmonary disease and bronchiectasis are common. You see elevated serum levels of α_1-fetoprotein and CEA.

For diagnosis in a child over 5 years of age, ataxia + telangiectasia + elevated α_1-fetoprotein make the diagnosis; but under the age of 5, remember that telangiectasias may not be present until later, so the diagnosis should still be considered without that classic finding.

How are these children immunodeficient? Children with A-T have defects in both humoral and cellular immunity. T-cell function is affected—the cells do not react to mitogens, and delayed hypersensitivity reactions are not present. The B cells are usually normal in number, but IgA and IgE levels are low. IgA deficiency is found in

Quiz

- What is the classic triad of Wiskott-Aldrich syndrome?
- What is distinctive about the platelets in Wiskott-Aldrich syndrome?
- Is IVIG required in the treatment of patients with Wiskott-Aldrich syndrome?
- What are the characteristic findings in ataxia-telangiectasia? (Don't think too hard!)
- For a child > 5 years of age, how is the diagnosis of ataxia-telangiectasia usually made?
- Children with ataxia-telangiectasia have a high incidence of which malignancies?
- What is Bloom syndrome?
- What chromosomal deletion is most commonly associated with DiGeorge syndrome?
- What are the characteristic findings in patients with DiGeorge syndrome?
- What are the characteristic cardiac lesions in patients with DiGeorge syndrome?
- Which endocrine abnormality is common in patients with DiGeorge syndrome?
- What disorder are infants at risk for if they have complete DiGeorge and have received nonirradiated blood products?

~ 70%. IgG deficiency may be found in ~ 50%, mainly due to a selective decrease in IgG2 and IgG4 subclasses. IgM and IgD are normal. In general, the neurologic problems are more disabling than the immune deficit.

Most ominous for A-T patients, however, is the high risk of malignancy, especially of the lymph system. When it occurs, almost all are lymphocytic leukemias or lymphomas.

Bloom Syndrome

Like A-T, Bloom syndrome is a chromosomal "instability" disorder. Bloom syndrome is associated with deficiency of DNA ligase I. It presents with small stature, telangiectasia, CNS abnormalities, and immunodeficiency. Bloom syndrome also has a high association with leukemias.

Nijmegen Breakage Syndrome

Nijmegen breakage syndrome is a rare AR disease. It is associated with a "bird-like" face and microcephaly, with normal or near-normal IQ. These children have combined cellular and humoral immunodeficiency and a high incidence of lymphoid cancers. Nijmegen breakage syndrome is due to a mutation in the Nijmegen breakage syndrome 1 gene (*NBS1*). This gene makes nibrin, which is responsible for the repair of double-stranded DNA breaks.

PRIMARY T-CELL IMMUNODEFICIENCIES

Overview

DiGeorge and Nezelof syndromes are sometimes defined as T-cell immunodeficiencies and sometimes as combined T- and B-cell immunodeficiencies. It is important to remember that normal B-cell function requires T-cell help; so the more severely affected the T cells, the more it also affects the B cells.

DiGeorge Syndrome

DiGeorge syndrome results from deficient T-cell development due to thymus absence or disorder. Individuals with DiGeorge syndrome have a variable degree of malformation in several areas, including the thymus, lymph system, heart, and parathyroid glands. Most with DiGeorge have heterozygous interstitial deletions of chromosome 22q11.2. This deletion is the most prevalent microdeletion syndrome and occurs in ~ 1 in 6,000 live births. A small group has monosomy 22 or a large deletion of the long arm of chromosome 22. DiGeorge can overlap in presentation with fetal alcohol syndrome and retinoic acid embryopathy. Infants with the **CHARGE** complex (**c**oloboma, **h**eart abnormalities, choanal **a**tresia, growth and development **r**etardation, **g**enital and **e**ar anomalies) may also have DiGeorge syndrome.

Clinically, DiGeorge presents with craniofacial abnormalities, including micrognathia, hypertelorism, a shortened philtrum, and low-set, dorsally rotated ears. Abnormalities of the heart include interrupted aortic arch, tetralogy of Fallot, transposition of the great vessels, double-outlet RV, and VSD. The parathyroid glands frequently are absent or reduced, and subclinical hypoparathyroidism is common. This may present as tetany. Other findings frequently include anomalies of the diaphragm, kidneys, eyes, and CNS. Intellectual disabilities are common.

The immune manifestations are variable. Most infants with the facial and cardiac features of DiGeorge syndrome have normal or near-normal immune function. In "complete" DiGeorge, T cells are absent and B cells are present, but the B cells cannot produce specific antibodies due to the lack of T-cell help. These infants can have immunodeficiency as severe as SCID; and, similar to SCID, infants with complete DiGeorge are at risk of GVHD (graft-versus-host disease) from nonirradiated blood and cells. More commonly, you will see patients with "partial" DiGeorge syndrome, with only partial T-cell depletion and normal B-cell function. In most patients with the partial form, the immune deficits improve with time. Severe deficits have been corrected with thymic transplants, but this treatment is reserved for those with complete DiGeorge. IVIG is useful if antibody production is poor.

Nezelof Syndrome

Nezelof syndrome is an autosomal recessive form of thymic hypoplasia, which leads to varying degrees of T-cell dysfunction.

PRIMARY B-CELL IMMUNODEFICIENCIES

Overview

B-cell deficiencies are the most common immunodeficiency category.

Some examples of B-cell deficiencies are:

- X-linked agamma/hypogammaglobulinemia
- Common variable immunodeficiency
- Hyper-IgM syndrome
- Duncan syndrome
- Transient hypogammaglobulinemia of infancy

X-linked Agammaglobulinemia

X-linked (Bruton's) agammaglobulinemia presents with recurrent bacterial infections in association with absent-to-low immunoglobulins of all classes. There are no, or minimal, immunoglobulin-carrying B cells in the peripheral circulation. However, B-cell precursors are normal in the bone marrow, but their development is arrested at a pre-B–cell stage. Only immature B cells are found in the marrow and circulation, and these cells cannot produce adequate antibodies.

X-linked agammaglobulinemia is due to a mutation in the gene *BTK* (at Xq22) that encodes for Bruton tyrosine kinase, which is necessary for B-cell development.

Boys with this disorder historically present late in the 1st year of life after all the placentally transferred IgG has been consumed. Encapsulated bacterial infections of the respiratory tract are common and include pneumonia, otitis, and sinusitis. Meningitis, sepsis, and osteomyelitis are not uncommon. Persistent and recurrent giardiasis can also occur. These children respond well to antibiotics, but recurrence is common for all of the infections. Because of powerful, modern oral antibiotics, boys with this disorder may not be recognized until after the 1st year of life, when it becomes apparent that you are frequently treating them with antibiotics for febrile illnesses.

IVIG is necessary to prevent the recurrent infections. These children also have a predisposition to enterovirus infections and are at high risk if given the live polio vaccine.

Lab findings are as expected with severe deficiency of all of the immunoglobulin classes. B lymphocytes are absent from the blood and from lymph tissue. Lymph nodes and tonsils are small or absent.

Give IVIG every month or more often, depending on the severity of the patient's disease and on the rate of consumption of the exogenous IVIG.

Common Variable Immunodeficiency

Patients with common variable immunodeficiency (CVID) have recurrent infections (usually sinopulmonary infections with encapsulated bacteria) and a deficiency of at least 2 classes of immunoglobulins (IgG, IgA, or IgM), and poor immunoglobulin function as demonstrated by Ig titers to vaccines (diphtheria/tetanus for protein and pneumococcal for polysaccharide). Although several genetic causes are recognized, most cases have an unknown genetic basis. The problem is that the B cells cannot differentiate—or have impaired differentiation—into plasma cells, which produce specific antibodies. Males and females are equally affected, and it is sometimes familial.

Common variable immunodeficiency can present at any age and has many different clinical manifestations. It is most often seen in the 2nd and 3rd decades and is very rare before the age of 6. Look for recurrent sinus and pulmonary infections. IgG levels are typically < 300 mg/dL, and IgA and IgM are < 50 mg/dL.

A sarcoid-like disease with noncaseating granulomas of the spleen, liver, lungs, and skin are common and may present as hepatosplenomegaly. A number of autoimmune conditions are seen in CVID, including idiopathic thrombocytopenic purpura (ITP), pernicious anemia, hemolytic anemia, malabsorption, and pancytopenia. Polyarthritis is frequently present. Amyloidosis and hemolytic-uremic syndrome are more common in patients with common variable immunodeficiency. A sprue-like illness is also very common. Diarrhea, malabsorption, steatorrhea, and protein-losing enteropathy occur in > 50% of patients.

Other associated findings:

- Incidence of lymphomas is also increased.
- *Giardia* infection is common.
- Chronic enteroviral meningitis is another well-described presentation.

Treat with IVIG and specific therapy for infectious complications.

Hyper-IgM Syndrome

Patients with hyper-IgM syndrome typically have a deficiency of IgA and IgG but normal or high IgM. There are X-linked and AR forms, with the X-linked being more common. The prognosis for the X-linked form is also poorer, with a high rate of malignancy by the 2nd decade of life.

X-linked hyper-IgM syndrome is due to abnormalities in the gene on the X chromosome coding for the ligand for CD40 (CD40L) on the T cell. CD40 (found on B cells, dendritic cells, and macrophages) and its ligand are important in T-cell–to–B-cell signaling, and, without them, immunoglobulin class-switching from IgM to other classes does not occur. AR hyper-IgM may be the result of defects in CD40 itself, or proteins required

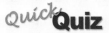

Quick Quiz

- For X-linked agammaglobulinemia, are immunoglobulin-carrying B cells prominent in the peripheral circulation?

- What mutation is responsible for X-linked agammaglobulinemia?

- Which type of infections is a child with X-linked agammaglobulinemia at risk for?

- What is characteristic about the lymph nodes and tonsils in patients with X-linked agammaglobulinemia?

- What is common variable immunodeficiency (CVID)?

- Which types of infection are common in patients with CVID?

- What would a biopsy of an enlarged spleen or liver commonly show in a patient with CVID?

- What type of GI disease is common in patients with CVID?

- What are the immunoglobulin findings in hyper-IgM syndrome?

- Which form of hyper-IgM syndrome—AR or X-linked—is more common?

- Which unusual pneumonia are children with hyper-IgM at risk for? What can you give for prophylaxis?

- Which disease can cause death or severe infections in patients with X-linked lymphoproliferative disease?

- What is transient hypogammaglobulinemia of infancy? Does it usually require treatment with IVIG?

for immunoglobulin class-switching such as activation-induced deaminase (AID) or uracil N-glycosylase (UNG).

Children with this disorder are susceptible to bacterial infections commonly associated with hypogammaglobulinemia, including recurrent sinopulmonary infections with encapsulated bacteria, giardiasis, and bacterial and viral meningitis. Also, the X-linked type is susceptible to *Pneumocystis jiroveci* pneumonia (formerly known as *P. carinii* pneumonia or PCP), which sometimes leads this disorder to be classified as a combined B- and T-cell disorder. A less common manifestation is chronic parvovirus infection, which results in red cell aplasia. On physical exam, it is common to find enlarged cervical lymph nodes and hepatosplenomegaly. Boys with X-linked disease frequently have neutropenia or autoimmune disease.

Aim therapy at correcting the hypogammaglobulinemia by giving IVIG and prophylactic antibiotics for pneumonia prophylaxis. Bone marrow transplant can be curative and is the most appropriate treatment for X-linked disease. The more optimistic prognosis in the AR disease tends to mitigate the need for transplantation.

X-linked Lymphoproliferative Disease (Duncan Syndrome)

X-linked lymphoproliferative disease causes severe or fatal infections with Epstein-Barr virus (EBV). EBV frequently causes fulminant hepatitis, B-cell lymphomas, agranulocytosis, aplastic anemia, or acquired hypogammaglobulinemia. How does this happen? EBV triggers a polyclonal expansion of T and B cells. The most common causes of death are hepatic necrosis and/or bone marrow failure due to NK cells and cytotoxic T cells infiltrating these organs. Patients who survive the initial EBV infection are both antibody-deficient and at risk for malignancy. A common malignancy is extranodal Burkitt-type lymphoma.

The defect involves a mutation of the *SH2D1A* gene found on chromosome Xq25. Patients typically do not have immune problems until exposure to EBV.

During the acute EBV "attack" and polyclonal expansion, steroids, immunosuppressants, and cytotoxic agents may be useful to stem the response. Currently, the only cure is allogeneic stem cell transplantation. Rituximab (anti-CD20 monoclonal antibody) may be useful to terminate EBV-driven lymphoproliferation.

Transient Hypogammaglobulinemia of Infancy

Transient hypogammaglobulinemia of infancy comes up most often in the workup of X-linked hypogammaglobulinemia. It is thought to be either a normal variant or an abnormal prolongation and accentuation of the physiological hypogammaglobulinemia that occurs naturally between 4 and 6 months of age. This is a diagnosis of exclusion! Normally, the term infant has an IgG level similar to the mother, which then falls gradually. The normal infant does not produce its own IgG until ~ 2–3 months of age. This dropping of maternal IgG and subsequent inadequate infant IgG production results in a physiologic hypogammaglobulinemia. The abnormal prolongation occurs when the infant's IgG production is delayed or muted. It is important to remember that Ig levels, like most immune laboratory markers, vary with age. Age-appropriate normal values should be used when evaluating for immunodeficiency.

Usually, these children have normal IgG levels by 3–4 years of age. A majority of them do not require IVIG, but consider this therapy in those with recurrent infections or markedly low IgG levels. Consider antibiotic prophylaxis in those with frequent respiratory and/or ear infections (amoxicillin or trimethoprim/sulfamethoxazole).

PHAGOCYTE DISORDERS

OVERVIEW

This group of disorders can be broken down into 3 types of problems:

1) Neutropenia (< 1,000 PMN, severe = < 100): Kostmann syndrome (AD), severe chronic neutropenia (AR), cyclic neutropenia

2) Chemotaxis defects: lymphocyte adhesion defect (LAD)

3) Killing defects: Job (hyper-IgE) syndrome, Chediak-Higashi syndrome, chronic granulomatous disease, specific granule deficiency

NEUTROPENIA

In general, it is much more dangerous to have an acute neutropenia, from leukemia or chemotherapy, than the chronic neutropenias described below.

Kostmann syndrome: a familial autosomal recessive form of severe chronic neutropenia due to mutation in *HAX1* gene.

Severe chronic neutropenia: an autosomal dominant form of neutropenia due to mutation in neutrophil elastase (ELA2).

Cyclic neutropenia: an autosomal dominant form of neutropenia in which the levels of neutrophils increase and decrease over time. It is also due to mutation in ELA2 (neutrophil elastase).

Treat all 3 disorders with G-CSF.

PHAGOCYTE CHEMOTAXIS DISORDERS

Leukocyte adhesion defect type 1 (LAD1): It is the reason we check, but it is definitely not the most common cause of, delayed umbilical cord separation. These patients have a baseline leukocytosis since they lack CD18, which would allow their cells to leave circulation and enter the tissues to fight off infection. They suffer recurrent necrotizing infections at places where the body interfaces with the environment (skin, mucosa, gut, lungs). When skin lesions heal, they leave characteristic cigarette paper scarring. For diagnosis, check CD18 by flow cytometry.

LAD2: Much less common than LAD1; caused by a defect in fucosylation of CD15s (Sialyl Lewis X), which is needed for the cell to roll along the endothelium of the blood vessel prior to the adhesion needed to enter the tissue. These patients also have intellectual disabilities, Bombay blood type, and poor growth.

PHAGOCYTE KILLING DEFECTS

Hyper-IgE syndrome (Job syndrome): A STAT-3 deficiency that produces defects in multiple systems, eczema, scoliosis, hyperextensibility, delayed dental exfoliation, fractures, and recurrent infections classically described as cold abscesses with *Staphylococcus*, *Haemophilus influenzae*, and *Streptococcus pneumoniae*. Patients also have post-infection pulmonary cysts (pneumatoceles). The characteristic appearance is an asymmetric face, broad nose, prominent forehead, triangular jaw, and 2 rows of teeth due to delayed dental exfoliation. They may also have elevated IgE (2,000–100,000 IU initially but may reduce to normal levels as they get older) and eosinophilia. Despite the fact that this entity is named hyper-IgE syndrome (HIES), elevated IgE is not needed to make the diagnosis, and high IgE levels can be found in other conditions.

Chediak-Higashi syndrome: Recurrent cutaneous and sinopulmonary infections, partial oculocutaneous albinism, mild intellectual disabilities, and progressive peripheral neuropathy. Diagnose by peripheral smear, which shows large neutrophil granules (giant granules) caused by the fusion of primary and secondary granules.

Chronic granulomatous disease (CGD): (Usually X-linked) chronic recurrent organ and skin abscesses—commonly *Staphylococcus aureus*, *Serratia marcescens*, *Burkholderia cepacia*, and *Aspergillus*. It is caused by a defect that prevents the generation of superoxide. Diagnosed by nitroblue tetrazolium (NBT) reduction interpreted visually: The yellow dye turns dark blue on cell activation. So, in the CGD patient, the yellow dye does not turn dark blue. Dihydrorhodamine (DHR) oxidation is now replacing NBT since it is interpreted by fluorescence with flow cytometry and thus requires less operator interpretation, making it less subject to human error. Follow with history, ESR, CT, and x-rays. Use prophylactic antibiotics, antifungals, and interferon-gamma. BMT can be curative.

Specific granule deficiency: Neutrophils have primary and secondary granules that normally fuse with the phagosome for killing. These patients lack either or both of these granules and have a phagocyte killing defect.

TOLL-LIKE RECEPTOR DISORDERS

Aside from defects in the actual receptors like TLR2, TLR4, etc., there are also NEMO, IRAK4, and NF-κB, which are all enzymes in the toll-like receptor signaling pathway. Without these enzymes, there is poor skin development and a decreased ability to activate the innate immune system, which leads to ectodermal dysplasia and recurrent infections.

COMPLEMENT DISORDERS

OVERVIEW

Complement disorders occur in association with over 30 of the different components of the complement system. However, only a few of these are common enough to discuss.

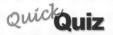
Quiz

- Terminal complement deficiency can lead to increased infection with which organism?
- What does the CH50 assay measure, and when is it used?
- Is hereditary angioedema an autosomal dominant or autosomal recessive disorder?
- What causes hereditary angioedema?
- How do patients with hereditary angioedema present?
- The combination of abdominal pain and extremity swelling in an adolescent make you think of what disease?
- Which drug is useful to terminate acute attacks in patients with hereditary angioedema?

COMPLEMENT CASCADE DEFICIENCIES

C1, C2, and C4 Deficiencies

C1, C2, or C4 deficiency causes decreased activation of complement via the classical pathway. Most of the complement proteins are inherited as autosomal recessive (AR) genes. Although the alternative pathway takes up some of the slack, these patients still have recurrent sinopulmonary infections (and ear infections when young) with encapsulated bacteria. In patients with 1 abnormal gene, complement blood levels are about 1/2 normal. In these patients, there is an increased incidence of rheumatoid diseases—especially SLE! C2 deficiency is the most common deficiency in North American Caucasians; thus, consider it in patients with early-onset SLE. This is because either these are important in removing immune complexes or their genes are somehow physically associated with genes that control immune responsiveness.

C3 Deficiency

C3 deficiency (complete absence) results in severe pyogenic infections with encapsulated bacteria, including *Streptococcus pneumoniae* and *Haemophilus influenzae*. With time, specific antibodies form against these organisms, and infections may become less frequent and less severe.

C5–C9 Deficiency

C5–C9 MAC deficiency is also called terminal complement deficiency. These terminal complements form the membrane attack complex (MAC) that is responsible for the lysis of *Neisseria* and other gram-negative bacteria. So, if you have a patient with invasive pneumococcal or meningococcal diseases, check for a complement deficiency. These patients must be immunized against encapsulated organisms.

Evaluation of Complement Disorders

The CH50 assay measures the total complement hemolytic activity of the classical pathway. A normal test shows that all factors (C1–C9) are present. Therefore, a CH50 is the 1st screening test to use to look for a complement deficiency! If the CH50 is low or absent, check for individual complement factors (C1–C9).

HEREDITARY ANGIOEDEMA

Overview

Hereditary angioedema (HAE) is an autosomal dominant (AD) disorder caused by a defect in C1 inhibitor enzyme (C1-INH) function with secondarily decreased C4 levels. Patients can have either a decreased C1 inhibitor enzyme (**Type I**) or a nonfunctioning C1 inhibitor enzyme (**Type II**). C1 inhibitor inactivates active C1 and is a major control point in the activation of the complement cascade, bradykinin-kinin system, and contact system. Without C1 inhibitor, there is ongoing consumption of C2 and C4, and there are low plasma C4 levels. Patients with hereditary angioedema have recurrent episodes of localized angioedema of distensible tissues, such as lips, eyelids, gastrointestinal tract, genitalia, and upper airway. Unlike angioedema and urticaria caused by IgE-mediated hypersensitivity reactions, hereditary angioedema does not cause urticaria. Bradykinin is thought to be the key mediator in the angioedema attacks.

Recurrent attacks of angioedema can begin anytime during childhood, and most people are diagnosed before their 20th birthday. Adolescents seem to experience an increased number and severity of attacks, and stress or trauma can trigger attacks. The swelling that occurs is nonpruritic and usually resolves within 5 days. Consider a diagnosis of hereditary angioedema in a patient with sudden onset of abdominal pain and extremity swelling. Laryngeal edema, leading to respiratory arrest, is the most life-threatening condition with this disorder.

Diagnosis

Screen by checking C4 levels. If C4 levels are low, diagnose by a decreased C1-INH functional assay. If the C1-INH level is also low, then it is Type I HAE. If the C1-INH level is normal, it is due to a nonfunctioning C1-INH enzyme, and it is Type II HAE.

Treatment

Purified C1-INH is the treatment of choice. Fresh frozen plasma can be used when C1-INH is unavailable. In the long term, attenuated androgens (danazol) increase C1-INH levels and decrease angioedema attacks! Purified C1-INH enzyme is available for the prevention and treatment of acute attacks.

ALLERGY & IMMUNOLOGY

VACCINE USE IN IMMUNOCOMPROMISED CHILDREN

Do not give live virus or live bacterial vaccines to children with congenital defects of their immune function, children receiving immunosuppressive therapy, or children undergoing (or having undergone) a bone marrow transplant.

The vaccines commonly asked about that fall into the live vaccine category are:

• Bacillus Calmette-Guérin (BCG)
• Oral poliovirus (OPV)
• Measles, mumps, rubella (MMR)
• Varicella vaccine
• Intranasal Influenza

Also, do not give OPV to household contacts of these children because the vaccine strain can be transmitted in the household to the immunocompromised child. It is fine, however, for the household contacts to receive MMR and varicella vaccines. There have been case reports of varicella vaccine strain transmission to immunocompromised children, but the resulting illness has generally been mild. In the case of a child in the house with SCID, varicella vaccine should probably be postponed in siblings until the SCID infant has some T-cell function after transplantation.

A new vaccine that poses a risk for severely immunodeficient patients is the live, cold-adapted, intranasal influenza virus vaccine. This vaccine strain is adapted to grow only at < 36° C, but because it replicates and is carried in the nasal cavity, it can be spread to contacts. Patients with profound B- or T-cell immunodeficiency would not be able to generate IgA antibody to clear the infection. Instead, use the inactivated influenza vaccine for contacts (including health care personnel) of immunodeficient patients.

The recent interest in smallpox vaccine (because of bioterrorism) has revived concern about this live virus vaccine in immunodeficient patients and also in patients with atopic dermatitis. Avoid giving this vaccine in these groups. As with other live virus vaccines that are shed from stool or skin, there is concern that the virus might pass to an immunodeficient host and cause severe disease. Do not give these vaccines to household contacts of immunodeficient patients or to health care workers with contact, unless contact can be avoided for the approximately 3 weeks required for the skin lesion to heal. Patients with atopic dermatitis are not immunodeficient in the sense discussed here, but they have altered barrier function and poor control and clearance of cutaneous viruses, including herpes simplex and vaccinia (smallpox vaccine virus). Use similar caution for contact with vaccine recipients.

As a rule, do not give live virus or bacterial vaccines to a child receiving 2 mg/kg or more of prednisone daily (total 20 mg), or every other day, for longer than 14 days. In general, a child should be off high-dose steroids for at least 3 months before you give these vaccines. However, many believe inhaled steroids are not immunosuppressive.

Children with HIV are a special group and, in general, should receive MMR and varicella vaccines at 12 months of age unless they are severely immunocompromised. Do not give OPV to these children. Also, remember that OPV should not be given to household contacts of a person with HIV. This has become a nonissue because IPV has replaced OPV in the United States for the most part.

ALLERGIC DISEASE

OVERVIEW

When we discuss allergies, we are typically discussing Type I hypersensitivity or IgE-mediated conditions. Some examples of allergic disease are anaphylaxis, urticaria, angioedema, asthma, rhinitis, atopic dermatitis, food allergy, drug allergy, insect allergy, and latex allergy. Not all forms of these diseases are IgE-mediated, but each of them does have an IgE-mediated form.

HYPERSENSITIVITY REACTIONS

The 4 Types of Hypersensitivity Reactions

All hypersensitivity reactions are immune-mediated tissue injury resulting in a variety of diseases: allergies, autoimmune disease, and a variety of other inflammatory diseases.

There are 4 types of hypersensitivity reactions (per Gell and Coombs):

Type I: IgE-mediated; immediate (anaphylactic, atopic)

Type II: IgG-mediated; cytotoxic

Type III: immune complex (antibody–antigen) mediated

Type IV: cell-mediated (further divided into IVa and IVb)

Type I: Immediate Hypersensitivity Reaction

Allergies

As mentioned above, the "classic" allergies are Type I hypersensitivity reactions. Examples: hives/urticaria, allergic rhinitis, allergic asthma, reaction to insect stings, drugs (PCN, etc.), latex, and foods (e.g., wheat, eggs, milk, peanuts, seafood).

Type I: Acute Response

The acute phase of immediate hypersensitivity reactions occurs within 1 hour after exposure—usually within minutes. Mast cell degranulation (especially producing histamine) is the cause of the symptoms. This reaction is IgE-mediated. These IgE antibodies are antigen-specific and occur only in response to previous exposure to the same allergen.

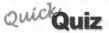

Quick Quiz

- What are the live viral or bacterial vaccines commonly used in children?

- A child is severely immunosuppressed; can his sister receive OPV? What about MMR?

- Which flu vaccine should be used for all health care workers who have the potential to come in contact with an immunosuppressed child?

- What is the highest dose of prednisone that a child can receive and concomitantly receive an MMR?

- Should a child with asymptomatic HIV receive the MMR vaccine?

- What is the mechanism of an immediate hypersensitivity reaction?

- When does the late phase of Type I hypersensitivity reaction occur? Why does it occur?

- At what antigen:antibody ratio does most immune-complex precipitation occur in a Type III hypersensitivity reaction?

The base (Fc portion) of IgE antibodies binds to a receptor on mast cells. This receptor is not specific, so there are many IgEs (each with its own antigen specificity) that can bind to a mast cell. No reaction occurs when IgE alone binds to the mast cell, but when IgE is attached to its specific allergen, degranulation of the mast cell can occur.

A certain allergen interacts with the allergen-specific receptor on the Fab portion of IgE, and, when the same antigen reacts with more than one IgE—thereby interlinking the 2—the mast cell is stimulated to degranulate and release mediators (especially histamine) and also to begin synthesizing and secreting other mediators (leukotriene C4, PGD2, and cytokines). Histamine is responsible for most of the acute symptoms.

Mast cells also release other products that have chemotactic effects, some of them enzymes (chymase and tryptase).

Review: Histamine interacts with 3 receptors: H_1, H_2, and H_3. Activation of the H_1 receptor causes the wheal and flare, bronchoconstriction, and pruritus. As you may recall, H_2 receptor activation results in increased gastric acid secretion. H_3 activation causes decreased histamine synthesis and release (negative feedback).

Type I: Late-Phase Response

Late-phase response: 3–12 hours after the immediate reaction is a late-phase response (LPR). This lasts hours to days and usually has an eosinophilic inflammatory infiltrate. Typically, there is an induration that has erythema, burning, and is occasionally pruritic. The LPR is probably one of the causes of the nonspecific airway hypersensitivity seen in asthma.

The LPR is a result of the initial, immediate IgE reaction stimulating the synthesis of cytokines. Basophils may also be involved with the late-phase response.

The probability of an LPR increases with the severity of the acute reaction.

Type II: Cytotoxic Hypersensitivity

Type II reactions occur when an IgG or IgM antibody binds to a fixed tissue antigen or cell receptor. These are autoantibodies.

Binding of the antibody results in target cell destruction by various means:

- Complement activation may cause cells to be lysed by the membrane attack complex.
- Complement activation may result in opsonization from the production of C3b. Phagocytes have a receptor for C3b.
- Phagocytes also have a receptor for the Fc portion of the antibodies and, therefore, may attack antibody coated cells.

Examples of target cell receptors are:

Target cell	Disease
Platelets	Thrombocytopenia
RBCs	Autoimmune hemolytic anemia
WBCs	Leukopenia

Examples of target fixed-tissue antigens are:

Target antigen	Disease
Component of the basement membrane (kidney and lung)	Goodpasture's
ACh receptor on muscle cells	Myasthenia gravis

Type III: Immune Complex Hypersensitivity

Any time you see a vasculitis, think of Type III hypersensitivity reaction. Type III reactions are also seen in Ig autoimmune diseases and in reaction to drugs.

Immune complexes (ICs) form when antibodies combine with antigen (self or foreign). A hypersensitivity reaction occurs when an antibody (usually IgG) reacts with a target antigen to form ICs, which precipitate and activate complement with subsequent small vessel inflammation and necrosis.

Remember: Just because an antibody reaction occurs and ICs are formed, it does not necessarily mean there will be precipitation. Significant precipitation occurs only when there is slight antigen excess in relation to antibody. When the antibody response initiates, there is a huge excess of antigens compared to antibodies (Ag:Ab >> 1). The ICs that are formed are small, soluble, and quickly cleared. Within 1–2 weeks, as exceedingly more antibodies are produced, a point is reached when there is only slight antigen excess, and the ICs interlace and become bigger and less soluble. These precipitate in the small vessels and activate complement, which starts a cascade causing the release of more cytokines and the gathering of more inflammatory cells. This process ultimately results in necrosis of the small vessels. The pathologic hallmark skin sign is leukocytoclastic vasculitis (hemorrhagic indurated lesions).

As the antigen is cleared, there comes a point when there is antibody excess. The formed ICs are large and quickly removed by circulating phagocytes (macrophages).

There are 2 animal models for what happens:

1) **Serum sickness (**a systemic reaction): A large amount of antigen is injected into a nonimmunized animal, and you see a similar necrotic vasculitis to the one just discussed.

2) **Arthus reaction** (a local reaction): The animal is 1st hyperimmunized—so there are many circulating IgG antibodies—and then given a small intradermal injection of the target antigen. All subsequent reaction occurs at the injection site, where many ICs are formed—inducing the complement cascade and inflammation. Within 4–6 hours, a painful indurated lesion appears and may progress to a sterile abscess.

Here are some examples of diseases in which Type III reaction plays a part.

Autoimmune diseases (and associated antigens):
• SLE (nuclear materials, such as ds-DNA, Smith antigen, and many others)
• Hashimoto thyroiditis (thyroglobulin)
• Pernicious anemia (intrinsic factor)
• Rheumatoid arthritis (rheumatoid factor)

External antigens:

• Hepatitis-antigen–associated serum sickness
• Tetanus and diphtheria immunization
• Local insulin reactions

Serum sickness and Arthus Type III hypersensitivity reactions are usually self-limited, and patients normally recover fully. Occasionally, corticosteroids are given.

Type IV: Cell-Mediated Hypersensitivity

Type IVa: Delayed-Type Hypersensitivity

Previously sensitized T cells interact with an antigen causing an inflammatory reaction. The reaction peaks in 24–72 hours—hence the common name: delayed-type hypersensitivity.

Tuberculin sensitivity and some types of contact dermatitis are examples of delayed hypersensitivity. There is also a delayed-type hypersensitivity component of asthma.

Don't confuse "delayed-type" IVa hypersensitivity reaction with the "late phase" of Type I!

Type IVb

Type IVb hypersensitivity reactions occur when cytotoxic T cells directly destroy target cells. Examples are allograft rejection and chronic hepatitis.

Type V: Autoimmune Stimulatory Hypersensitivity

The term Type V hypersensitivity reaction is used by some to indicate when the autoimmune IgG has a stimulatory effect on a receptor (as distinguished from Type II, which is destructive). It is not part of the Gell and Coombs's classification. Examples are:

• Graves disease, where there is IgG with a stimulatory effect on the TSH receptor
• Myasthenia gravis, where antibodies block ACh receptors on the postsynaptic neuromuscular junction

ALLERGIC DISORDERS

Oftentimes, these disorders occur together in "atopic" individuals. A given patient could have asthma, eczema, rhinitis, conjunctivitis, food allergy, and urticaria. In fact, it is prudent to look for additional diseases when you find one of them.

Anaphylaxis

Etiology and Presentation

Anaphylaxis is an IgE-mediated, Type I immediate systemic hypersensitivity reaction to an allergen. A similar reaction that is not IgE-mediated is known as "anaphylactoid." It is not possible to clinically distinguish between anaphylactoid reactions and anaphylaxis. Anaphylaxis is more common in adults than in children. Girls are more at risk for anaphylaxis caused by intravenous muscle relaxants, aspirin, and latex. Boys are more at risk from insect stings.

The list of allergens known to produce anaphylaxis is enormous. Antibiotics (especially penicillin) are one of the most frequent causes. Latex has been a problem mainly in high-exposure populations (such as patients with spina bifida or urogenital malformations). Anesthesia agents are another common cause of anaphylaxis. Insulin, blood products, antisera, and IVIG have all been implicated. Foods are also common causes. A nice mnemonic for this is **WEMPS** (**w**heat, **e**ggs, **m**ilk and soy, **p**eanuts and tree nuts, and **s**eafood).

Anaphylactoid reactions are most commonly due to aspirin, NSAIDs, and radiographic contrast.

Anaphylaxis is a result of a huge activation of IgE-sensitized mast cells by the allergen. Histamine release occurs within 5–10 minutes after exposure to the allergen, and histamine remains at high serum levels for at least an hour. Histamine interacts with specific receptors and causes increased heart rate, vascular permeability,

Quick Quiz

- A tuberculin test is an example of which type of hypersensitivity reaction?

- What is the difference between a Type II and a Type V hypersensitivity reaction?

- Know the difference between Type II, Type III, and Type IV hypersensitivity reactions.

- What are the most common manifestations of anaphylaxis?

- Know how to treat anaphylaxis—both mild and severe.

vasodilatation, smooth muscle contraction, sensory nerve irritation, and coronary artery vasospasm. Multiple other mediators are released; some, such as leukotrienes and prostaglandins, may have vascular effects. The complement pathway may be activated. The cumulative effect of all of these mediators is vasodilatation, hypotension, and loss of intravascular fluid volume. This can then be followed by vasoconstriction and myocardial depression with severe hypotension.

Anaphylaxis usually begins within 5–30 minutes after antigen exposure but can be delayed up to 2 hours. Urticaria and angioedema are the most common manifestations of anaphylaxis (see Image 6-1 and Image 6-2), followed by flushing and respiratory tract symptoms in approximately 50% of those affected. Absence of skin findings does not rule out anaphylaxis. The effects of respiratory tract edema can be life-threatening. Clinically, this presents as stridor. Hypotension and shock are also fairly common. Cardiac arrest can occur without any of the other symptoms. GI complaints occur in ~ 33% of patients.

Ensure that patients with a serious history of allergy or anaphylaxis have a self-injectable epinephrine device, such as an EpiPen® or Twinject®, available for immediate administration at the 1st sign of symptoms or exposure.

Anaphylaxis can also be caused by the byproducts of activated C3, C4, and C5 (anaphylatoxins), which, like IgE, cause the release of the cytoplasmic granules from mast cells (+/– basophils). The released cytoplasmic granules cause an immediate hypersensitivity reaction. ASA/NSAIDs, physical stress, and certain chemicals (sulfites that cause asthma, opiates) can be causes of non-IgE–mediated anaphylaxis.

Note that ASA-induced anaphylaxis is a separate syndrome from ASA-induced urticaria; both of these are separate from ASA-induced asthma, which is often associated with rhinosinusitis and polyps.

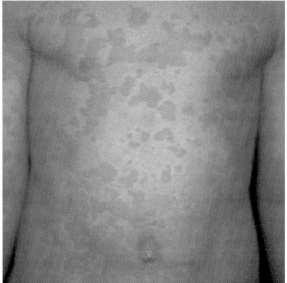

Image 6-1: Urticaria

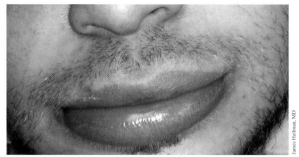

James Heilman, MD

Image 6-2: Angioedema

Treatment of Anaphylaxis

General treatment strategy for immediate hypersensitivity diseases is: **A**voidance of the allergen, and give **A**ntihistamines (occasionally steroids) and **A**llergen-specific immunotherapy (**3 As**). The immunotherapy may take 6 months to show an effect, with maximal effect in 3 years. Patients at high risk, such as beekeepers, should also get an epinephrine autoinjector kit (EpiPen, Twinject). Effective immunotherapy causes an increase in T-regulatory cell secretion of IL-10 and blocking antibodies of the IgG isotype, among many other effects.

Severe: In patients with stridor or swelling of the lips and tongue, the 1st step is to protect the airway. Endotracheal intubation may be necessary.

Patients with evidence of hypotension or shock should immediately be given a bolus of normal saline intravenously. In addition, give epinephrine 0.01 mg/kg (max 0.5 mg) IM; repeat every 15–20 minutes as needed. EpiPens have 0.3 mg and EpiPen Jr.® has 0.15 mg.

Note: There are 2 forms of epinephrine:

1) 1:1,000 for IM use. It is 1 mg/1 mL so 0.3 mg is 0.3 mL, which is lower volume and more appropriate for IM.

2) 1:10,000 for IV use. It is 1 mg/10 mL so 0.3 mg is 3 mL, which is higher volume and more appropriate for IV.

It is very important not to confuse the 2 forms because doing so can lead to serious over- or underdosing.

Ensure that the patient is recumbent. Start an IV so that boluses of normal saline or more epinephrine can be given as needed. Epinephrine is an alpha and beta adrenergic agonist that causes bronchial relaxation, vasoconstriction, and decreased vascular permeability. The effect of epinephrine is blunted in patients on beta-blockers, so these are relatively contraindicated in patients at risk of anaphylactic reaction. Glucagon or vasopressin injections may be used in patients on beta-blockers during anaphylaxis if the response to epinephrine is poor. However, epinephrine is always 1st line therapy.

Parenteral H_1 and H_2 antagonists (usually diphenhydramine and cimetidine, respectively) may also be given. Inhaled albuterol may be given if bronchospasm is present. Steroids may help prevent the delayed (late-phase) reactions.

Urticaria

Acute urticaria: superficial, blanching, transient, pruritic lesions. Consider anaphylaxis, and, if suspicion is high enough, treat appropriately. If the patient has isolated urticaria, you may treat initially with just antihistamines.

Chronic urticaria: when the urticaria lasts longer than 6 weeks. Prior to the identification of the important role of autoimmunity in chronic urticaria, the majority (~ 80%) were considered to have idiopathic urticaria. In other words, the causative agent was not found in the majority of cases. More recently, we have identified a large component of autoimmunity in these patients. Now, about 60% of these previously identified chronic idiopathic urticaria (CIU) patients are identified as autoimmune. ~ 45% are allergic to their own IgE receptors, ~ 5% are allergic to their own IgE, and ~ 10% have antithyroid antibodies. These patients also have a strong association with autoimmune diseases like autoimmune hypothyroidism, hyperthyroidism, SLE, and RA. ~ 20% of such patients have their autoimmune diagnosis before they develop CIU, and the other 80% develop their autoimmune disease afterward.

It is not recommended to send any routine labs (CBC, BMP, ESR, C3, C4, ANA, etc.) in the initial workup unless guided by history and physical exam. Other causes to consider besides autoimmunity are infections, neoplasms, and physical urticarias such as urticaria due to cold, heat, pressure, vibration (vibratory), sun light (solar), and water (aquagenic).

Other urticarias:

- **Acquired cold urticaria** is generally mediated by IgE, and less commonly by cryoglobulin. When cryoglobulin or cold agglutinins are identified, underlying diseases like Hepatitis B or C should be considered and investigated. Shock may occur if the patient is immersed in cold water! Test with a 5-minute skin ice-cube challenge test.

- **Familial cold urticaria** is an autosomal dominant inherited inflammatory disease characterized by urticaria, myalgias, fever, and joint pain after cold exposure.

- **Cholinergic urticaria** is precipitated by heat (e.g., hot shower, hot day, exercise). Usually presents as punctate lesions, which are very pruritic.

- **Immediate pressure urticaria** is seen with severe dermatographism and may develop around the waistline.

- **Delayed pressure urticaria** typically causes swelling and burning (not itching) of palms and soles several hours after carrying a load for a while or walking long distances.

- **Urticarial vasculitis** can clinically resemble chronic urticaria. However, patients report hives lasting > 24 hours in a fixed location (in contrast to chronic urticaria, which resolves in minutes to hours or migrates continually). Other red flags include residual ecchymosis, hyperpigmentation, or purpura. Diagnose with skin biopsy.

- Also see urticaria pigmentosa under Mastocytosis on page 6-24.

Angioedema

Angioedema often occurs with urticaria, either chronic or acute; and again, anaphylaxis should be considered and treated if the suspicion is high enough.

With angioedema alone, consider hereditary angioedema (see earlier description).

Asthma

The current guidelines contain more than 400 pages, protecting it from ever being read by most docs! We have boiled it down into a few paragraphs here, and there is much greater detail in Respiratory Disorders, Book 4.

Asthma is a chronic inflammatory disorder of the airways, characterized by recurrent episodes of acute reversible airflow obstruction, cough (especially at night), wheeze, chest tightness, and shortness of breath. The chest x-ray is usually normal or hyperinflated. Infiltrates or opacifications on chest x-ray should make one consider a different diagnosis.

Treatment options for asthma are broken down into 2 major categories:

1) **Relievers**: Short-acting beta-agonists; e.g., albuterol or levalbuterol

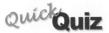

Quick Quiz

- Which antihypertensive agent is relatively contraindicated in a patient at risk for anaphylaxis? Why?
- What is the most common cause of chronic urticaria?
- Which lab tests should be routinely sent for the workup of chronic urticaria?
- What are the 2 domains of asthma control, and what are their significance?
- In reference to asthma control, what is the rule of 2s for patients < 12 years old?
- What are some common physical signs of allergic rhinitis?
- Nasal polyps are indicative of what disease in young children?

2) **Controllers**:
- Inhaled corticosteroids; e.g., budesonide or fluticasone
- Leukotriene receptor antagonists; e.g., montelukast.
- Long-acting beta-agonists; e.g., formoterol or salmeterol (Note: When given alone, they increase morbidity but when paired with an inhaled corticosteroid, they reduce morbidity, so they should always be paired in combination with an inhaled corticosteroid.)

Severity: At the 1st visit, severity should be assigned as intermittent, mild persistent, moderate persistent, or severe persistent.

Control: At subsequent visits, the level of control should be assessed as well controlled, not well controlled, or very poorly controlled. The domains of control are broken down into 2 categories:

1) **Impairment**: symptom frequency (number of episodes per week or month during the day or night)
2) **Risk**: morbidity (number of hospital admissions or emergency department visits in the last year)

In general, patients are considered well controlled (or intermittent at the 1st visit) if they follow the rule of 2s:

Impairment: ≤ 2 episodes per week during the day, and ≤ 2 episodes per month during the night
Risk: < 2 ED visits or hospitalizations per year

For patients under 12 years of age, this rule of 2s is even more conservative:

Impairment: < 2 episodes per week during the day, and < 2 episodes per month during the nigh
Risk: < 2 ED visits or hospitalizations per year

The asthma predictive index (API) can be applied to wheezing children < 3 years to assess their risk of continuing to wheeze and of having asthma. To satisfy this prediction of being high-risk for developing asthma, they need to have 1 major criterion *or* 2 of the minor criteria:

- **Major Criteria** (1 of the following):
  - One of the parents has asthma.
  - The child has physician-diagnosed eczema.

    or

- **Minor Criteria** (2 of the following):
  - The child has physician-diagnosed allergic rhinitis.
  - The child has wheezing apart from colds/URIs.
  - The child has eosinophilia.

If the child has a negative API, it is unlikely that the child will develop asthma by 6 years of age (negative predictive value 95%).

Allergic Rhinitis and Conjunctivitis

Signs and Symptoms

What exactly happens to cause allergic rhinoconjunctivitis? First, allergens are inhaled into the nose. Those that are water-soluble diffuse through mucus in the nose and interact with allergen-specific IgE on the surface of mast cells. This initiates cellular activation and results in the release of histamine and other mediators. Histamine and these other mediators then produce their local symptoms of congestion and runny nose and abate fairly quickly. But several hours later, the symptoms recur, due to the appearance of helper T cells and eosinophils in response to the cytokines released in the initial response. From this develops the chronic inflammation in allergic rhinitis and the common chronic symptoms.

After allergic rhinitis occurs, nasal congestion is the most common symptom reported, along with itchy nose, throat, and ears. Sneezing also occurs frequently and is accompanied by clear coryza. Fever is not a feature of allergic rhinitis. Eye findings can include excessive/frequent lacrimation and red conjunctiva.

Nasal polyps (Image 6-3) develop in adolescents over time but are very rare in children; if you see them in younger children, consider another diagnosis, such as cystic fibrosis.

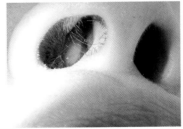

Image 6-3: Nasal polyp

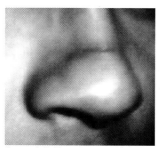

Image 6-4: Transverse nasal crease

Other physical findings are dark circles under the eyes—so-called allergic shiners—which are very nonspecific and due to chronic venous congestion. The "nasal salute" occurs with frequent rubbing of the nose and may progress to a transverse nasal crease (Image 6-4). Dennie-Morgan lines (Image 6-5) are folds below the eyes due to edema and frequently accompany allergic shiners. Mouth breathing is common, and the tonsils/adenoids are often enlarged in allergic rhinitis. The nasal mucosa is usually swollen and pale. "Cobblestoning" of the posterior oropharynx is common and is due to chronic postnasal drainage.

In allergic conjunctivitis, it is common to find bilateral conjunctival injection, periorbital edema, and excessive tearing.

Don't forget that it is easy to examine the nasal secretions for eosinophils. This is suggestive, but not pathognomonic, for allergic rhinitis.

Avoidance of Specific Triggers

Clues in the child's history generally steer you in the right direction as far as the etiology for the allergic reaction. Seasonal changes vs. year-round patterns can be helpful in narrowing down the etiology. Tree pollens are highest in the spring, grass pollens in the early summer, and weeds in the fall. Mold may be high year-round (e.g., in southern climates) or diminished considerably by snow.

Once skin testing or a RAST has determined which allergens are likely causing the disease process, you can suggest specific measures aimed at reducing exposure to those allergens. For example, dust mites are a common source. Impermeable, zippered covers on mattresses, box springs, and pillows considerably reduce the amount of dust mite allergen in the room by trapping the allergen in its main reservoirs! If coupled with laundering of all bed linens at least every other week, dust mite allergen recovery from the bed surfaces is reduced by as much as 90%.

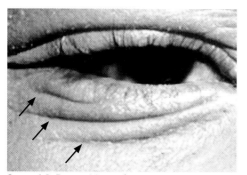

Image 6-5: Dennie-Morgan lines

Secondary considerations for mite reduction include removal of upholstered furniture, heavy draperies, and carpeting, and also humidity control. Dust mites require a relative humidity > 50% to be most viable, so suggest measures to reduce in-home humidity. Interestingly, use of home air filtration systems does not help with dust mites because few of their allergens are airborne.

Cat and dog dander are another major source of allergens in the home, with cat dander usually creating a much more severe response. Both dog and cat allergens are found in saliva and dander. Removal of the pet is the best means of reducing allergen burden, but dog allergen levels can be detectable at 4–5 months after such removal. Cat allergen levels last even longer! HEPA filters reduce airborne levels of cat and dog allergens.

Medications

H1 antihistamines are the 1st line therapy for allergic rhinitis. They function by blocking the interaction between histamine and the H_1 histamine receptor. If antihistamines are used before an allergen exposure, they will prevent the development of allergic symptoms. Used after exposure, their effect gradually alleviates symptoms as less histamine is able to interact with the H_1 histamine receptor.

Early histamine blockers (diphenhydramine, chlorpheniramine, and hydroxyzine) have the major side effect of sedation. This is due to the ability of these drugs to cross the blood-brain barrier and interact with dopamine, serotonin, and acetylcholine receptors in the brain. The interaction with acetylcholine receptors also results in the blurry vision and dry mouth sometimes seen with the older antihistamines. Recently developed 2nd generation antihistamines (cetirizine, fexofenadine, loratadine, desloratadine) do not cross the blood-brain barrier as much, and are more specifically aimed at the H_1 receptor and not the other receptors.

Other Medications

Leukotriene receptor antagonists also reduce allergic symptoms by blocking the vascular and proinflammatory actions of leukotrienes released in the allergic reaction.

Recent newer ocular agents, such as lodoxamide and olopatadine, have histamine-blocking properties as well as mast-cell stabilization.

Steroids are very potent antiinflammatory agents, and they prevent the late phase of the allergic response and provide relief of many symptoms. Intranasal corticosteroids are the most effective agent for nasal allergy and do not have the systemic side effects seen with oral prednisone. These topical steroids are the most effective medicines for allergic rhinitis and are the treatment of choice for **NARES** (**n**on-**a**llergic **r**hinitis with **e**osinophilia **s**yndrome).

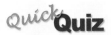

Quick Quiz

- Which pollens are highest in the spring? Early summer? Fall? Year-round?

- Do home air filtration systems help with dust mites allergies?

- True or false? If a dog or cat is removed from a living environment, the pet's allergens are gone by 2 months.

- Do intranasal corticosteroids have systemic side effects?

Allergen Immunotherapy

Allergen immunotherapy, or desensitization, is generally the last resort in therapy for allergies. Prescribe environmental control and medications 1st and, if there is no improvement over time, then consider immunotherapy.

Immunotherapy involves giving increasing doses of allergens via the subcutaneous route to induce alteration in the immune response to the allergen. As mentioned above, effective immunotherapy causes an increase in T-regulatory cell secretion of IL-10 and blocking antibodies of the IgG isotype, among many other effects.

It usually takes 1 year before beneficial effects occur, and this is most effective for individuals with a limited number of specific allergens. Systemic and even anaphylactic reactions can occur during therapy, so you must carefully monitor and evaluate these patients.

Atopic Dermatitis

Atopic dermatitis is one of the many types of eczema. Typically it presents as a dry, pruritic, scaly rash on the flexor surfaces (cubital fossae, axilla, inguinal area, behind the ears, around the eyes, almost anywhere that the skin creases).

In infants, atopic dermatitis has a slightly different pattern of distribution, presenting on the scalp, face, and extensor surfaces rather than on the flexor surfaces like older children.

1/3 of patients with atopic dermatitis also have food allergies. So avoidance of the trigger (if one can be identified) is one component of therapy.

Treatment is done in a layered approach:

1) **Moisturizers**: The 1st level is aggressive application of moisturizers like Cetaphil®, Vanicream®, Aquaphor®, Eucerin®, or Crisco® shortening. These should be applied multiple times a day and after every time the patient gets wet (showers, baths, sweating, swimming). Moisturizers are less effective if applied to dry skin.

2) **Immunomodulatory creams**: The 2nd level is the use of topical corticosteroids or topical calcineurin inhibitors (pimecrolimus or tacrolimus). This should be applied to problem areas of the skin to decrease inflammation. Although topical corticosteroids are 1st line antiinflammatory agents, they can cause skin atrophy, so avoid use on the face and the axilla. Topical calcineurin inhibitors do not cause skin atrophy.

3) **Antihistamines**: The 3rd level option. It is important to break the scratch-itch-scratch cycle. Again, 1st generation antihistamines are more effective than later-generation ones, but they have some degree of sedation. This may actually be useful for patients who can't sleep because they are constantly scratching their skin at night.

4) **Wet wraps**: The 4th level option, if frequent moisturizing, immunomodulatory creams, and antihistamines are not enough. Take the patient's pajamas or a towel, make it slightly damp with room temperature water, and cover the areas that are most affected while the patient sleeps. This does 3 things:
   - Keeps the skin moist.
   - Prevents trauma from the patient scratching in their sleep.
   - As the water evaporates, the wrap remains cool and decreases the sensation of pruritus.

5) **Oral corticosteroids**: The 5th level option. If the rest of the interventions are ineffective, then a 5-day burst of corticosteroids usually calms down the disease acutely so better control can be achieved.

6) **Antibiotics**: The 6th level option. If the patient is still uncontrolled or shows signs of infection, such as impetigo, treat with topical or oral antibiotics to decrease the damage that is being done by the infection. Most patients with atopic dermatitis are colonized with *Staphylococcus aureus*, and superinfection is fairly common.

Food Allergy

The most common food allergies in children are:

- **W**heat: IgE-mediated reaction, which makes it different from celiac disease (see Gastroenterology & Nutrition, Book 4)
- **E**ggs: Most common in atopic dermatitis
- **M**ilk and soy
- **P**eanuts and tree nuts
- **S**eafood: crustacean shellfish and fish

If the history is consistent with anaphylactic episodes, then the patients should be prescribed an epinephrine autoinjector (EpiPen, Twinject) and trained on how to use it.

Patients should also be trained on how to avoid the food they are allergic to. They should be told how to ask the right questions in restaurants and how to read food labels to avoid exposure.

Most children (85%) outgrow their allergy to wheat, eggs, milk, and soy. In contrast, allergies to peanuts, tree nuts, shellfish, and fish tend to be more persistent. Only 20% of children with peanut allergy outgrow their allergy.

Adverse Drug Reactions

Drug reactions are fairly common, but few are due to immune responses. Many are idiosyncratic; the rest are mostly due to drug overdose, drug-drug interactions, or drug side effects.

There are 4 general immune responses/hypersensitivities with drugs:

Type I: Specific IgE-hypersensitivity reactions.

Type II: Antibody-mediated hemolysis by the binding of the drug to the surface of RBCs.

Type III: Antibody:antigen precipitation resulting in serum sickness.

Type IV: Drug-induced, delayed-type hypersensitivity reaction mediated by T lymphocytes and monocytes.

Timing of the reaction can be a clue to the type of reaction elicited. For example, if a drug is given intravenously and an immediate reaction occurs (within an hour), an IgE-mediated process is likely. Or, if reaction is delayed up to 72 hours, a delayed-hypersensitivity reaction is indicated. Skin reactions are the most common and generally are maculopapular or morbilliform eruptions (Image 6-6). Urticaria is suggestive of an IgE-mediated process. More severe skin manifestations include Stevens-Johnson syndrome (Image 6-7), toxic epidermal necrolysis, fixed drug reactions, and photosensitivity. These manifestations generally appear more than 72 hours after exposure to the drug.

Besides skin manifestations, other problems can occur, including fever, arthritis, and vasculitis as well as GI, neurologic, and pulmonary findings. Prior exposure to the drug is necessary for an immunologic reaction to occur, but prior exposures need not have induced an allergic reaction.

Laboratory testing is usually not helpful. Peripheral blood eosinophilia is suggestive but not conclusive of a drug allergy. Penicillin skin testing may be helpful, but skin testing for other drugs has not been reproducible.

Penicillin is composed of benzylpenicillin; this is 95% of the tissue-bound penicillin. Benzylpenicillin is known as the major determinant of penicillin and is used in skin testing initially. However, not all individuals with penicillin allergy are identified because minor determinants also can induce allergy. In fact, the 2 minor determinants, benzylpenicilloate and benzylpenicilloic acid, are responsible for most of the anaphylaxis occurring due to penicillin allergy. Therefore, it is important to include these in penicillin allergy testing. Also, note that even those who have a negative reaction to the 3 antigens could still have an urticarial or delayed hypersensitivity reaction on subsequent administration of penicillin.

For any drug causing an allergic reaction, the key is to stop the drug. If anaphylaxis is occurring, use epinephrine, antihistamines, and corticosteroids if necessary. Penicillin cross-reacts with cephalosporins at a rate of 1–3%, so patients with a non-life-threatening penicillin allergy can usually safely get cephalosporins. On the other hand, patients with life-threatening penicillin allergies should get prior desensitization before getting cephalosporins.

Desensitization is a relatively safe procedure done in the hospital using gradually increasing doses of penicillin (oral is preferred). The process is completed in 4-12 hours.

Desensitization is necessary if the drug is the only known clinically effective therapy. Desensitization is likely to be effective only if the drug reaction is due to an immediate hypersensitivity mechanism (i.e., IgE-mediated). A common test question involves a pregnant woman with syphilis or a person with neurosyphilis. Both require desensitization and then treatment with penicillin.

In a children's hospital, the major indication for desensitization is for use of penicillins or cephalosporins in drug-allergic children with cystic fibrosis and multiple, drug-resistant *Pseudomonas* disease. Also, remember that desensitization works only for that particular episode, and subsequent administrations down the road will require repeat desensitization.

Vancomycin hypersensitivity, or the "red man syndrome," is one of the more famous adverse reactions to the drug. One treats it by lowering the infusion rate, not by decreasing the dose.

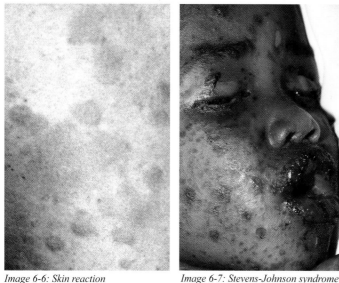

Image 6-6: Skin reaction   *Image 6-7: Stevens-Johnson syndrome*

Quick **Quiz**

- If a drug is given intravenously and there is an immediate reaction, what is the likely type of hypersensitivity reaction? What if the reaction is delayed up to 72 hours?

- A child with cystic fibrosis has a life-threatening pneumonia with a very resistant strain of *Pseudomonas*. The only effective drug is a cephalosporin. He has had life-threatening anaphylactic reactions to penicillin in the past. What can be done to give him this lifesaving drug?

- What pediatric conditions are associated with a higher risk of latex allergy?

- Which foods have known clinically relevant cross-reactivity with latex?

- Can you do valid skin-prick testing with a child who is on antihistamines?

Insect Allergy

Insects from the *Hymenoptera* order, such as hornets, bees, wasps, yellow jackets, and fire ants, are the most common cause of insect allergy.

Location of nests:

- **Hornet** nests are found attached to the outside of trees or shrubs.
- **Bee** nests are found inside of trees, in natural hollows.
- **Wasps** (legs dangle when flying) are found on the outside of buildings attached to eaves, window sills, or wood decks.
- **Yellow jacket** nests are found inside cracks of old buildings, inside walls, or in the ground of gardens or golf courses.
- **Fire ant** nests are mounds of dirt with a hole in the top.

A large, local reaction to a sting or bite does not increase the risk of anaphylaxis, and further workup is not necessary. Of course, anaphylaxis itself does require workup—usually skin tests (because reliance on history to identify the correct stinging insect is notoriously unreliable).

Anaphylaxis from insect stings should be followed up subsequently with immunotherapy (allergy shots).

Latex Allergy

Latex allergy has been a frequent cause of anaphylaxis in children in hospitals and among health care workers. Latex allergy is uncommon in children unless they have conditions that give them a high exposure rate to latex, like spina bifida or congenital urologic problems.

For children with spina bifida, the main risks are number of surgeries, total serum IgE, presence of a VP shunt, and a personal history of atopy. Multiple surgeries at an early age appear to be the highest risk factor for all children (not just those with spina bifida).

Latex allergy is due to sensitization to proteins—primarily hevein—on the surface of the latex products.

Interestingly, there is cross-reactivity between several fruits and vegetables with latex. While these patients can show a high IgE level to multiple fruits, vegetables, and nuts, the main ones that show clinical relevance **PKB PACT** (PeeKaBoo PACT) are:

- **P**apaya, **k**iwi, **b**anana (fruits)
- **P**otato, **a**vocado, **c**hestnut, **t**omato (nuts and vegetables)

Patients with spina bifida have more cross-reactivity to potato, and health care workers have more cross-reactivity to kiwis, bananas, and avocados.

You can test for latex allergy in several ways. Questioning about prior reactions is very helpful. Skin-prick testing and a RAST may rule out latex sensitivity because a negative test pretty much rules out latex allergy as causative. Unfortunately, skin-test reagents are not commercially available.

Treat by providing a latex-free environment, which many hospitals and clinics have adopted.

Allergy Testing and Other Laboratory Tests

Skin Testing

Skin testing for immediate hypersensitivity can be helpful to determine which specific allergens a child is allergic to. How does it work? You prick the skin with a small drop of an extract of a specific allergen (mites, pollens, animal dander, mold, drugs, foods, etc.); this is called epicutaneous testing. In some cases, you might use a needle to make a small injection into the skin. This is the intradermal technique. If the allergen is recognized by allergen-specific IgE on the mast-cell surface, the mast-cell IgE receptors undergo cross-linking, which leads to mast-cell activation and degranulation. Essentially, you have initiated a localized IgE-mediated (Type I) hypersensitivity reaction. The activation of the mast cells causes a release of histamine and other products. The histamine then binds to type-specific histamine receptors and causes local vasodilatation and increased vascular permeability, resulting in a wheal. Additionally, an axonal reflex occurs, producing the surrounding erythema, known as the "flare." The wheal and flare develop within 15–20 minutes and then quickly resolve.

For valid skin testing, the patient cannot be on antihistamines because these may mute the response and give a false-negative reaction. Patients should be off these agents for a minimum of 72 hours before you begin skin testing. A positive control with histamine is useful to detect the presence of antagonism. Steroids do not block skin testing for immediate hypersensitivity but may interfere with delayed hypersensitivity!

Laboratory Testing

Specific laboratory testing is quite varied. A common, nonspecific finding in most people with allergic tendencies is an elevated eosinophil count. Blood eosinophils may run ~ 1–3% in normal individuals. An absolute number > 350 cells/mm^3, or > 5%, is considered elevated. Eosinophils in secretions are also common; a Hansel stain of nasal secretions from a child with allergic rhinoconjunctivitis may have up to 10% eosinophils.

Elevated IgE levels are also common in those with atopy, but some individuals with allergies do not have elevated IgE levels. Other diseases can result in elevated IgE levels, so proceed with caution. These other hyper-IgE conditions include Job/Hyper-IgE syndrome, Omenn syndrome, Wiskott-Aldrich syndrome, parasitic infections, neoplasia (Hodgkin's in particular), allergic bronchopulmonary aspergillosis, Churg-Strauss syndrome, and cystic fibrosis.

A radioallergosorbent test (RAST) is another method to determine allergen-specific IgE in serum. The benefits of a RAST are that antihistamines do not interfere with results, and allergen provocation is not a problem since this is an *in vitro* test. However, the test is not as accurate, must be sent to a lab, and, unlike skin testing, a return visit is needed to discuss test results. A RAST involves a solid-phase support to which allergens are bound and then incubated in the patient's serum. After washing unbound allergens from the solid-phase support, a radiolabeled human IgE antibody is incubated with the solid-phase support and then washed again. The amount of radiolabeled human IgE antibody bound to the support is proportional to the amount of allergen-specific IgE in the patient's serum.

Remember: Both skin testing and a RAST are only suggestive evidence for sensitivity to a particular item, but a negative skin-prick test is strong evidence against allergy to an item.

Serum Sickness

Serum sickness is a Type III hypersensitivity reaction. The interaction of IgG (sometimes IgM) and a foreign antigen produces the reaction (not IgE-mediated). It usually takes 6–12 days for the reaction to occur, but it can take up to 3 weeks.

Serum sickness differs from IgE-mediated hypersensitivity reactions in that serum sickness does not require prior exposure to an antigen (prior sensitization) for a reaction to occur. Thus, serum sickness can develop on the initial exposure.

Originally, serum sickness was most commonly due to administering heterologous serum (like equine antitetanus). Today, serum sickness is most commonly due to antibiotics, most frequently cefaclor and penicillin. Also, antithymocyte globulin, antilymphocyte globulin, OKT3 monoclonal antibodies, and stings from *Hymenoptera* (bees, wasps, and some ants) can cause serum sickness.

If previous exposure has occurred, reaction may occur as quickly as 1–3 days postexposure. Usually, an antigen-antibody complex forms, and for most individuals, these are cleared easily by the reticuloendothelial system. However, if the antigenic burden is too high, intravascular immune complexes form, which precipitate in joints, renal glomeruli, and blood vessel walls. These immune complexes then activate the classic complement pathway, which leads to further problems such as vascular injury, influx of neutrophils, and eventual tissue injury or death. IgE may be elevated as a result of serum sickness, although IgE is not the mediator of serum sickness.

Clinically, patients may present with fever, skin rashes, joint pain, lymph node swelling, muscle aches, and proteinuria. Skin findings are nearly universal and include itching, redness, urticaria, and angioedema. Arthralgia and arthritis can involve multiple joints, especially the knees, ankles, fingers, and toes. GI complaints are common and include nausea and vomiting. Symptoms last ~ 7–10 days and then resolve spontaneously.

Treatment is to stop the offending agent. Nonsteroidals can be helpful for fever and muscle/bone pain. Diphenhydramine or hydroxyzine help relieve urticaria and itching. If other interventions are not helpful, you can start prednisone at 1–2 mg/kg/day.

Mastocytosis

Mastocytosis is a rare disorder characterized by abnormal mast cell proliferation and accumulation in various organs. The degree of involvement determines the extent of the disease:

- **Cutaneous mastocytosis** results from increased mast cells in the dermis. It causes urticaria pigmentosa, which is diagnosed by formation of a wheal on gentle stroking of the macule (Darier sign).
- **Systemic mastocytosis** also has increased mast cells in the tissues (so patients also have abdominal symptoms, flushing, and fatigue besides the urticaria pigmentosa).
- **Malignant mastocytosis** causes severe systemic symptoms, but often no skin changes. Signs include hepatosplenomegaly and lymphadenopathy.

Diagnosis: Because tryptase is a by-product of mast cells, tryptase levels will be elevated (> 20) in all types of mastocytosis. Perform skin biopsy for isolated cutaneous mastocytosis. If there is evidence of systemic or malignant involvement, then bone marrow biopsy is recommended.

Treatment: Stay away from cold, heat, alcohol, ASA, and opiates. Oral cromolyn may help for GI symptoms. Various chemotherapy regimens have been used in the treatment of systemic and malignant mastocytosis. Unfortunately, chemotherapy has not been particularly successful.

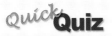

Quiz

- A child with allergic rhinitis is skin-prick tested for dust mites. The test is negative. Does this finding make dust mite an unlikely etiology for her symptoms?
- How does serum sickness differ from immediate hypersensitivity reactions?
- What agents most commonly cause serum sickness?
- What type of hypersensitivity reaction is serum sickness?
- How long does it take for a serum sickness reaction to occur?
- How do patients with serum sickness present?

PREVENTION OF ATOPIC DISEASE

In 2008, the AAP published guidelines reviewing the nutritional options during pregnancy, lactation, and the 1st year of life that may affect the development of atopic disease.

Know:

- Maternal dietary restrictions during pregnancy do not prevent the development of atopic disease.
- Breastfeeding for at least 4 months prevents or delays the occurrence of atopic dermatitis, cow milk allergy, and wheezing in early childhood.
- In infants at high risk of atopy who are not breastfed, the onset of atopic disease may be delayed or prevented by the use of hydrolyzed formulas.
- There is no evidence that delaying the introduction of solids after 4 to 6 months of age prevents the occurrence of atopic disease. In fact, there is even some evidence that the delayed introduction of foods like peanuts may increase the prevalence of food allergies.
- Use of soy-based formulas does not prevent atopic disease.

FOR FURTHER READING

THE IMMUNE SYSTEM

Murphy K, et al. *Janeway's Immunobiology*, 7th Ed. Taylor & Francis Group, 2008.

Turvey SE, Broide DH. Innate immunity. *J Allergy Clin Immunol.* 2010 Feb;125(2 Suppl 2):S24–S32.

Bonilla FA, Oettgen HC. Adaptive immunity. *J Allergy Clin Immunol.* 2010 Feb;125(2 Suppl 2):S33–S40.

IMMUNODEFICIENCIES

Bonilla FA, et al. Practice parameter for the diagnosis and management of primary immunodeficiency. *Ann Allergy Asthma Immunol.* 2005 May;94(5 Suppl 1):S1–S63.

McCusker C, Warrington R. Primary immunodeficiency. *Allergy Asthma Clin Immunol.* 2011 Nov 10;7 (Suppl 1):S11.

Moses S. Primary immunodeficiency. *Family Practice Notebook.* 2007.

Notarangelo LD. Primary immunodeficiencies. *J Allergy Clin Immunol.* 2010 Feb;125(2 Suppl 2):S182–S194.

Oliveira JB, Fleisher TA. Laboratory evaluation of primary immunodeficiencies. *J Allergy Clin Immunol.* 2010 Feb;125(2 Suppl 2):S297–S305.

Tangsinmankong N, et al. The immunologic workup of the child suspected of immunodeficiency. *Ann Allergy Asthma Immunol.* 2001 Nov;87(5):362–369.

McKusick VA. Immune defect due to absence of thymus. Record created 1986; updated 2012 (Carol).

Conley ME, et al. Primary B cell immunodeficiencies: comparisons and contrasts. *Annu Rev Immunol.* 2009;27:199–227.

Cunningham-Rundles C, et al. Clinical and immunologic analyses of 103 patients with common variable immunodeficiency. *J Clin Immunol.* 1989 Jan;9(1):22–33.

Yong PF, et al. Hypogammaglobulinaemia. *Immunol Allergy Clin North Am.* 2008 Nov;28(4):691–713.

Durandy A. Autosomal recessive form of hyper-IgM syndrome (HIGM2). *Orphanet Encyclopedia.* 2002.

PHAGOCYTE DISORDERS

Davies EG, Thrasher AJ. Update on the hyper immunoglobulin M syndromes. *Br J Haematol.* 2010 Apr;149(2):167–180.

Davis SD, et al. Job's syndrome. Recurrent, "cold," staphylococcal abscesses. *Lancet.* 1966 May 7;1(7445):1013–1015.

TOLL-LIKE RECEPTOR DISORDERS

Sabroe I, et al. Toll-like receptors in health and disease: complex questions remain. *J Immunol.* 2003 Aug 15;171(4):1630–1635.

VACCINE USE IN IMMUNOCOMPROMISED CHILDREN

National Center for Immunization and Respiratory Diseases. General recommendations on immunization—recommendations of the Advisory Committee on Immunization Practices (ACIP). *MMWR Recomm Rep.* 2011 Jan 28;60(2):1–64. Erratum in: *MMWR Recomm Rep.* 2011 Jul 29;60:993.

Pickering LK, et al. Immunization programs for infants, children, adolescents, and adults: clinical practice guidelines by the Infectious Diseases Society of America. *Clin Infect Dis.* 2009 Sep 15;49(6):817–840.

Tamma P. Vaccines in immunocompromised patients. *Pediatr Rev.* 2010 Jan;31(1):38–40.

ALLERGY & IMMUNOLOGY

ALLERGIC DISORDERS

Adkinson F Jr, et al (eds). *Middleton's allergy: principles and practice*, 7th Ed. Mosby, Inc., 2008.

Ghaffar A. Hypersensitivity reactions. *Microbiology and Immunology On-line*. University of South Carolina School of Medicine. 2010.

Rajan TV. The Gell-Coombs classification of hypersensitivity reactions: a re-interpretation. *Trends Immunol*. 2003 Jul;24(7):376–379.

Simons FE. Anaphylaxis. *J Allergy Clin Immunol*. 2010 Feb;125(2 Suppl 2):S161–S181.

Lemanske RF Jr, Busse WW. Asthma: clinical expression and molecular mechanisms. *J Allergy Clin Immunol*. 2010 Feb;125(2 Suppl 2):S95–S102.

Dykewicz MS, Hamilos DL. Rhinitis and sinusitis. *J Allergy Clin Immunol*. 2010; 125:S103–S115.

Fonacier LS, et al. Allergic skin diseases. *J Allergy Clin Immunol*. 2010 Feb;125(2 Suppl 2):S138–S149.

Caubet JC, et al. Educational case series: mechanisms of drug allergy. *Pediatr Allergy Immunol*. 2011 Sep;22(6):559–567.

Khan DA, Solensky R. Drug allergy. *J Allergy Clin Immunol*. 2010 Feb;125(2 Suppl 2):S126–S137.

Joint Task Force on Practice Parameters; American Academy of Allergy, Asthma, and Immunology; American College of Allergy, Asthma, and Immunology; Joint Council of Allergy, Asthma, and Immunology. Drug allergy: an updated practice parameter. *Ann Allergy Asthma Immunol*. 2010 Oct;105(4):259–273.

Joint Task Force on Practice Parameters; American Academy of Allergy, Asthma, and Immunology; American College of Allergy, Asthma, and Immunology; Joint Council of Allergy, Asthma, and Immunology. Stinging insect hypersensitivity: a practice parameter update 2011. *J Allergy Clin Immunol*. 2011 Apr;127(4):852–854.e1–e23.

Golden DB. Stinging insect allergy. *Am Fam Physician*. 2003 Jun 15;67(12):2541–2546.

PREVENTION OF ATOPIC DISEASE

American Academy of Pediatrics. Committee on Nutrition and Section on Allergy and Immunology. Effects of early nutritional interventions on the development of atopic disease in infants and children: the role of maternal dietary restriction, breastfeeding, timing of introduction of complementary foods, and hydrolyzed formulas. *Pediatrics*. 2008 Jan;121(1):183–191.

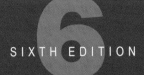
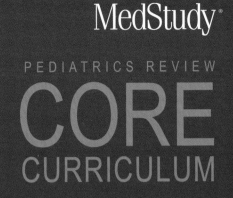

SIXTH EDITION

DERMATOLOGY

DERMATOLOGY

Section Editor:

K. Robin Carder, MD
Pediatric Dermatology of Dallas, P.A.
Dallas, TX

Medical Editor:

Yasmine Subhi Ali, MD, MSCI, FACC, FACP
President, Nashville Preventive Cardiology, PLLC
Nashville, TN

Table of Contents
Dermatology

NEONATAL DERMATOLOGY

APLASIA CUTIS

Aplasia cutis is a congenital absence of skin that usually occurs only in a small localized area, most commonly on the scalp (Image 7-1). However, ~ 20% have underlying skull abnormalities. If it occurs in multiple places on the top of the scalp, look for trisomy 13. Larger or midline defects can have underlying bony defects or vascular abnormalities. If it occurs as a midline defect, look for spinal dysraphia!

Midline scalp lesions that are encircled by thicker, darker hair ("hair collar sign") are suggestive of cranial dysraphism.

Neonates with large areas of aplasia cutis congenita on the lower extremities are likely to have the congenital blistering disorder, epidermolysis bullosa. Infants with epidermolysis bullosa typically have multiple bullae and erosions distributed over the face, trunk, and extremities, which are apparent at the time of birth.

RASHES

Milia

These are 1–2-mm, firm, white papules that appear at the surface of pilosebaceous units, most commonly on the face. These tiny, epidermal inclusion cysts generally resolve spontaneously over several months and require no treatment.

Sebaceous Hyperplasia

Seen in approximately 50% of term newborns, this is the most important condition in the differential diagnosis of milia. Typically, several pinpoint, white-to-yellowish, fine papules are present on or around the nose and upper lip (Image 7-2). Sebaceous hyperplasia is caused by increased androgen stimulation in utero and generally resolves spontaneously during the first few weeks of life.

Neonatal Acne

Neonatal acne (also known as neonatal cephalic pustulosis) is generally apparent within the first 2–4 weeks of life. Look for the distribution of many small, 1–2-mm, dusky pink papules and pustules on the face and scalp (Image 7-3). Note: Comedones are lacking in neonatal acne. The etiology of this self-limited condition is controversial; some experts consider this to be a hyposensitivity reaction to the presence of *Malassezia furfur* (also known as *Pityrosporum*). Neonatal acne usually resolves spontaneously within the first 1–2 months of life. Neonatal acne can resemble miliaria rubra or cutaneous candidiasis.

Infantile Acne

In contrast, infantile acne normally becomes evident at ~ 2–4 months of age and is caused by androgenic stimulation of the sebaceous glands. In addition to papules and pustules, there are typically open and closed comedones distributed over the face (Image 7-4). Acne cysts or nodules can also occur. The condition, more commonly seen in boys, usually resolves over 6–12 months. Rarely, infantile acne can be due to pathologic causes of androgen excess, such as congenital adrenal hyperplasia, adrenal tumors, or precocious puberty. Because infantile acne can be more persistent, and occasionally results in scarring, treatment with topical benzoyl peroxide or antibiotics can be beneficial. For extensive comedonal lesions, topical retinoids (tretinoin or Retin-A Micro®) can be helpful. For more severe inflammation with the concern of scarring, use oral erythromycin (oral tetracyclines are contraindicated in young children); case reports have shown efficacy of oral isotretinoin for severe cases.

Epstein Pearls

These are small, benign, whitish-yellow papules on either side of the raphe on the hard palate of the newborn. These are essentially intraoral milia and resolve without treatment.

Bohn Nodules

These are small, benign retention cysts in the mouths of infants.

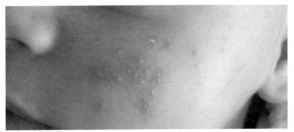

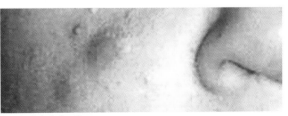
Image 7-3: Neonatal acne

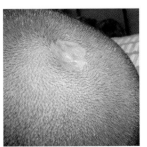
Image 7-1: Aplasia cutis

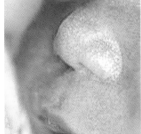
Image 7-2: Sebaceous hyperplasia

Image 7-4: Infantile acne

DERMATOLOGY

Found on the alveolar ridges, these lesions generally resolve spontaneously during the first several months of life.

Miliaria

These are cutaneous changes associated with sweat retention and extravasation of sweat occurring at different levels of skin. Usually, it is due to overheating.

Miliaria rubra (prickly heat) occurs when the sweat glands are blocked and the sweat escapes into the epidermis, producing red papulovesicles (Image 7-5).

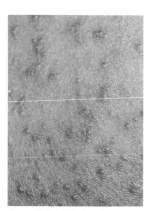

Image 7-5: Miliaria rubra

Miliaria crystallina also occurs with blocked sweat glands. The sweat escapes just beneath the surface, producing noninflammatory vesicles that look like "clear droplets."

Erythema Toxicum

This is a common, self-limited, urticarial condition occurring in the first few days of life; rarely is it present at birth. It consists of small pustules filled with eosinophils (Image 7-6). The pustules are surrounded by a red wheal. It comes and goes, and it appears at different sites.

You see erythema toxicum primarily in term infants, and it typically resolves spontaneously within 1 week after birth. For reasons we don't understand, erythema toxicum is almost never seen in significantly premature infants.

Transient Neonatal Pustular Melanosis (TNPM)

This is always present at birth with pustules that transform into scaly, hyperpigmented macules of uniform

Table 7-1: Tzanck and Gram Stain Findings in Neonatal Eruptions		
Disease	**Type of WBC**	**Bacteria Present**
Miliaria	PMNs	No
Erythema toxicum	Eos	No
Transient neonatal pustular melanosis	PMNs	No
Bullous impetigo	PMNs	Gram-positive cocci in clusters

size (Image 7-7). TNPM is seen in 2–5% of African-American neonates.

Tzanck smear will show neutrophils. Because these subcorneal pustules can easily rupture, you may not see them after the initial cleaning of the infant. Rupture of the pustules leaves small superficial erosions with a collarette of scale, which leave small hyperpigmented macules that can persist for several months.

One last time … to reiterate Tzanck smear or Gram stain findings in neonatal eruptions, see Table 7-1.

A FEW INFECTIOUS RASHES

Rashes that are infectious in etiology are discussed briefly here; a fuller discussion can be found in Infectious Disease, Book 2.

Neonatal Candidiasis

This is seen in 4–5% of neonates born through a yeast-infected birth canal. Characteristically, it is a beefy-red, moist dermatitis with satellite papules in the genital area, which occurs after the 1st week of life. Oral thrush can also develop. KOH shows budding yeasts with pseudohyphae. Topical therapy with anticandidals is effective. If neonatal candidiasis is difficult to treat, suspect immunosuppression.

Image 7-6: Erythema toxicum

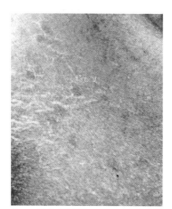

Image 7-7: TNPM

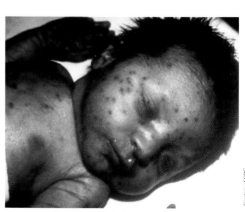

Image 7-8: Congenital rubella

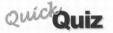

- If aplasia cutis occurs in multiple areas of the scalp, what genetic disorder should you suspect?
- What are milia?
- Describe sebaceous hyperplasia.
- How does neonatal acne differ from infantile acne?
- What are Epstein pearls?
- What is miliaria rubra?
- What WBC is found in erythema toxicum?
- What WBC is found in TNPM?

Impetigo Neonatorum

Staphylococcus aureus is present as a skin colonizer in > 30–40% of newborns. Illness can begin within the first few days-to-weeks of life. Disease can range from localized bullous impetigo to generalized staphylococcal scalded skin syndrome. The exotoxins (if present) of the staphylococci determine the extent of the disease. Gram stain and culture confirm diagnosis.

Congenital Rubella

This can present with macular or slightly raised, purple lesions, especially on the abdomen and trunk; it is also referred to as "blueberry muffin" syndrome (Image 7-8).

Herpes Simplex

This can cause a few vesicles or a more generalized eruption with grouped vesicles on a red base. Frequently, you will see these at the site of fetal scalp monitors or the presenting part (Image 7-9).

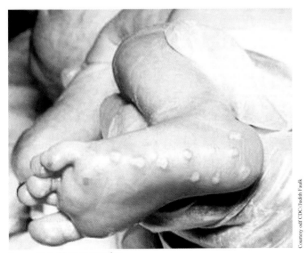

Image 7-9: Herpes simplex

Congenital Syphilis

The rash is usually pink and maculopapular and later turns brown or can become vesiculobullous, even hemorrhagic. Frequently, the rash involves the palms and soles.

Listeria monocytogenes

This organism can cause petechiae, pustules, or purple, miliary granulomas of the skin; and affected infants are quite ill.

LESIONS DUE TO VASCULAR ABNORMALITIES

Infantile Hemangiomas

These occur in ~ 2.5% of neonates. The initial appearance can resemble a port-wine stain, bruise, or hypopigmented patch. Approximately 10–12% of Caucasian infants have one develop by age 1 year. The ratio of affected females to males is 3:1. Around 30–50% of affected babies have a clinically apparent hemangioma at birth, with the remaining hemangiomas generally appearing within the first 1–2 months. Initially, the lesion can be either a discrete white macule with central telangiectasia or a red macule. Within a few days-to-weeks, the lesion rapidly becomes elevated and enlarged. The size, shape, and color vary from a bright red superficial tumor to a deeper bluish tumor. Occasionally, the deeper hemangiomas can be skin-colored. Hemangiomas typically proliferate rapidly during the first 6 months of life and then stabilize between 6 and 10 months, usually reaching their largest size by 1 year of age. Shrinkage or involution often begins in the child's 1st or 2nd year. Around 50% of hemangiomas have involuted by 5 years of age and 90% by 9 years of age (Image 7-10), but some discoloration or scarring can remain.

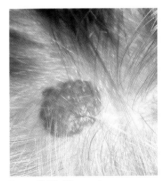

Image 7-10: Hemangioma

While some infantile hemangiomas do not require therapeutic intervention, there are several potential complications and associations to be aware of. Look for ulceration, the most common complication; this occurs most often in rapidly growing hemangiomas during the first several months of life. The perineum and lip are the most common sites of ulceration, particularly for larger lesions. Ulceration can be a significant cause of morbidity for the affected infant and can result in infection, bleeding, scarring, and severe pain. Treatment includes topical barrier ointments, topical and/or systemic antibiotics, protective dressings, pulsed dye laser therapy, or oral propranolol.

Regarding the other hemangioma complications: It all depends on location!

Potentially problematic locations and their possible complications include:

- Periorbital lesions: ~ 80% risk of ocular complications, including astigmatism, amblyopia, refractive errors, and, occasionally, blindness.
- Beard lesions (mandible, chin, submental): Watch for signs of subglottic hemangioma, including stridor, cough, or swallowing or respiratory difficulties. This usually occurs during the first 6 months of life and is more likely to be associated with bilateral lesions.
- Ear: Risk of obstruction in the external auditory canal, which can cause a conductive hearing loss and, if persistent, can impact/delay the development of normal speech.
- Nose and lip: These hemangiomas have a greater tendency to ulcerate. Furthermore, these anatomic locations carry an increased risk of significant cosmetic deformity.
- Midline lumbosacral region: Hemangiomas in this region carry an increased risk of spinal dysraphism, particularly when associated with other markers of dysraphism, such as hypertrichosis, sacral dimple or skin tag, or deviated intergluteal cleft. Evaluate infants with these findings for underlying spinal cord abnormalities. MRI scan is the best test to rule out spinal dysraphism, but, in some centers, lumbosacral ultrasound is done first. GU anomalies also have been reported with large, lumbosacral hemangiomas.
- Multiple cutaneous hemangiomas (> 5): Can occur with visceral hemangiomas, especially of the liver and GI tract. Most infants with > 5 have a benign self-limited course, but a subset have severe, disseminated, visceral involvement. These infants are at risk for high-output congestive heart failure, hepatic complications (including jaundice and coagulopathy), GI hemorrhage, and thyroid abnormalities.

PHACE syndrome occurs with large, segmental facial hemangiomas:

- **P**osterior fossa abnormalities (Dandy-Walker syndrome)
- **H**emangioma (generally large, cervicofacial lesions involving cranial nerve V1 distribution)
- **A**rterial anomalies (typically intracerebral arterial anomalies)
- **C**ardiac defects, especially coarctation of the aorta
- **E**ye abnormalities (microphthalmia)

Historically, large, rapidly growing hemangiomas were associated with Kasabach-Merritt syndrome (aggressive, vascular tumor associated with thrombocytopenia, consumptive coagulopathy and high-output congestive heart failure). More recent studies indicate that Kasabach-Merritt syndrome is associated with other less common vascular tumors; these include kaposiform hemangioendothelioma or tufted angioma, rather than true infantile hemangiomas.

Not all hemangiomas require therapy. Proliferating lesions in problematic locations can require intervention with oral propranolol (quickly becoming the treatment of choice) or systemic corticosteroids. Vincristine is a second-line agent for severe or refractory lesions. Historically, α-interferon has been used for function-threatening or life-threatening hemangiomas; however, recent reports of spastic diplegia have dampened the enthusiasm of many clinicians for this therapeutic intervention.

Nevus Simplex

Nevus simplex (a capillary malformation) is also known as salmon patch, angel kiss (on the glabella), or stork bite (on posterior hairline). You will see these pink-to-red blanching macules on half of all newborns (Image 7-11). Most facial lesions fade with time, while nuchal patches persist. These are dilated, superficial vessels probably resulting from vasomotor immaturity. Be careful to distinguish these from the next lesion, nevus flammeus!

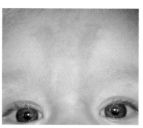

Image 7-11: Nevus simplex

Nevus Flammeus (Capillary Malformation)

Port-wine stains—sometimes called nevus flammeus—are capillary malformations and occur in ~ 0.3% of newborns. They usually appear as pink, red, or violaceous patches that persist throughout life and grow proportionally with the child (Image 7-12). The lesions can lighten or darken slightly over time, and some darken and thicken in adulthood.

Port-wine stains involving the ophthalmic branch of the trigeminal nerve (V1) can occur with Sturge-Weber syndrome, which consists of an ipsilateral cerebral vascular malformation that can cause neurologic complications, including:

- Seizures
- Intellectual disabilities
- Contralateral hemiplegia
- Characteristic ophthalmologic findings, particularly choroidal vascular anomalies and glaucoma

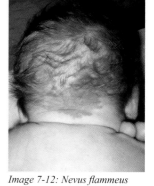

Image 7-12: Nevus flammeus

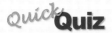

Quiz

- What complications should you watch out for if hemangiomas occur in the periorbital area? In the beard area?

- Infants born with port-wine stains in the V1 distribution are at risk for what syndrome? How do you screen for this entity?

- Port-wine stains of the lower extremity predispose to what syndrome?

- When should you remove a nevus sebaceous?

Screen infants born with port-wine stains in the V1 distribution, especially bilateral, for Sturge-Weber syndrome using an ophthalmologic examination and radiologic imaging of the head. Radiologic abnormalities may not appear on initial imaging. Potential abnormalities include:

- Leptomeningeal vascular malformation
- Calcifications of the leptomeninges and the underlying white matter
- Cerebral atrophy
- Enlarged choroid plexus

Note, however: The majority (90%) of V1 port-wine stains are not associated with Sturge-Weber syndrome.

Infants with port-wine stains in the V2 distribution are also at risk for developing glaucoma; thus, monitor regularly. Additionally, lesions in the V2 distribution are at an increased risk for soft tissue or bony overgrowth of the area underlying the capillary malformation, which can result in orthodontic challenges.

Infants with port-wine stains of the lower extremities are at risk for Klippel-Trenaunay syndrome. A child with this syndrome presents with a vascular malformation (mixed capillary-venous-lymphatic) of an extremity, with associated soft tissue and/or limb overgrowth, and with development of venous varicosities. Limb overgrowth is generally progressive in nature. Parkes-Weber syndrome is similar but associated with more marked limb overgrowth—in both length and girth. The skin is characterized by capillary stains, but there are also multiple arteriovenous fistulae that you can see on ultrasound with color Doppler. These patients usually have a more problematic clinical course and can develop high-output cardiac failure and marked limb overgrowth.

Pulsed dye laser therapy can be helpful in the management of capillary malformations. Multiple treatments are generally required but can result in considerable fading of the port-wine stain over time.

PIGMENTED LESIONS

Nevus Sebaceous

Nevus sebaceous is considered a type of epidermal nevus—a localized lesion seen most commonly on the scalp and occasionally on the face. It consists of a yellow- to salmon-colored, hairless plaque that often has a waxy texture (Image 7-13). The lesions are typically flat at birth and stable during childhood; however, during puberty, the nevus sebaceous becomes much thicker—often verrucous—in texture as a response to hormonal changes. Biopsy of the lesion during this stage often shows an abundance of sebaceous glands with absent or very deformed

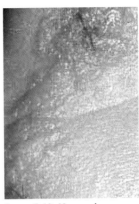

Image 7-13: Nevus sebaceous

hair follicles. The risk of basal cell carcinoma within a nevus sebaceous was previously estimated at 10–15%! In recent years, some have questioned this statistic and believe that what were previously interpreted as basal cell carcinomas were actually benign hair follicle tumors. Nevertheless, most experts advocate prepubertal removal of a nevus sebaceous.

Nevus Spilus

Nevus spilus (speckled lentiginous nevus) is relatively common and can be congenital or acquired. It presents as a well-demarcated, tan or light-brown, non-hairy patch, usually on

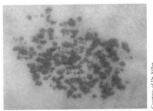

Image 7-14: Nevus spilus

the trunk, face, or extremities. Characteristically, these patches tend to develop multiple, small, dark macules and papules throughout the lesion and can resemble a chocolate chip cookie (Image 7-14). These lesions have a minimal future risk of neoplastic change into melanoma. Because they are often large, you would normally not excise the lesion prophylactically unless a worrisome clinical change warrants it.

Congenital Melanocytic Nevi

Congenital melanocytic nevi represent collections of melanocytes (pigment cells) in the skin that are typically present at birth or within the first few months of life (Image 7-15). The nevi are generally classified based on the adult size of the lesion:

- Small: < 1.5 cm (found in 1–2% of newborns)
- Medium: 1.5–20 cm (present in ~ 0.6% of newborns)
- Large: > 20 cm (rare; present in ~ 0.02% of newborns)

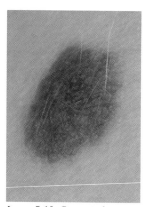

Image 7-15: Congenital melanocytic nevi

The future risk of melanoma within small or medium congenital melanocytic nevi remains unclear, but the risk appears to be small, and malignant change is rare before puberty. However, there is a 6–8% lifetime risk of developing melanoma within a large, congenital melanocytic nevus. The risk appears to be substantial during the first 5 years of life, in contrast to the risk in small and medium lesions, which, again, is primarily postpubertal.

The small- to medium-sized lesions usually present as well-demarcated, raised, uniformly pigmented lesions. Colors can range from tan to brown to black. They also can develop coarse dark hairs. Typically, you can identify the large lesions, and they are most common on the trunk. On exams, look for key words like "coat sleeve," "stocking," "cape-like," "bathing trunk," or "garment-type" descriptions! Increased hair growth, irregular borders, and uneven pigmentation are not unusual; thus, they warrant close observation for clinical changes. Large lesions located over the scalp, midline neck, or spine can be associated with leptomeningeal involvement. This is known as neurocutaneous melanosis.

The initial radiographic findings can be very subtle (and easily missed) by those unfamiliar with these types of lesions. If the melanocytic nevi occur over the midline scalp or spine, consider spinal dysraphism and Dandy-Walker malformation—in addition to neurocutaneous melanosis. Patients with symptomatic neurocutaneous melanosis carry a very poor prognosis. The need for baseline radiologic imaging to screen for neurocutaneous melanosis in large melanocytic nevi of the midline spine or scalp, or multiple congenital melanocytic nevi, remains controversial. Some experts recommend baseline MRI of the head and spine in high-risk infants.

Mongolian Spots

Mongolian spots generally are present at birth and seen in > 90% of African-American and Native American babies; occurrence is < 10% in Caucasians (Image 7-16). Clinically, they are flat and brownish–to–blue- or slate-gray. They are poorly circumscribed and can range in size from

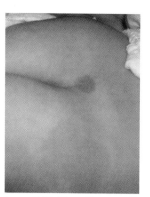

Image 7-16: Mongolian spots

a few millimeters to > 10 cm. The most common sites are the lumbosacral region, back, flanks, and shoulders. Most disappear or fade over 7–13 years. No therapy is necessary.

Nevus of Ota

Nevus of Ota is most commonly seen in African-American or Asian infants. They present as unilateral, irregularly speckled areas of bluish-gray discoloration on the face—specifically on the periorbital area, temple, forehead, cheek, nose, an/or sclera (Image 7-17). These are different from Mongolian spots in that they don't clear with time. Rarely, cutaneous and ocular melanoma can occur within these lesions, so periodic ophthalmologic and skin exams are recommended, as well as biopsy of darker or atypical areas that can suggest malignant change; if they present as a cosmetic problem, laser therapy is effective.

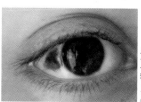

Image 7-17: Nevus of Ota

Courtesy of Dr. Luninsky

Nevus of Ito

Nevus of Ito is similar to Nevus of Ota, except for the areas of distribution: shoulder, upper extremity, or neck.

Café-au-lait Spots

Café-au-lait spots appear in 10–20% of the average population. They are generally flat, tan lesions, ranging in size from a few millimeters to 10–20 cm (Image 7-18). Having 1 or 2 lesions is normal, but large (> 3 cm) or multiple lesions can indicate a neurocutaneous syndrome. The borders are regular; some say they look like the coast of California (hmmm … before or after the earthquake?). They can be present at birth and tend to increase in size and number during childhood. They are not induced by sunlight (like freckles) but will darken with sun exposure. On the exam: Look for the Crowe sign—small, grouped, freckle-like, café-au-lait spots measuring 1–4 mm in the axilla or groin. These are indicative of neurofibromatosis Type 1!

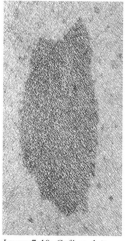

Image 7-18: Café-au-lait

Other associations with café-au-lait spots are neurofibromatosis Type 2, McCune-Albright syndrome, Watson syndrome, and occasionally tuberous sclerosis.

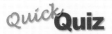

Quick Quiz

- In an infant with a large (> 20 cm) congenital melanocytic nevus, at what age range is there a substantial risk of melanoma?

- A "bathing-trunk" nevus should make you think of what diagnosis?

- Describe neurocutaneous melanosis.

- What is Crowe sign?

- What diseases are associated with café-au-lait spots?

- X-linked recessive ichthyosis is associated with what genitourinary abnormality in boys?

Supernumerary Nipples

Supernumerary nipples are fairly common and occur along the embryologic milk lines of the chest and abdomen. They can be accompanied by breast tissue. Smaller lesions usually require no treatment. Surgically excise larger lesions with apparent glandular tissue—because they can increase during puberty and be a source of embarrassment for the child (or leave them as is, so the child could star as an evil scientist in a James Bond movie); and because breast carcinoma has been reported in these lesions. Reports conflict on whether accessory nipples are associated with an increased risk of renal or urogenital anomalies; consider screening with a renal ultrasound.

GENETIC SKIN DISORDERS

ICHTHYOSES

Ichthyosis Vulgaris

Ichthyosis vulgaris is the most common form of the ichthyoses and occurs in 1/250. It is autosomal dominant (AD) and is due to loss of function mutations in the gene encoding filaggrin. Most commonly, ichthyosis occurs after age 3 months on the extensor surfaces of the extremities as fine white scales without redness (Image 7-19). You will also see increased skin markings on the palms and soles (hyperlinear). Ichthyosis typically improves in hot, humid climates and during the summer months. It is commonly associated with atopic dermatitis. Treatment is irritant avoidance and use of emollients and keratolytic products.

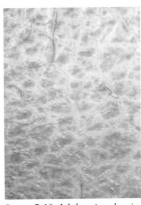

Image 7-19: Ichthyosis vulgaris

X-Linked Recessive Ichthyosis

X-linked recessive ichthyosis occurs in 1/2,000–6,000 boys and usually becomes apparent at birth or during the first few months of life. The scales are more pronounced than in the AD form and tend to be bigger and darker. The trunk is involved, but the palms and soles are unaffected. It typically affects the neck and ears but spares the antecubital and popliteal fossa. It is due to the absence of the microsomal enzyme steroid sulfatase. Males can have associated undescended testes with underdeveloped penis and scrotum; check for this in all patients you suspect of having X-linked recessive ichthyosis.

Lamellar Ichthyosis and Nonbullous Congenital Ichthyosiform Erythroderma

These two conditions classically present as the "collodion baby." These newborns appear with taut, shiny skin that is similar to a cellophane (collodion) membrane. The eyelids and lips are everted (ectropion and eclabium). They can have digital contractures. The membrane sheds during the first few weeks of life with proper treatment, but many develop lamellar ichthyosis or congenital ichthyosiform erythroderma. Classic lamellar ichthyosis and congenital ichthyosiform erythroderma are considered polar phenotypes along a clinical spectrum of autosomal recessive (AR) ichthyosis. Lamellar ichthyosis is characterized by generalized large, dark plate-like scaling and minimal-to-no appreciable erythema. Congenital ichthyosiform erythroderma presents with smaller, fine scales and generalized pink erythema. Many patients have intermediate clinical findings. In addition to the cosmetic ramifications of these disorders, these patients have in common the tendency to develop skin infections (especially fungal) and impaired sweating with heat intolerance, and can struggle with malnutrition and growth delay, especially earlier in life.

The genetic causes of these disorders have not been fully elucidated. Genetic mutations in the transglutaminase 1 and two lipoxygenase genes have been identified so far.

GENETIC PIGMENTATION DISORDERS

Oculocutaneous Albinism

Albinism occurs in most patients due to a genetic mutation in either the gene that codes for tyrosinase—important for melanin synthesis—or in the gene that codes for P protein, which leads to an abnormal transport of melanin to keratinocytes. These are primarily AR disorders with decreased pigmentation of the skin, hair, and eyes. Photophobia, nystagmus, and poor visual acuity are common.

Those with the tyrosinase-negative form have the most eye abnormalities, which do not improve with age; those with the P protein-deficient form can develop some pigmentation as they age.

DERMATOLOGY

Hermansky-Pudlak Syndrome

The Hermansky-Pudlak syndrome is a rare AR disorder with albinism, mild bleeding diathesis, and tissue storage of ceroid material. Epistaxis and prolonged bleeding are common due to platelet storage pool defects. The ceroid material deposits in the lungs, GI tract, and renal tubule cells.

Chediak-Higashi Syndrome

This syndrome is due to a *LYST* gene defect and presents with a silvery sheen to the skin and hair due to the accumulation of giant melanosomes, along with the inability to transport melanin granules to epidermal cells. EBV triggers the "accelerated phase" with atypical lymphocytes, pancytopenia, and organ infiltration. Long-term survival requires bone marrow transplantation.

GENETIC SKIN AND TUMOR SYNDROMES

Type 1 Neurofibromatosis

Type 1 neurofibromatosis (von Recklinghausen disease) is an autosomal dominant (AD) disorder with multiple café-au-lait spots and neurofibromas. This disorder is covered in Genetics, Book 3.

Tuberous Sclerosis

Tuberous sclerosis is another AD neurocutaneous disorder and is associated with facial angiofibromas (adenoma sebaceum), ash-leaf spots, shagreen patch, and periungual fibromas. It is also discussed further in Genetics, Book 3.

Gorlin Syndrome

Gorlin syndrome (basal cell nevus syndrome) is an AD disorder due to mutations of the "patched" gene—a tumor suppressor gene that controls cell growth and patterning. These children develop basal cell carcinoma in childhood and have dysmorphic facies, palmoplantar pits, and skeletal defects. The basal cell carcinomas can be very subtle in appearance and resemble small skin tags or melanocytic nevi. Jaw cysts also are common and can become malignant. These patients have a tendency to develop ovarian tumors, as well as other malignancies, including medulloblastoma.

Peutz-Jeghers Syndrome

Peutz-Jeghers syndrome is another AD defect; this one is due to mutations in the serine threonine kinase *STK11* gene. It presents with gastrointestinal polyposes and hyperpigmented macules of the mucosa, perioral areas, digits, palms, and soles. It is covered in Gastroenterology & Nutrition, Book 4.

OTHER NEUROCUTANEOUS DISORDERS

Incontinentia Pigmenti

Incontinentia pigmenti is an X-linked dominant disorder that is lethal in males. In females, the skin manifestations generally clear by adulthood—so a careful history of a mother with recurrent miscarriages is important. There are 4 stages of skin manifestations:

1) Patterned blistering that follows the lines of Blaschko (the routes of embryonic cell migration; it is not always obvious that this is a Blaschko-like pattern during the blistering stage). The blistering has a predilection for the extremities and is typically apparent within the first few weeks of life. The blisters often have erythematous background skin.
2) Verrucous papules occur after the first 2–6 weeks of life and persist for months.
3) Hyperpigmented linear swirl patches occur along the lines of Blaschko at 3–6 months and then persist for years.
4) Hypopigmented patches replace the hyperpigmentation in affected adult women.

Note: Not all patients pass through each cutaneous stage, and some patients have lesions of different stages concurrently. Skin biopsy can help confirm the clinical diagnosis.

Cicatricial alopecia occurs in ~ 1/3 of patients. Delayed eruption of teeth occurs in ~ 2/3 of patients. The teeth are usually abnormal in appearance and can be peg- or cone-shaped; often, the child is missing teeth (Image 7-20). Strabismus is a common eye association. Around 7% become blind due to retinal neovascularization and detachment. Seizures occur in > 10%.

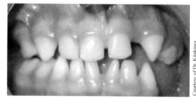
Image 7-20: Incontinentia pigmenti

Ataxia Telangiectasia

Ataxia telangiectasia is an AR disorder due to a mutation in the *ATM* gene, which prevents DNA synthesis from proceeding after radiation damage. Ataxia develops early. Telangiectasias develop after the ataxia on the bulbar conjunctiva, between ages 2 and 6 years. The telangiectasias subsequently develop on the eyelids, cheeks, ears, and flexor forearms. Patients have progressive neurologic deterioration and recurrent sinopulmonary infections.

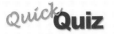

Other Disorders

Menkes syndrome is an X-linked recessive disorder due to copper transport abnormalities. Fabry disease is also an X-linked recessive disorder. Both are discussed in Metabolic Disorders, Book 3.

EPIDERMOLYSIS BULLOSA

Epidermolysis bullosa (EB) is a group of wide-ranging dermatologic disorders due to defects in the strength of skin, resulting in skin fragility and blistering after mechanical trauma. There are more than 30 distinct genetic forms that fall under 3 main subtypes: simplex, junctional, and dystrophic; each is distinguished by the level of blistering.

EB simplex is an AD disorder and occurs when the blister is located through the basal keratinocytes (lowermost layer of epidermal cells). EB simplex is due to defects in keratin genes 5 and 14. The blisters typically heal without scarring. EB simplex subtypes are usually the least severe forms of this disorder and can be localized to the extremities and sites of frequent trauma or friction.

Junctional EB is AR and results in a defect in the hemidesmosomes or anchoring filaments, with the cleavage plane through the epidermal-dermal junction. This form is due to many genetic etiologies. Blistering is severe and can occur spontaneously or after trauma. In the most severe Herlitz subtype (due to mutations in the Laminin 5 gene), death by sepsis is common at < 6 months of age.

Dystrophic EB occurs when the cleavage plane lies below the basement membrane zone in the upper dermis. It is due to defects in the genes that encode Type VII collagen. An AD form results in blistering in localized areas of the knees, elbows, and dorsum of the hands. An AR form results in generalized blistering with extensive scarring, along with the potential for development of squamous cell carcinoma by adolescence. Patients with the recessive dystrophic form of EB usually develop a severe, chronic anemia.

Strictures of the esophagus are common in recessive dystrophic EB, and dietary therapy is paramount. Over time, the progressive scarring of the fingers and toes causes pseudosyndactyly ("mitten deformities") of the hands and feet.

Skin biopsy is required for diagnosis.

Never apply tape or other adhesives to the skin of patients with EB disorders. Secondary infection is common.

Registry data in 2009 showed that those with EB are at increased risk for squamous cell carcinoma in adolescence and adulthood.

GENETIC DISORDERS OF THE DERMIS

Ehlers-Danlos Syndrome

Ehlers-Danlos syndrome is discussed in Genetics, Book 3.

Cutis Laxa

Cutis laxa is a disorder of decreased or absent elastic tissue. It can be AR, AD, X-linked recessive, or acquired. It can present with pendulous folds of redundant skin at birth (recessive form), or it can develop later in life (dominant). Those with severe disease have pulmonary emphysema, bladder or GI diverticula, and inguinal or umbilical hernias. The acquired form occurs after penicillin or isoniazid administration and is commonly progressive.

Pseudoxanthoma Elasticum

Pseudoxanthoma elasticum has both AR and AD forms. Yellow papules develop on the axilla, groin, and neck—and then become wrinkled. The areas have been described as "plucked chicken skin." GI bleeding, claudication, and angina pectoris occur with this disease.

GENETIC DISORDERS OF THE HAIR, NAILS, SWEAT GLANDS, SEBACEOUS GLANDS, AND TEETH

Hypohidrotic Ectodermal Dysplasia

Hypohidrotic ectodermal dysplasia is the most common form of ectodermal dysplasia and is X-linked recessive. Females may or may not be affected depending on which X chromosome is activated. Facies are characteristic with frontal bossing; flat malar ridges; depressed nasal root; thin upper lip; large, "pouting" lower lip; small chin; and prominent ears. Pegged teeth are common. Periorbital wrinkling and increased pigmentation are common. Sweating is almost absent, which leads to heat stress or fevers. Secretions from the nose, eyes, and mouth are lacking as well.

Hidrotic Ectodermal Dysplasia (Clouston Syndrome)

Hidrotic ectodermal dysplasia is an AD disorder with hair and nail hypoplasia. Additionally, there is palmar-plantar keratoderma. Sweating is normal.

Monilethrix

Monilethrix is a rare hair structure abnormality. The hairs have a beaded appearance microscopically. Hair grows 2–3 cm and then breaks off. It is due to mutations in hair keratins.

GENETIC IMMUNODEFICIENCIES

The immunodeficiencies of X-linked agammaglobulinemia, SCID, Wiskott-Aldrich syndrome, CGD, leukocyte adhesion deficiency, and hyper-IgE syndrome are all associated with skin manifestations. They are discussed in Allergy & Immunology, Book 2.

GENETIC DISORDERS OF AGING

Progeria (Hutchinson-Gilford Syndrome)

Progeria is a rare AR disorder with premature aging occurring as early as 1 year of age. Growth failure is severe, and the child appears "aged." Atherosclerosis is common by adolescence. The skin is thin, and you can easily see the veins. Total alopecia and nail dystrophy occur. Characteristically, the child has a squeaky voice, bird-like face, and a hunched-over shuffling gait. Death occurs due to cardiovascular disease during the teenage years.

DISORDERS OF PIGMENTATION

NEVI

Freckles

Freckles (ephelides) are small, light-brown, pigmented macules. They are benign and generally limited to sun-exposed areas of the skin; they darken with sun exposure.

Acquired Melanocytic Nevi

Acquired melanocytic nevi, or pigmented moles, are made up of groups of melanocytes at the dermal-epidermal junction or in the dermis. They begin to appear in the preschool years, and another crop can develop during adolescence.

Junctional nevi occur only in the epidermis along the dermal-epidermal junction. They are flat and brown-to-black, with even pigmentation and are most common on sun-exposed areas. In time, they evolve into compound nevi, which are raised and pink to dark brown. Eventually, they can evolve into intradermal nevi, which are dome-shaped or pedunculated and composed of groups of dermal melanocytes at the dermal-epidermal junction. Hairs can develop in compound or intradermal nevi.

Excision of acquired melanocytic nevi may be recommended if they:

- Become painful
- Become pruritic
- Ulcerate
- Change significantly in size
- Change in color
- Change in shape
- Are bothersome, such as getting nicked while shaving

Halo nevus occurs when a ring of depigmentation develops around a nevus. Halo nevi require no special intervention unless atypical findings occur (see above).

Dysplastic nevi (atypical moles) appear on sun-exposed areas. They have irregular borders with nonuniform color. They are larger than ordinary nevi, > 5 mm in diameter. A single dysplastic nevus has a low risk of malignancy, but an adolescent with multiple dysplastic nevi is at increased risk for malignant melanoma, especially if there is a relevant family history.

Spitz nevi (spindle and epithelioid cell nevi) are dome-shaped, red-brown to brown-black, and often occur on the face. Spitz nevi are rarely malignant.

Congenital melanocytic nevi were discussed at the beginning of this section, along with Nevus of Ota, Nevus of Ito, and Mongolian spots.

PIGMENT CHANGES

VITILIGO

Vitiligo is acquired macular depigmentation (Image 7-21). It usually occurs in healthy people, but rarely, it can also be part of the AR polyglandular deficiency, in which case any of the following can occur: DM, Graves disease, Addison's/adrenal insufficiency, hyper/hypothyroidism, hypoparathyroidism, pernicious anemia, and vitiligo. If you see a patient with vitiligo and endocrine abnormalities, think of this AR deficiency!

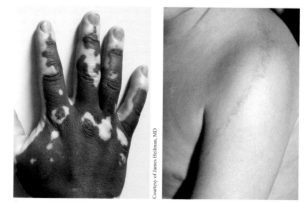

Image 7-21: Vitiligo   *Image 7-22: Lichen striatus*

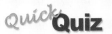

Quick Quiz

- In which layer of skin do junctional nevi occur?
- What are the reasons to remove an acquired melanocytic nevus?
- What is vitiligo? What disorders are associated (rarely) with vitiligo?
- Describe lichen striatus. What is the recommended treatment, if any?
- Which type of patient has acanthosis nigricans?
- Which skin areas are affected by atopic dermatitis in infants? In older children?
- Patients with atopic dermatitis are at high risk for what skin infections?

LICHEN STRIATUS

Lichen striatus is common in childhood and presents with a linear group of small, pink to skin-colored papules that slowly flatten leaving a hypopigmented streak that resolves within several months to a few years. It is asymptomatic, self-limited, and occurs most commonly on an arm or leg (Image 7-22).

LICHEN NITIDUS

Lichen nitidus is a benign, self-limited condition with multiple, 1–2-mm, flat-topped, skin-colored papules that can be asymptomatic or slightly pruritic. The papules can occur anywhere on the body including the face and genitalia. Some debate whether lichen nitidus is a clinical variant of lichen planus.

ACANTHOSIS NIGRICANS

Acanthosis nigricans is hyperpigmented skin with a thickened, velvety appearance, most noticeable in the skin folds (Image 7-23). It rarely is familial. You tend to see it in obese patients, and it is associated with hyperinsulinemia. On exams, look for hyperpigmented skin that involves the axilla or neck of an obese child or adolescent. These patients have an increased risk of developing diabetes; thus screen for hyperglycemia, hyperlipidemia, and hypertension. In adults, it can be associated with GI cancer.

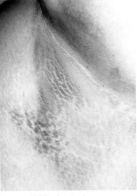
Image 7-23: A. nigricans

HYPERPIGMENTATION IN GENERAL

Diffuse hyperpigmentation can occur in biliary sclerosis, scleroderma, Addison disease, hemochromatosis (a grayish/bronze coloration), and with the use of busulfan. Other causes include primary biliary cirrhosis, porphyria cutanea tarda, malabsorption/Whipple syndrome, pellagra (niacin deficiency), B_{12} deficiency, and folate deficiency.

Hyperpigmentation in sun-exposed areas is common with use of amiodarone and phenothiazines and seen with porphyria cutanea tarda. Hyperpigmentation is diffuse but darker in sun-exposed areas in pellagra, biliary sclerosis, and scleroderma. Methotrexate can cause a reactivation of sunburn.

COMMON SKIN PROBLEMS

ATOPIC DERMATITIS

Clinical Manifestations

Atopic dermatitis has 3 stages: infant, childhood, and adult (least common).

In infants, the lesions are most commonly on the cheeks and extensor surfaces of the extremities, with scalp and trunk involvement also seen (Image 7-24). Older children have disease in the antecubital fossa, popliteal fossa, and back of the neck, with ankles, wrists, and the back of the hands and feet also commonly affected. Some report that Asian and African-American children can have more severe disease.

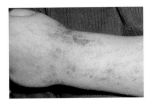
Image 7-24: Atopic dermatitis

The adult/adolescent phase has continued flexural involvement with chronic hand and foot dermatitis. Periocular involvement is common. Pruritus is significant at any age.

Other clues to diagnosis:

- Double or triple creases under the lower eyelid (Dennie-Morgan folds)
- Obvious sparing around the nose ("headlight sign")
- Small fissures at the base of the ear lobe
- Increased skin markings on palms and soles
- Dry skin (xerosis)

Children with atopic dermatitis are at high risk for widespread skin infection with molluscum contagiosum and herpes simplex (eczema herpeticum). Widespread HSV infection can present with a sudden worsening of the eczema with an outbreak of multiple vesicles. Because the child is likely to scratch the vesicles, they will open early in disease evolution and result in some patients presenting with widespread punctate erosions. The affected child often has an associated fever and

DERMATOLOGY

other systemic symptoms. There is frequently a history of a cold sore in the affected patient or a family member. Patients with eczema herpeticum usually require hospitalization and treatment with IV acyclovir. Patients with periorbital lesions must have a prompt ophthalmologic evaluation to help prevent the development of herpetic keratitis. This condition can recur in susceptible individuals.

It is common for *S. aureus* to colonize in these children as well. Impetigo can be severe. Colonization and infection with MRSA has increased markedly in recent years and presents a therapeutic challenge in many moderate-to-severe atopic patients.

Treatment

The most important therapy is to decrease skin dryness. You can do this by suggesting emollients and avoiding bathing with strong alkaline soaps. Most pediatric dermatologists recommend daily short baths, followed by immediate application of a bland emollient. Encourage patients to avoid products with fragrances. In general, lotions are not very useful; heavy creams and petrolatum-based ointments are typically more effective in controlling the xerosis of atopic patients. Avoidance of fragrance-containing soaps, laundry detergents, and fabric softeners can also be helpful. In dry months or environments, room humidifiers can help. Unless the eczema is severe or persistent, most children do not require food avoidance or dietary investigation.

Treat the inflammatory component with topical corticosteroids. Ointments work better than creams because of the better emolliency. Use of 1% hydrocortisone ointment is adequate for many mildly affected patients. For more severe flares, you may need medium-to-high potency topical steroids. Topical steroids are usually effective within 5–14 days in patients with mild-to-moderate atopic dermatitis. Avoid oral or systemic steroids because they increase the likelihood of rebound flares, as well as have severe long-term side effects.

More recently, a new class of medications, known as topical immunomodulators/calcineurin inhibitors, has become available. This group includes tacrolimus (Protopic®) ointment and pimecrolimus (Elidel®) cream. These medications are approved as 2nd line therapy for management of atopic dermatitis in children > 2 years of age. The topical immunomodulators have some advantages over topical steroids in that they do not tend to cause thinning of the skin, and there is not the concern of systemic glucocorticoid side effects from absorption. However, long-term safety data on this new class of medications is very limited in regards to potential carcinogenicity from regular use. Furthermore, they are much more expensive than many commonly used topical corticosteroids. A black box warning was mandated by the FDA in 2006: "Although a causal relationship has not been established, rare cases of malignancy (skin and lymphoma) have been reported in patients treated with topical calcineurin inhibitors."

Tacrolimus appears to be the stronger of the 2 agents and is comparable to a mid-potency topical steroid. It is best used for moderate atopic dermatitis or as maintenance therapy for more severe disease. Furthermore, it can be systemically absorbed, so use it with caution on widespread disease, extensive excoriations, and on younger children. Pimecrolimus does not appear to be absorbed systemically to the same extent. It is probably comparable in efficacy to a low-potency topical steroid, and, therefore, it is best used in mild atopic dermatitis as maintenance therapy rather than for acute exacerbations.

You can control itching with antihistamines. Oral antibiotics may be required for superinfection but are not recommended for routine prophylactic use.

Aim treatment at controlling the disease process, as there is no "cure." Most children improve with age, and 40–50% are disease-free by adolescence.

Other skin disorders are more common in children with atopic dermatitis and include the following:

Pityriasis alba is common in school-age children and presents with areas of hypopigmentation with a fine scale. It most commonly affects the cheeks and extensor extremities. It likely represents a form of postinflammatory hypopigmentation at sites of dry skin or mild eczema and is more apparent in children with darker skin. It often becomes more readily visible in the summer because the affected skin does not tan normally.

Keratosis pilaris is a manifestation of the dry skin associated with atopic dermatitis. It is characterized by many < 1-mm, dry, rough, skin-colored to pink, follicular papules distributed symmetrically over the cheeks, backs of the upper arms, and the anterior thighs. In severe cases, this condition can be more widespread. Treatment consists of avoiding irritants (dyes and perfumes) and regular use of emollients and keratolytic agents (lactic acid, urea, topical retinoids). This condition runs in families and generally improves some with age.

Juvenile plantar dermatosis presents with redness, cracking, and fissuring of the weight-bearing part of the soles. It is aggravated by occlusive footwear (boots, sneakers) and can be confused with tinea pedis. Treat by applying petrolatum for lubrication and an absorbent powder. Sometimes, a moderate topical steroid is required.

Dyshidrotic eczema (pompholyx) presents with eczema of the palms, soles, and sides of the digits. Look for small, firm, "tapioca-like" vesicles on the lateral edges of the fingers. It is very itchy, and if fissuring occurs, it can be quite painful. Emollients and potent topical steroids are helpful.

SEBORRHEA

Seborrheic dermatitis manifests as erythema, has a greasy scale, and commonly occurs in infants. It usually begins within 2 months of birth. It can be mild and occurs on the scalp vertex with patches of greasy,

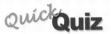

Quiz

- What is the 1st and most significant therapy measure to carry out in a child with atopic dermatitis?
- What is the best pharmacologic therapy for children with mild atopic dermatitis?
- What are recent, 2nd line therapies for atopic dermatitis?
- Describe pityriasis alba.
- How does seborrheic dermatitis manifest?
- If seborrheic dermatitis is really severe, what disorder should be in your differential?
- Why don't 5-year-olds have seborrheic dermatitis?
- Describe allergic contact dermatitis.
- What is a common presentation of allergic contact dermatitis to nickel?

yellowish scales known as "cradle cap" (although some grandmothers seem to add an "r" before the letter "a" in cap!). Cradle cap can be more severe and spread to the forehead and cheeks. Most cases resolve in several weeks to months (Image 7-25).

Treat severe cases with 1% hydrocortisone cream or daily shampooing of the scalp. Shampoos with selenium sulfide or ketoconazole can be helpful. Emollient use can also help remove scales.

If the seborrheic dermatitis is extremely severe, consider the possibility of Langerhans cell histiocytosis (formerly known as histiocytosis X), especially if atrophy, ulceration, or petechiae are present. A skin biopsy and special staining are generally diagnostic.

In older children and adolescents, the seborrheic dermatitis manifests as "dandruff." It also can cause redness and scaling on the eyebrows and paranasal areas. It responds well to zinc or tar shampoo. Seborrhea can usually be managed successfully with a low-potency

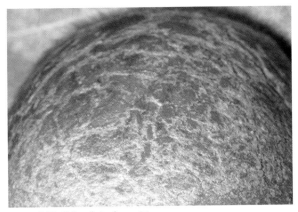

Image 7-25: Seborrheic dermatitis

topical steroid (e.g., hydrocortisone), and it can be helpful to concurrently use a topical antifungal cream (e.g., ketoconazole).

What about kids between ages 1 and 9? They normally don't get seborrheic dermatitis, because you have to have active sebaceous glands. More commonly, tinea capitis and head lice cause itching in this age group. For noninfectious causes, atopic dermatitis and psoriasis are most common in this age group. However, because puberty seems to be occurring earlier, seborrhea can be seen in children as young as age 7–9 years.

INTERTRIGO

Intertrigo is an irritant dermatitis caused by maceration and friction and usually is found in the skin folds of obese patients. It can be secondarily infected by *Candida albicans*. Occasionally, an inverse subtype of psoriasis can be confused with intertrigo.

CONTACT DERMATITIS

Contact dermatitis can be caused by a chemical irritant or an allergic reaction. Image 7-26 shows contact dermatitis due to material in a sandal.

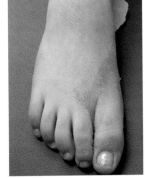

Image 7-26: Contact dermatitis

Primary irritant contact dermatitis is due to the direct effects of a chemical or physical substance. The most common primary irritants are detergents, acidic products, soaps, urine, and feces.

Allergic contact dermatitis is due to a delayed hypersensitivity reaction in the skin. Patients first become sensitized to the antigen after one or several exposures. After sensitization, and upon re-exposure, the skin develops a pruritic lesion within 1–4 days. The most common allergens are nickel, chromium, neomycin, bacitracin, and oleoresin (poison oak, poison ivy, and poison sumac). Know: Poison ivy is not spread by fluid contained in the vesicular or bullous lesions! Nickel allergy is localized at the area the contact occurs, such as from earrings, bracelets, zippers, or metal snaps or clasps. Around 20% of individuals with ear piercings have nickel sensitization. Jewelry with stainless steel or 22K gold is usually safe. Treatment for allergic contact dermatitis consists of cool compresses (Burow solution = aluminum acetate, 1:20), topical glucocorticoids, and emollients. If severe, such as poison ivy dermatitis on the face, give systemic glucocorticoids for 14 days (shorter courses can lead to rebound flaring). A common presentation of allergic contact dermatitis to nickel in children is the presence of an infraumbilical eczematous plaque, often associated with widespread id reaction on the extensor extremities.

DERMATOLOGY

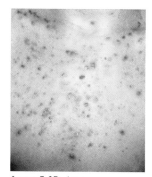

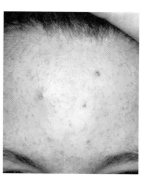

Image 7-27: Acne   *Image 7-28: Acne*

ACNE VULGARIS

The clinical manifestations of acne vulgaris are open and closed comedones and inflammatory papules, pustules, or nodules on the face, shoulders, chest, and back. Propionibacterium acnes is a normal resident of the pilosebaceous unit and overgrows within a blocked sebaceous follicle. Severity of acne is genetically determined. Most have generally thought that foods and poor hygiene do not contribute to acne formation, but recent literature suggests that high-glycemic or "Western" diets can contribute. (See Image 7-27 and Image 7-28.)

A majority of adolescents can be treated with topical medications of 3 types:

1) Benzoyl peroxide products—which have both bactericidal and comedolytic effects

2) Antibiotics

3) Retinoids—which are particularly effective for comedonal acne

Topical therapy most often involves tretinoin (Retin-A®), benzoyl peroxide (2.5–10%), and topical erythromycin or clindamycin. Oral therapy is usually with tetracycline, doxycycline, minocycline, or erythromycin. TMP/SMX is occasionally used but carries a higher risk of serious allergic reactions, including Stevens-Johnson syndrome and toxic epidermal necrolysis. Several oral contraceptives are also approved for the management of acne.

Isotretinoin (Amnesteem®, Claravis™, Sotret®) is highly effective in resistant cases but is also a powerful teratogen. Only clinicians experienced with the management of severe acne, knowledgeable of the side-effect profile, and who understand appropriate monitoring of isotretinoin therapy should prescribe this drug. Generally, adolescent females must be on 2 forms of effective birth control. Serious side effects include pseudotumor cerebri (especially if used with tetracyclines), depression/suicidal ideation, hypertriglyceridemia, elevated liver enzymes, potential for developing inflammatory bowel disease, and, rarely, decreased night vision and skeletal issues.

ACNE ROSACEA

Acne rosacea is seen most commonly in middle-aged patients, but it can occasionally be seen in adolescents.

It presents with acne-like lesions, erythema, and telangiectasias on the central face. Even before the lesions appear, patients can have a flushing reaction to various stimuli (alcohol, stress, exercise, heat, and sun exposure). Once the rosacea manifests, the flush can become permanent. Rhinophyma (big nose) occurs primarily in adult patients. Treat with oral tetracyclines, topical metronidazole, or sulfacetamide preparations.

ALOPECIA

Alopecia Areata

Patients present with this common disorder with the sudden appearance of round or oval patches of hair loss on the scalp and, sometimes, other body sites as well (Image 7-29). Generally, it occurs in school-age children, but you can see it in infants. Alopecia areata is rarely associated with autoimmune diseases, mainly Hashimoto thyroiditis, Type I DM, and vitiligo.

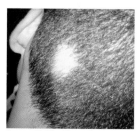

Image 7-29: Alopecia areata

Short, tapered hairs, which are thinner proximally, are known as "exclamation point hairs." You can usually observe these in areas of active disease, and they can resemble the broken-off hairs of tinea capitis. However, redness, scaling, and lymphadenopathy are generally absent in alopecia areata, in contrast to tinea capitis.

Alopecia areata can present in 2 ways:

1) Patchy alopecia areata; regrowth potential is good.

2) Alopecia totalis (loss of all scalp hair) or universalis (loss of all scalp and body hair); hair is less likely to regrow.

Diagnosis is clinical, but scalp biopsy will show a peribulbar lymphocytic infiltrate. Pitting of the nails can be a helpful clinical clue to the diagnosis. Therapy includes topical, intralesional, or systemic steroids; topical minoxidil; or topical immunotherapy.

Trichotillomania

Trichotillomania is the compulsive pulling, twisting, or breaking of one's own hair (Image 7-30). "Moth-eaten" appearance is common. There are often well-defined patches of hair loss, with hairs of varying lengths, but rarely complete alopecia. The eyelashes and eyebrows can also be affected. Differentiate

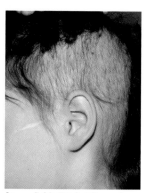

Image 7-30: Trichotillomania

DERMATOLOGY

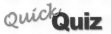

Quiz

- What are some of the serious side effects of isotretinoin?
- Describe alopecia areata.
- How does alopecia areata contrast with tinea capitis?
- Define trichotillomania.
- Describe traction alopecia.
- What is telogen effluvium?
- What is the most common cause of hair breakage in African-American patients?
- Define hidradenitis suppurativa.
- In what disease are Koplik spots found?
- What disease should you consider when finding melanotic pigmentation of the lips and buccal mucosa?

trichotillomania from alopecia areata, tinea capitis, and secondary syphilis. Behavioral modification and antidepressants, such as fluoxetine, can be helpful.

Traction Alopecia

Traction alopecia is common in girls who wear tight ponytails or braids. Hair thinning is usually seen at the scalp margin and the temporal areas in particular. There can be associated inflammation with the development of papules or pustules along the hairline. Over time, chronic traction can cause scarring.

Telogen Effluvium

Telogen effluvium is hair loss that occurs 6 weeks to 4 months after a severe stress to the body. It can be seen following childbirth, acute fever, surgery, crash dieting, stress, thyroid disorders, with certain medications, or after stopping oral contraceptives. Sudden stress causes the hair shaft to go into "hibernation," or the telogen growth phase. In several months, when the growing phase of the hair begins again, it falls out. Total alopecia does not occur with this; instead, you typically see a diffuse thinning of the hair.

You can diagnose this condition by "the hair-pull test." The hair-pull test is, in essence, very simple. You pinch a group of about 30 hairs between your thumb and forefinger and give a sharp tug. Repeat this in a few different areas over the scalp. Anagen, or growing hairs, should remain rooted in place while telogen hairs come out easily. It is normal for 1–2 hairs to be removed each time because about 10% of hair is in the telogen phase, but if 4–5 hairs come out, then telogen effluvium is likely. Of course, the test depends a lot on the person doing the pulling.

Trichorrhexis Nodosa

Trichorrhexis nodosa is the most common cause of hair breakage in African-American patients. It follows chemical treatments. The hairs break off easily and may not recover for 2–4 years.

Other Causes of Alopecia

Other causes of alopecia include tinea capitis (which is the most common cause of alopecia in children) nutritional deficiencies, hypothyroidism, and syphilis.

HIDRADENITIS SUPPURATIVA

Hidradenitis suppurativa is a chronic, inflammatory, scarring process involving apocrine glands of the axilla and inguinal region. This disease occurs in both sexes, and often there is a positive family history. The patient usually presents with inflammatory papules and pustules in these intertriginous regions; in more severe instances, there can be abscesses and draining sinuses. Sometimes, you also can see open or closed comedones. This disease is difficult to control and can be more problematic in obese individuals. Treatment modalities include topical and systemic antibiotics, such as erythromycin or the tetracycline family, as well as topical benzoyl peroxides and antibacterial soaps. Severe cases can be amenable to surgical excision of the apocrine glands.

MOUTH FINDINGS

The most common, problematic mouth findings are:

- Hyperpigmented (blue-black) gingiva: seen in Addison disease.
- Koplik spots: small, white vesicles on an erythematous base, which are found on the palate in patients with measles. These normally precede the skin lesions by several days.
- Hairy leukoplakia most commonly occurs in patients with AIDS. It appears as areas of ribbed whiteness along the sides of the tongue. This is due to Epstein-Barr virus in the superficial layers of the tongue's squamous epithelium.
- Peutz-Jeghers syndrome (multiple intestinal hamartomatous polyps): Rule out in patients with melanotic pigmentation (freckles) on the lips and buccal mucosa.
- Beefy red tongue and angular cheilitis: associated with glucagonomas.
- Macroglossia (big tongue): associated with primary amyloidosis, acromegaly, trisomy 21, congenital hypothyroidism, Beckwith-Wiedemann syndrome, metabolic storage disease, congenital vascular tumors, and congenital malformations of the tongue.
- White lesions: candidiasis, hairy leukoplakia (AIDS), lichen planus. Lichen planus also causes ulceration.

- "Geographic tongue" has the appearance of migratory, denuded red patches. It is benign and usually asymptomatic. It can be associated with psoriasis.
- "Strawberry tongue": associated with scarlet fever and Kawasaki disease (mucocutaneous lymph node syndrome).
- "Bald tongue": atrophy that is associated with pellagra, iron deficiency anemia, pernicious anemia, and xerostomia (salivary gland problems, as seen in Sjögren syndrome, lymphoma, mumps, sarcoidosis; occasionally idiopathic).

CUTANEOUS DRUG REACTIONS

OVERVIEW

Drugs that can produce harmful skin changes include:

- **Penicillin** (PCN):
  - Immediate hypersensitivity reaction; anaphylaxis (IgE)
  - Delayed hypersensitivity reaction, immune complex reaction/vasculitis, or morbilliform eruption
- **Tetracycline/Doxycycline**: photosensitivity.
- **NSAIDs**: urticaria/angioedema in 1%, asthma in 0.5%; can cause photosensitivity.
- **Phenytoin**:
  - Hypersensitivity syndrome: purpuric rash, fever, facial edema, lymphadenopathy, and organ involvement (such as hepatitis)
  - Various skin reactions, including Stevens-Johnson syndrome and toxic epidermal necrolysis
  - Hypertrophied gums
- **Glucocorticoids**: skin changes, including striae, atrophy, and acne-like lesions.
- **Warfarin** (Coumadin®): necrotic skin patches appearing 3–10 days after starting warfarin.
- **Radiocontrast dye**: urticaria/erythema (1/15) and anaphylaxis (1/1,000). There is a 30% repeat-reaction incidence in an individual with a previous reaction to contrast dye. The repeat reaction can be very serious and, rarely, can lead to TEN (described next). Prophylaxis with diphenhydramine and glucocorticoids (start 13 hours prior) decreases this reaction significantly.

TOXIC EPIDERMAL NECROLYSIS

Toxic epidermal necrolysis (TEN) typically presents as a sloughing away of skin but occurs at a deeper level than staphylococcal scalded skin syndrome (SSSS; subepidermal). In contrast to SSSS, patients with TEN do poorly. It is typically caused by a hypersensitivity reaction to a drug, especially sulfa antibiotics and the aromatic anticonvulsants: phenytoin, phenobarbital, or carbamazepine. TEN is generally accompanied by skin tenderness and significant mucous membrane involvement of the eyes and lips, similar to Stevens-Johnson syndrome.

Treatment consists of discontinuation of the offending drug, monitoring for internal organ involvement, and supportive care—many recommend IVIG therapy. Most agree that systemic steroids should not be used in this clinical setting, although randomized, controlled studies are lacking.

INFLAMMATORY SKIN DISEASES

PSORIASIS

Among initial presentations of psoriasis, 35% occur in children < 20 years of age. The most common form of psoriasis has well-defined, erythematous skin lesions with distinctive, mica-like (silvery) scales. It is usually symmetrical and occurs on knees, elbows, sacral area, and scalp. Koebner phenomenon (outbreak in the area of an abrasion) is common and often has a linear configuration.

Guttate psoriasis is common in childhood and presents with sudden onset of many small, scaly papules and plaques on the face, trunk, and extremities (Image 7-31). It can be induced by streptococcal pharyngitis or perianal streptococcal disease.

Infants rarely have psoriasis, but if it occurs, it typically presents in the diaper area and can sometimes be quite extensive, resembling candidal or severe seborrheic dermatitis.

There are 2 severe cutaneous types of psoriasis:

1) Erythrodermic psoriasis

2) Pustular psoriasis

Erythrodermic psoriasis is an exfoliative reaction in which the entire surface of the skin becomes red, warm, and scaly; patients are unable to control body temperature (hypo-/hyperthermia is common). Dehydration, hypoalbuminemia, and anemia of chronic disease are common sequelae. The erythroderma and psoriasis of any type are often precipitated/exacerbated by sunburn, infection (virus, strep pharyngitis), and drugs (especially antimalarials, gold, lithium, and beta-blockers). It is controversial whether alcohol exacerbates psoriasis, but many feel it does. Treatment usually includes acitretin

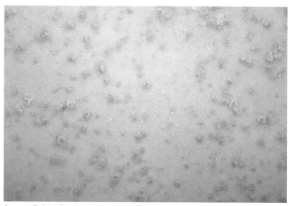

Image 7-31: Guttate psoriasis of the back

Quick Quiz

- What is the significance of "geographic tongue"?
- "Strawberry tongue" is associated with what diseases?
- Define Koebner phenomenon.
- What is erythrodermic psoriasis?
- Pitted nails with onycholysis are specific for what disorder?
- What antibody is found in neonates with neonatal lupus and congenital heart block?
- Describe skin findings in sarcoidosis.

(Soriatane®)—and sometimes methotrexate or biologics (TNF-alpha inhibitors) in refractory cases.

Pustular psoriasis has many small pustules, often coalescing to form "psoriatic pustular lakes of pus." There are 2 forms:

1) The localized form affects only the palms and soles and is associated with DIP joint arthritis.

2) The rare, generalized form (von Zumbusch) can occur with the erythrodermic type, it is often triggered by oral steroids, and treatment is most often acitretin.

Nail changes: Most specific (but seldom seen in children) is an "oil drop" sign (glycoprotein deposition) in nails. Ice pick-like pitting of the nails is common. These pits are usually in small groups on the nail. Thickened nails and onycholysis (separation of distal nail from the nail bed) are also common in psoriasis. Pitted nails in association with onycholysis are fairly specific for psoriasis. Nail pitting can also be seen in alopecia areata, but there is no associated onycholysis.

Treatment: Plaques are commonly treated with topical steroids, calcipotriene (a synthetic vitamin D_3 analog), tazarotene gel (Tazorac®, a retinoid), tar, and anthralin, often in combination with UVB (290–320 nm) phototherapy. "PUVA" (oral psoralen + UVA light [320–400 nm]) is also very effective but is associated with increased skin cancer and generally not recommended for children. Methotrexate and cyclosporine are used for widespread psoriasis, especially with arthritis. Acitretin is used for the severe forms of all types, but is teratogenic, so menstruating females must avoid pregnancy for at least 2 years after ending treatment. TNF-alpha inhibitors have been used for treatment of severe disease, but, in August 2009, the FDA required a black box warning for increased risk of leukemia and other malignancies in children and adolescents on these medications.

CUTANEOUS LUPUS

Subacute cutaneous lupus erythematosus can sometimes be seen in teenagers. Most have a positive speckled ANA. Anti-Ro (SS-A) antibodies are seen in 70–95% and anti-La (SS-B) in a lesser percentage. It often has a negative anti-dsDNA and negative anti-Sm.

Anti-Ro antibodies cross the placenta and can cause congenital heart block and cutaneous lupus lesions in infants. This condition is referred to as neonatal lupus and is the most common cause of congenital heart block. Neonatal lupus typically involves either the skin or the heart, but normally not both organs. Most affected infants have anti-Ro antibodies, but a few have anti-U1RNP (anti-nRNP) antibodies. The most common cutaneous findings are periorbital erythema (often referred to as raccoon eyes) and round or annular, often atrophic-appearing, patches and plaques. These lesions are generally most prominent in a photodistribution that includes the face and scalp, but they also can occur on the trunk and extremities. The lesions can be annular, scaly, and resemble tinea corporis.

The cutaneous lesions usually resolve spontaneously within several months, but can leave residual telangiectasias or atrophic scarring. Treatment is conservative with photoprotection, topical steroids, and emollients. Other potential systemic manifestations include cholestatic liver disease and thrombocytopenia in a minority of patients.

It is important to note that more than 50% of mothers who pass on this condition do not carry an established diagnosis of collagen vascular disease. Those mothers who do have a known rheumatologic disorder most often have lupus erythematosus, rheumatoid arthritis, or Sjögren syndrome and have a positive anti-SSA/Ro antibody. If you suspect an infant has neonatal lupus, check for the anti-SSA/Ro, anti-SSB/La, and anti-nRNP antibodies.

Differential diagnosis includes cutaneous fungal infection and psoriasis. Active SLE (see Rheumatology, Book 5) typically has a peripheral ANA pattern.

Patients with discoid lupus usually have a negative ANA, negative anti-dsDNA, and negative anti-Sm; but 95% have a positive lesional-direct immunofluorescence (DIF)!

CREST

CREST syndrome can present with calcinosis cutis (small tender nodules on the fingers), Raynaud phenomenon, esophageal dysmotility, sclerodactyly (sclerosis of the fingers), and telangiectasias. CREST syndrome is rare in children.

SARCOIDOSIS

Sarcoidosis is a noncaseating granulomatous disease that often affects the lungs, lymph nodes, eyes, and skin. It is most common in African-Americans. Scar sarcoidosis presents as granulomatous changes in a healing skin wound (laceration, tattoo, old scars). Sarcoidosis is a recognized cause of erythema nodosum (see next). It is the 2nd greatest mimic of other diseases (1st is syphilis); it can mimic anything but a vesicular eruption.

Lupus pernio presents with violaceous plaques or tumors on the cheeks, nose, and ears, which can be scarring/disfiguring. It is associated with upper respiratory tract involvement with sarcoid, has a slow onset, and almost never resolves!

The best prognosis of the sarcoid skin changes is with erythema nodosum or the small papules. Treat cutaneous sarcoid with intralesional/topical steroids; occasionally, antimalarials, azathioprine, and methotrexate. Dapsone is ineffective.

Erythema Nodosum

Erythema nodosum consists of red, tender, warm nodules that usually appear on the shins (Image 7-32). It is one of the most common types of panniculitis (inflammation of the fat). Although sarcoidosis is one of the causes of erythema nodosum, other more common causes in pediatrics include infection (TB, streptococcal, deep fungal), drugs (especially oral contraceptives, sulfas, and penicillins), and inflammatory bowel disease. Erythema nodosum can also be idiopathic. In addition to identifying and addressing the underlying cause, treatment includes rest and elevation of the lower extremities and nonsteroidal antiinflammatory agents. Oral systemic corticosteroids are rarely needed and are generally not recommended.

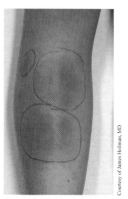

Image 7-32: E. nodosum

Courtesy of James Heilman, MD

DERMATOMYOSITIS

Dermatomyositis (see Rheumatology, Book 5): Buzz phrase is a periorbital heliotrope rash (+/– periorbital edema). The upper eyelids are scaly, dusky pink-to-violet with edema and sometimes a malar (lupus-like "butterfly") rash; it can sometimes mimic a facial allergic reaction.

Gottron papules are also seen in dermatomyositis. These are flat-topped, reddish-to-violaceous, sometimes scaly papules (some claim it looks like "cigarette paper" crinkling of the skin) over the knuckles (MCP, PIP, and/or DIP). Gottron papules are the most specific finding of dermatomyositis. Patients often describe it simply as a "rash" or "eruption" over the knuckles. These lesions can have a psoriasiform appearance, with similar lesions on the elbows and knees. Calcinosis cutis and ulceration can also be seen and are a bad prognostic sign.

Livedo reticularis is nonspecific; it is seen in dermatomyositis but also in cutaneous polyarteritis nodosa, SLE, cholesterol embolism (atheroembolism), and there is a fairly common benign idiopathic type.

Treatment: glucocorticoids; add immunosuppressives or antimalarials if needed for skin changes. In older patients, dermatomyositis can indicate cancer (usually GI).

REACTIVE ARTHRITIS

Reactive arthritis causes pustular or thick, red-to-yellowish scaly papules/plaques on the palms and soles (keratoderma blennorrhagica) and penis (circinate balanitis). See Rheumatology, Book 5.

VASCULITIS

The main cutaneous reaction with vasculitis is palpable purpura. If a child presents with arthralgias, abdominal pain, and palpable purpura, think Henoch-Schönlein purpura. See Rheumatology, Book 5 for complete coverage of vasculitis.

PYODERMA GANGRENOSUM

Pyoderma gangrenosum is an inflammatory ulcer that usually occurs on the legs. It is often associated with inflammatory bowel disease. It can also occur with rheumatoid arthritis, leukemia, monoclonal (IgA) gammopathy, and chronic, active hepatitis. Although a skin biopsy is not diagnostic, it serves to exclude other causes of ulceration. Treating the colonized bacteria generally does not help. Treat with biologic dressings, dapsone, systemic steroids, or other immunosuppressive agents, including cyclosporine.

VITAMIN DEFICIENCIES

HYPERPIGMENTATION

Deficiencies of B₁₂, folate, and niacin (pellagra) can cause hyperpigmentation.

ZINC DEFICIENCY

Zinc deficiency causes a red, eczematous, sometimes erosive or vesicular rash that typically involves the perioral, periocular, or paranasal skin, extensor surfaces of the hands/feet, and perineum/scrotum (Image 7-33).

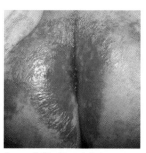

Image 7-33: Zinc deficiency

Quiz

- Define erythema nodosum.
- What is the classic facial rash of dermatomyositis?
- How does zinc deficiency manifest dermatologically?
- How is a Wood's lamp helpful in the diagnosis of erythrasma?

Zinc deficiency can occur as an acquired or inherited disorder—acrodermatitis enteropathica. This is an AR disorder with impaired absorption of zinc from the intestine. Diagnose by finding low-plasma zinc concentrations. Treatment with zinc supplementation results in rapid improvement.

ERUPTION SEEN IN CYSTIC FIBROSIS

A similar, but usually more extensive periorificial eruption can also be seen in infants with cystic fibrosis. These scaly, red eruptions generally involve perioral and perineal skin but can become more generalized. They are typically associated with significant edema due to low protein and albumin levels. You commonly see these eruptions in association with FTT and anemia. The eruptions generally resolve rapidly with improvement in the nutritional status of the patient. Patients with protein malnutrition (Kwashiorkor disease) can have similar erosions on the intertriginous areas and oral commissures, but they have diffuse desquamation with a "peeling or flaky paint" appearance.

BIOTIN DEFICIENCY

Biotin deficiency can present with skin changes very similar to zinc deficiency and, like zinc deficiency, it can also occur as an acquired or genetic disorder. There is a late infantile form known as biotin-responsive multiple carboxylase deficiency due to biotinidase deficiency. This deficiency presents with rash and alopecia. CNS symptoms are common and include ataxia, seizures, and developmental delay. Biotin levels are usually low but can be in the normal range, so do a trial of biotin if patient history and examination suggest this disorder.

ESSENTIAL FATTY ACID DEFICIENCY

Essential fatty acid deficiency commonly presents with eczematous dermatitis. You can observe dry, eczema-like skin and hypopigmentation in children with protein malnutrition.

BACTERIAL

Note

Also see Infectious Disease, Book 2, where many of the images are displayed as well.

Erythrasma

Erythrasma is a well-defined, brown-to-reddish, slightly scaly patch, which you generally find in the axillae, groin, and toe webs. In obese female adolescents, it also is seen under the breasts. Although gram-positive *Corynebacterium minutissimum* is frequently isolated from the lesion (especially after it has become scaly or macerated), it appears to be polymicrobial in origin. Differentials are fungal infection and intertrigo (an irritant dermatitis in the skin folds of obese patients).

Diagnosis: It will fluoresce bright red with the Wood's lamp. Treat with oral or topical erythromycin +/− an "-azole" antifungal cream.

Streptococcus pyogenes

Streptococcus pyogenes (group A strep) is an occasional cause of impetigo—a skin infection confined to the epidermis. (Most cases are due to *S. aureus*.)

Ecthyma starts as an impetigo and then becomes deeper, causing shallow ulcerations.

Intertrigo is most common in infants and young children (Image 7-34). It is due to friction of opposing skin surfaces and moisture. Commonly, intertrigo occurs in the folds of the neck, axillae, and inguinal areas. It has a distinctive foul odor, and there are no satellite lesions. It responds well to topical/oral antibiotics depending on the severity.

Perianal dermatitis (also can be caused by *S. aureus*) is most common in boys (70%) between 6 months and 10 years of age (Image 7-35). Only 10% have symptomatic concurrent pharyngitis. Familial spread is common (siblings bathing together). 80% present with pruritus, 50% with rectal pain/burning (often leading

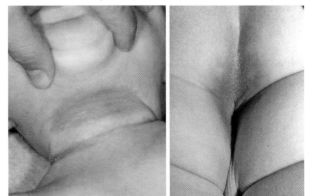

Image 7-34: Streptococcal intertrigo   Image 7-35: Perianal dermatitis

DERMATOLOGY

to constipation due to pain with defecation), and 33% with blood-streaked stools. Perianal dermatitis can trigger guttate psoriasis. Therapy is a 10-day course of oral penicillin. Recurrence rates are high at nearly 50%.

Erysipelas is an explosive, superficial cellulitis (caused by group A strep), usually confined to the dermis; it spreads quickly through skin lymphatics. A clear demarcation line of swelling and redness indicates the extent of infection (Image 7-36). It normally starts from a superficial abrasion or break in the skin, leading to erythema, swelling, and fever. Common sites of involvement are the lower legs, face, umbilical stump (omphalitis), and sites of circumcision or insect bites. Clinically, this can resemble an acute allergic contact dermatitis.

Necrotizing fasciitis (streptococcal gangrene) is a deep cellulitis involving the subcutaneous fat and fascia. Unlike erysipelas, it does not have a distinct border and can be difficult to diagnose early. Also, the infection can be polymicrobial (group A strep + anaerobes). Mortality is high, even with appropriate medical and surgical intervention.

Scarlet fever causes "scarlatina"—a fine, red, sandpaper-like rash with desquamation of the skin commonly occurring during healing.

Streptococcal toxic shock syndrome causes symptoms similar to staphylococcal TSS (described next). Even with high-dose IV PCN (or clindamycin, which can have some therapeutic advantages), mortality is ~ 30%!

Penicillin is far and away the best treatment for a known group A strep infection. Give oral PCN (x 10 days) or IM benzathine PCN. Give erythromycin for PCN-allergic. Clindamycin is often added to PCN when there is serious infection, such as necrotizing fasciitis or toxic shock.

Staphylococcus aureus

S. aureus is responsible for several skin syndromes:

- It is by far the most common cause of impetigo—this starts as an erythematous, vesicular lesion that quickly becomes pustular and crusty ("honey-colored crust").

- Bullous impetigo usually occurs in young children and presents with the acute onset of large, loose bullae. These bullae rupture quickly, leaving shallow erosions (Image 7-37). It is due to a toxin-producing strain of *S. aureus*. Bullous impetigo is a localized form of staphylococcal scalded skin syndrome.

- Patients with staphylococcal scalded skin syndrome (SSSS) present with tender, red, peeling skin due to circulating toxins from localized staph infection or colonization generally occurring on the mucous membranes of the nose, conjunctiva, and nasopharynx. (These are the best sites for bacterial culture—not the skin!) Skin changes are similar to those seen in toxic epidermal necrolysis (which is noninfectious and a side effect of drugs), so consider it during the workup. The skin in SSSS separates much more superficially than in TEN through the granular layer of the epidermis—and, therefore, SSSS is a much less serious disorder.

- *S. aureus* is the main culprit in toxic shock syndrome (TSS), which presents with abrupt development of hypotension and shock. Patients have a diffuse, scarlatiniform rash, followed by desquamation of the palms and soles.

- Staphylococcal scarlet fever can mimic streptococcal scarlet fever.

- Staph is also a common cause of furuncles and folliculitis.

Neisseria gonorrhoeae

Disseminated gonococcal infection causes a few (generally < 12) papular petechial lesions that become pustular—usually around the joints. Culture of skin exudate is usually negative. Culture is generally positive when taken from the site of infection (typically genital).

Neisseria meningitidis

Meningococcemic skin signs start as macular or petechial lesions and evolve to large purpura. The affected skin rapidly becomes necrotic.

Pseudomonas

Pseudomonas causes a variety of skin infections. It is the cause of "hot tub folliculitis." Normal chlorine levels prevent the growth and possibility of infection with this organism. The pustules from hot tub folliculitis resolve without treatment in 1 week. Pseudomonal septicemia causes small, dark-centered (necrotic) papules. In a very ill, neutropenic patient, this papule can evolve to ecthyma gangrenosum—a necrotic ulcer with an erythematous rim.

Pasteurella multocida

Animal bites: *Pasteurella multocida* often causes infection from dog and cat bites (multiple bacteria cause human bite infections). Treatment: Thoroughly clean/lavage

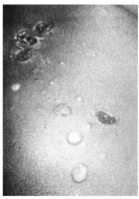

Image 7-36: Erysipelas   Image 7-37: Bullous impetigo

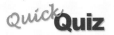

Quick Quiz

- Define erysipelas.
- How does bullous impetigo present in young children?
- How does SSSS differ from toxic epidermal necrolysis?
- How may disseminated gonococcal infection present?
- What is the etiology of ecthyma gangrenosum?
- What is the organism responsible for infection in cat bites?
- Describe the rash of Lyme disease.
- What causes molluscum contagiosum?

and give AM/CL (amoxicillin-clavulanate) as prophylaxis as described in Infectious Disease, Book 2.

RICKETTSIAL

Rocky Mountain spotted fever is usually heralded by several days of fever; then the patient gets small lesions that progress in distribution from peripheral to central, and in type from macular to petechial to purpuric.

SPIROCHETAL

Lyme disease is characterized by erythema migrans. This typically is an enlarging (> 1 week), annular erythematous patch or plaque with a clear center. By definition, the lesion must be at least 5 cm; occasionally, the center is not clear (Image 7-38). Also see Infectious Disease, Book 2.

A chancre indicates primary syphilis. Diffuse, scaly papule/plaques on the palms and soles, trunk, penis, and mucosal surfaces suggest secondary syphilis. Gummas occur in tertiary syphilis.

VIRAL

Warts

Warts (verrucae) are caused by any 1 of > 80 types of human papillomaviruses (HPV):

- Verruca vulgaris is the common wart. You can treat it with liquid nitrogen, topical salicylic acids, etc. (Image 7-39).
- Verruca plana is the flat wart.
- Verruca plantaris is the plantar wart. It is typically caused by HPV-1, -2, or -4. Treatment can consist of salicylic acid, liquid nitrogen, chemo vesicants, or pulsed dye laser.
- Condyloma acuminata are the anogenital warts. They are often caused by HPV-6 and -11 and, sometimes, by HPV-16, -18, and -31—the HPVs associated with cancer of the cervix. Treat with podophyllin 25% in a tincture of benzoin, trichloroacetic acid, or liquid nitrogen. Podophyllin is teratogenic, so do not give it to pregnant patients. Newer treatments are topical imiquimod (Aldara®) and sinecatechins (Veregen®).

Molluscum Contagiosum

Molluscum contagiosum is caused by a pox virus. It consists of smooth, umbilicated pearly papules (Image 7-40). The lesions vary in size from < 1 mm to several millimeters and are skin-colored to pink. It usually occurs in children but is also seen in the pelvic area of sexually active young adults. It is common in patients with AIDS. It can be sexually transmitted in adults. Molluscum contagiosum usually resolves spontaneously within 6–18 months. It is not unusual for children to develop a surrounding eczematous dermatitis, and the lesions often become inflamed shortly before they resolve. Treatment modalities are suboptimal but include chemo vesicants, liquid nitrogen, or curettage. In many instances, it is best to await spontaneous resolution.

Rubella

Rubella (German measles, 3-day measles) is benign, except when it occurs in pregnant women. Congenital rubella results in a variety of serious birth defects: heart malformations, ocular defects, microcephaly, intellectual disabilities, deafness, TTP, and bone problems.

DERMATOLOGY

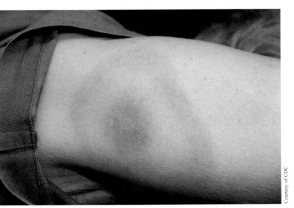

Image 7-38: Erythema migrans

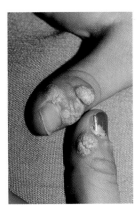

Image 7-39: Verruca vulgaris

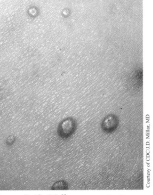

Image 7-40: Molluscum contagiosum

Measles

Measles (rubeola) has several stages. The prodromal stage lasts 3–4 days with fever, malaise, sinus discharge, and a hacking cough. Koplik spots often appear on the palate 1–2 days before the onset of rash. The red maculopapular rash (Image 7-41) starts on the forehead and quickly spreads downward, with the densest concentration of lesions from the forehead to the shoulders.

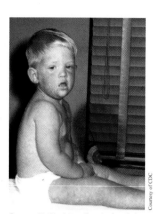

Image 7-41: Measles (rubeola)

Varicella Zoster

Varicella-zoster virus (VZV) causes two diseases: chickenpox and herpes zoster (shingles). Herpes zoster is reactivation of VZV in a person who has had chickenpox.

Chickenpox: Only 10% of cases occur in persons > 15 years old. Rash starts as maculopapular and rapidly progresses to vesicles, then to scabbed lesions. These tend to come in "crops" over 2–4 days (Image 7-42).

The herpes zoster skin manifestation presents as grouped vesicles with a dermatomal distribution. Topical acyclovir is not effective, although oral/IV acyclovir does help. Oral famciclovir and valacyclovir are also effective, but there is less experience with these agents in the pediatric population. Shingles can occur in both immunocompetent and immunocompromised children. The risk of developing pediatric zoster (as opposed to zoster in adulthood) is increased in children who had varicella during the 1st year of life or *in utero*. While it is associated with significant pain during—and even preceding—the outbreak, postherpetic neuralgia is very uncommon in children.

In the immunocompromised, treat both chickenpox and herpes zoster with IV acyclovir. Establish diagnosis promptly with a Tzanck smear (or DFA), and confirm by a viral culture.

FUNGAL

Tinea

These include: tinea capitis (scalp ringworm usually due to *Trichophyton tonsurans* or *Microsporum canis*), tinea corporis (common ringworm [Image 7-43]), tinea cruris (jock itch—differential diagnoses includes moniliasis, which has satellite lesions), tinea pedis (athlete's foot), and tinea unguium/onychomycosis (nails).

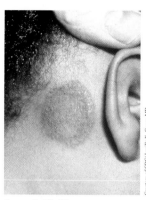

Image 7-43: Ringworm

Candida

Candidiasis of the mouth (thrush) causes white, semiadherent plaques on the tongue/mucosa/soft palate. Vaginal candidiasis has similar plaques with cheesy discharge.

Tinea Versicolor

Tinea versicolor (pityriasis versicolor) is caused by *Malassezia globosa*. It causes no initial symptoms but results in hypopigmented to reddish-brown, coalescing macules, usually on the upper torso and upper arms (Image 7-44). Lesions do not fluoresce red with a Wood's lamp, as erythrasma does, although they can sometimes have a yellowish fluorescence. This condition can lead to significant postinflammatory hyper- or hypopigmentation despite effective treatment. Furthermore, there is a tendency for tinea versicolor to recur, especially during warmer, more humid seasons.

Treatment of Fungal Infections

Most fungal skin infections are controlled by topical antifungal creams. Use miconazole, clotrimazole, and topical terbinafine (Lamisil®). Tinea capitis and tinea unguium require oral therapy. Potential therapeutic options for tinea capitis include griseofulvin, fluconazole,

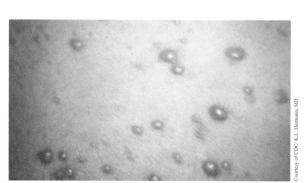

Image 7-42: Chickenpox

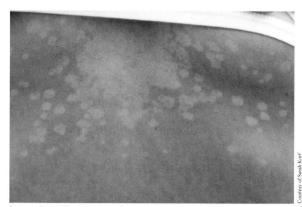

Image 7-44: Tinea versicolor

Quick Quiz

- What causes tinea versicolor?
- What causes scabies?
- How do infants and younger children differ from adolescents and adults in the presentation of scabies?
- Describe the appropriate therapy for scabies.

terbinafine, and itraconazole. Griseofulvin is the most common agent used, and lab work is not necessary for routine dosing of normal children.

Treat tinea versicolor with imidazole creams, selenium sulfide shampoo, ketoconazole shampoo, or oral fluconazole.

PARASITIC

Lice

Pediculus humanus capitis/corporis is a head or body louse. *Phthirus pubis* is the pubic louse ("crabs").

Treatment:

- Body lice: permethrin 5% cream or 1% lindane cream or lotion. Lindane creates the potential for neurotoxicity, and many do not recommend its use anymore.
- Head lice: Currently, many begin with over-the-counter permethrin cream 1% (Nix® cream rinse), because it is over-the-counter and least expensive; however, resistance is rising to > 50% in some areas of the U.S. The more toxic drugs, 1% lindane shampoo and pyrethrin + piperonyl butoxide (RID®, etc.), do not kill the eggs and require another treatment 1 week later. In the U.S., resistance is growing against all preparations. Malathion (0.5%) is highly effective (and has some egg-killing ability) and is approved for children ≥ 6 years of age. Benzyl alcohol 5% lotion (Ulesfia®) was approved in 2009 as an alternative to the pesticides. It has the advantage of not having neurotoxic effects.

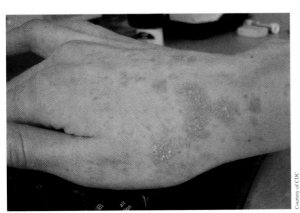

Image 7-45: Scabies burrow

- "No-nit" policies requiring children to be free of nits before the return to school are not effective and are not recommended by the 2012 Red Book. Treat infested household members, but those uninfested do not require prophylactic therapy. Children should not be excluded from school or sent home early from school because of head lice. Treatment of dogs, cats, or other pets is not indicated because they do not play a role in transmission of human head lice.
- Pubic lice: permethrin 1% or 5% cream or pyrethrin + piperonyl butoxide; lindane shampoo not recommended as first-line therapy.

Body lice live in clothes and are on the body only when they are feeding. The only treatment required is bathing and clean clothes, but topical pyrethrin + piperonyl butoxide or topical permethrin can also be used.

Scabies

Scabies is caused by a mite (*Sarcoptes scabiei*) that tunnels into the skin to lay eggs. It is spread by skin-to-skin contact (does not live > 48 hours without a host!). Infants and small children with scabies often have a distinct clinical appearance. Whereas adults usually have lesions most prominently on the wrists, ankles, and interdigital spaces, children often have widespread cutaneous lesions. Most infants have significant papules, vesicles, or pustules on the palms and soles. Often with careful inspection, you can identify burrows (curvilinear papules) (Image 7-45). Lesions can be generalized over the trunk and can often have an urticarial appearance or can become impetiginized. Even after treatment, postscabies nodules (especially in intertriginous areas) and pruritus can persist.

Treat affected infants and children with 5% permethrin, applying from the neck down (include scalp for infants) for 6–8 hours. Repeat this treatment in 1 week. Also, encourage all household members to be treated and to take special laundry precautions. Any items that cannot be washed and dried in a hot dryer should be placed in a plastic bag for 72 hours, because the mite cannot live without a human host. In infants < 2 months, use precipitated sulfur (6%) in petrolatum for 3 successive nights.

BLISTERING LESIONS

PEMPHIGUS VULGARIS

Pemphigus vulgaris probably has a multifactorial etiology with a common autoimmune result. There is an antibody against the epidermal desmoglein proteins. This causes acantholysis (the separation of epidermal cells from each other due to decreased cohesion), which results in the formation of large, loose bullae that peel off and leave denuded skin. Oral mucosal involvement is common and often is the 1st manifestation of this serious disorder. Any cutaneous area can be affected. Nikolsky sign is epidermal sliding with digital pressure on the skin and indicates the acantholysis that causes the symptoms. (Nikolsky sign is also seen in toxic epidermal necrolysis and staphylococcal scalded skin syndrome [SSSS].) Treatment with high-dose glucocorticoids +/– cyclosporine, azathioprine, mycophenolate mofetil, dapsone, methotrexate, rituximab, and sometimes IV immunoglobulin has been successful in this life-threatening disorder.

PORPHYRIA CUTANEA TARDA

Porphyria cutanea tarda (PCT) is the most common type of porphyria. It causes hyperpigmentation and tense blisters in sun-exposed areas, milia, skin fragility, and increased facial hair. PCT is caused by congenital or acquired decreased activity of uroporphyrinogen decarboxylase, which allows a buildup of phototoxic porphyrins in the skin. Symptoms can be induced by ingestion of estrogen or alcohol! Many patients have associated hepatitis C. Lab results usually show an increased serum Fe, Hct, ALT, and AST. For screening, check for increased urinary coproporphyrins and uroporphyrins. The urine of affected patients can show pink fluorescence with Wood's lamp examination.

PHOTOSENSITIVITY REACTIONS

Know that the most common causes of photosensitive reactions are medications such as thiazides, tetracycline, doxycycline, phenothiazine, sulfonamides, quinolones, and piroxicam (Feldene®). Rule these out first.

DERMATITIS HERPETIFORMIS

Dermatitis herpetiformis is a skin disease in which very pruritic vesicular lesions occur, usually on the extensor surfaces of the extremities, and mid-to-lower back, caused by IgA deposition (Image 7-46). It often occurs with celiac disease (gluten-sensitive enteropathy).

ERYTHEMA MULTIFORME

Erythema multiforme (EM) consists of well-defined, dusky red macules or papules that evolve into target shapes (Image 7-47). Palms and soles are frequently involved, and mucous membranes can be affected. The "target" or "iris-shaped" lesions are pathognomonic for EM and are characterized by a central blister or zone of necrosis/crusting. Lesions can be edematous or bullous. These fixed lesions last for several days before resolving spontaneously. They are often confused with the annular plaques of urticaria.

Historically, EM, which is caused by a preceding herpes simplex virus infection, was called EM minor, and Stevens-Johnson syndrome (SJS) was called EM major. SJS is associated with *Mycoplasma* infections or medications and causes severe involvement of 2 or more mucous membranes; less than 10% of EM cases are thought to be due to medications. Many now consider EM and SJS to be separate entities and do not consider SJS to be a more severe form of EM.

It is important to be able to differentiate between EM and urticaria, which can be quite similar in appearance. Urticarial reactions are much more common than EM in the pediatric population. In general, individual lesions in urticaria resolve in < 24 hours (are not fixed), lack blistering or central necrosis, and continue to come/go over days to weeks. It can be helpful to outline several lesions to help follow their progression: If the lesions have resolved in < 24 hours, it is not EM. Furthermore, the lesions of urticaria are often very bizarre in shape and haphazardly distributed; EM lesions are usually round or oval, well-demarcated, and symmetrically distributed over the extensor surfaces.

ROUND LESIONS

GRANULOMA ANNULARE

Granuloma annulare is an annular, but not scaly, ringworm-like plaque, which usually appears on the distal portion of the extremities (Image 7-48). Lesions can be solitary or multiple. It often occurs in children and young adults. Granuloma annulare is usually asymptomatic and self-limited, disappearing within months to a few years. It is frequently misdiagnosed as tinea corporis (ringworm), but granuloma annulare is not scaly. A subcutaneous form of granuloma annulare can resemble rheumatoid nodules, both clinically and histologically.

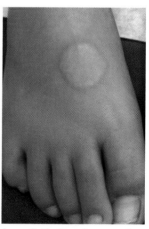

Image 7-48: Granuloma annulare

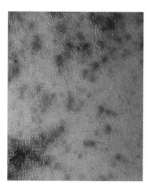

Image 7-46: D. herpetiformis

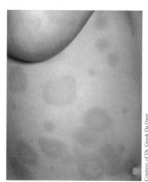

Image 7-47: E. multiforme

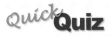

- What is Nikolsky sign? In what disorders is it seen?
- What is the most common type of porphyria?
- What antibiotics are involved in photosensitivity reactions?
- Describe the lesion of erythema multiforme.
- What is the difference between EM and Stevens-Johnson syndrome? Name an infection most commonly associated with each.
- Describe the rash of pityriasis rosea.

NUMMULAR ECZEMA

Nummular eczema consists of round (nummular = coin-shaped), weepy-to-lichenified plaques that are more common on the lower legs in adults, but can occur anywhere in children. Like other forms of eczema, it is very pruritic. It has no pathologic significance but can be more difficult to treat than other forms of eczema. Rule out fungal infection.

PITYRIASIS ROSEA

Pityriasis rosea is common in children and young adults. It presents as multiple small, oval, pink, slightly scaly, minimally pruritic plaques scattered symmetrically on the trunk and proximal extremities, parallel to the ribs in a "Christmas tree" pattern (Image 7-49). A larger "herald patch" often precedes subsequent lesions by 1–2 weeks (Image 7-50) and is often confused with tinea. It probably has a viral etiology (possibly human herpesviruses 6 and 7). The disease is self-limited, usually lasting 4–8 weeks. Consider secondary syphilis in the differential diagnosis for adolescents. Treatment is symptomatic. Note that pityriasis (tinea) versicolor has no relationship with pityriasis rosea.

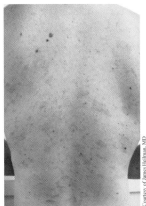

Image 7-49: Pityriasis rosea　　*Image 7-50: Herald patch*

FOR FURTHER READING

NEONATAL DERMATOLOGY

Ely JW, Seabury Stone M. The generalized rash: part I. Differential diagnosis. *Am Fam Physician*. 2010 Mar 15;81(6):726–734.

Ely JW, Seabury Stone M. The generalized rash: part II. Diagnostic approach. *Am Fam Physician*. 2010 Mar 15;81(6):735–739.

O'Connor NR, et al. Newborn skin: part I. Common rashes. *Am Fam Physician*. 2008 Jan 1;77(1):47–52.

Su J. Common rashes in neonates. *Aust Fam Physician*. 2012 May;41(5):280–286.

McLaughlin MR, et al. Newborn skin: part II. Birthmarks. *Am Fam Physician*. 2008 Jan 1;77(1):56–60.

Metry D, et al. Consensus Statement on Diagnostic Criteria for PHACE Syndrome. *Pediatrics*. 2009 Nov;124(5):1447–1456.

GENETIC SKIN DISORDERS

Schalock PC. Overview of pigmentation disorders. *The Merck Manual for Health Care Professionals*. 2012.

Boyd KP, et al. Neurofibromatosis type 1. *J Am Acad Dermatol*. 2009 Jul;61(1):1–14; quiz 15–16.

Wee SA, Fangman B. Tuberous sclerosis. *Dermatol Online J*. 2007 Jan 27;13(1):22.

Leger M, et al. Nevoid basal cell carcinoma syndrome. *Dermatol Online J*. 2011 Oct 15;17(10):23.

Jabbari A, et al. Incontinentia pigmenti. *Dermatol Online J*. 2010 Nov 15;16(11):9.

PIGMENT CHANGES

Moses S. Hyperpigmentation. *Family Practice Notebook*. 2010.

Shapiro J, et al. Practical management of hair loss. *Can Fam Physician*. 2000 Jul;46:1469–1477.

MOUTH FINDINGS

Gonsalves WC, et al. Common oral lesions: part I. superficial mucosal lesions. *Am Fam Physician*. 2007 Feb 15;75(4):501–507.

Gonsalves WC, et al. Common oral lesions: part II. masses and neoplasia. *Am Fam Physician*. 2007 Feb 15;75(4):509–512.

VITAMIN DEFICIENCIES

Finner AM. Nutrition and hair: deficiencies and supplements. *Dermatol Clin*. 2013 Jan;31(1):167–172.

Gehrig KA, Dinulos JG. Acrodermatitis due to nutritional deficiency. *Curr Opin Pediatr*. 2010 Feb;22(1):107–112.

Moses S. Hyperpigmentation. *Family Practice Notebook*. 2010.

Bernstein ML, et al. Cutaneous manifestations of cystic fibrosis. *Pediatr Dermatol*. 2008 Mar–Apr;25(2):150–157.

DERMATOLOGY

SKIN INFECTIONS

Usatine RP, Sandy N. Dermatologic emergencies. *Am Fam Physician*. 2010 Oct 1;82(7):773–780.

Empinotti JC, et al. Pyodermitis. *An Bras Dermatol*. 2012 Mar–Apr;87(2):277–284.

Stulberg DL, et al. Common bacterial skin infections. *Am Fam Physician*. 2002 Jul 1;66(1):119–124.

Mullegger RR. Dermatological manifestations of Lyme borreliosis. *Eur J Dermatol*. 2004 Sep–Oct;14(5):296–309.

Mulhem E, Pinelis S. Treatment of nongenital cutaneous warts. *Am Fam Physician*. 2011 Aug 1;84(3):288–293.

Centers for Disease Control and Prevention. Sexually transmitted diseases treatment guidelines: genital warts. 2010.

Pasqualotto AC, Denning DW. New and emerging treatments for fungal infections. *J Antimicrob Chemother*. 2008 Jan;61 Suppl 1:i19–i30.

Pearson RD. Approach to parasitic infections. *The Merck Manual for Health Care Professionals*. 2009.

American Academy of Pediatrics. Council on School Health and Committee on Infectious Diseases. Head lice. *Pediatrics*. 2010 Aug;126(2):392–403.